D1423798

BRITISH MEDICAL ASSOCIATION

0994534

OXFORD MEDICAL PUBLICATIONS

# Inherited Cardiac Disease

# Oxford Specialist Handbooks in Cardiology
# Inherited Cardiac Disease

*EDITED BY*

## Dr Perry Elliott

Reader in Inherited Heart Disease/Honorary Cardiologist
The Heart Hospital
University College Hospital
London, UK

## Dr Pier D. Lambiase

Consultant Electrophysiologist and Cardiologist
The Heart Hospital
University College Hospital
London, UK

## Professor Dhavendra Kumar

Consultant in Clinical Genetics/Lead
Clinician for Cardiovascular Genetics
Institute of Medical Genetics
University Hospital of Wales
Heath Park
Cardiff, UK

**OXFORD**
UNIVERSITY PRESS

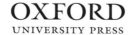
BMA LIBRARY
WITHDRAWN
BRITISH MEDICAL ASSOCIATION

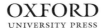

# OXFORD
UNIVERSITY PRESS

Great Clarendon Street, Oxford OX2 6DP.

Oxford University Press is a department of the University of Oxford.
It furthers the University's objective of excellence in research, scholarship,
and education by publishing worldwide in

Oxford  New York

Auckland  Cape Town  Dar es Salaam  Hong Kong  Karachi
Kuala Lumpur  Madrid  Melbourne  Mexico City  Nairobi
New Delhi  Shanghai  Taipei  Toronto

With offices in

Argentina  Austria  Brazil  Chile  Czech Republic  France  Greece
Guatemala  Hungary  Italy  Japan  Poland  Portugal  Singapore
South Korea  Switzerland  Thailand  Turkey  Ukraine  Vietnam

Oxford is a registered trade mark of Oxford University Press
in the UK and in certain other countries

Published in the United States
by Oxford University Press Inc., New York

© Oxford University Press, 2011

The moral rights of the author have been asserted
Database right Oxford University Press (maker)

First published 2011

All rights reserved. No part of this publication may be reproduced,
stored in a retrieval system, or transmitted, in any form or by any means,
without the prior permission in writing of Oxford University Press,
or as expressly permitted by law, or under terms agreed with the appropriate
reprographics rights organization. Enquiries concerning reproduction
outside the scope of the above should be sent to the Rights Department,
Oxford University Press, at the address above

You must not circulate this book in any other binding or cover
and you must impose this same condition on any acquirer

British Library Cataloguing in Publication Data
Data available

Library of Congress Cataloging-in-Publication-Data
Data available

Typeset by Glyph International, Bangalore, India
Printed in China
on acid-free paper through
Asia Pacific Offset

ISBN 978–0–19–955968–8

10 9 8 7 6 5 4 3 2 1

Oxford University Press makes no representation, express or implied, that the
drug dosages in this book are correct. Readers must therefore always check the
product information and clinical procedures with the most up-to-date published
product information and data sheets provided by the manufacturers and the most
recent codes of conduct and safety regulations. The authors and publishers do not
accept responsibility or legal liability for any errors in the text or for the misuse or
misapplication of material in this work. Except where otherwise stated, drug dosages
and recommendations are for the non-pregnant adult who is not breastfeeding.

# Foreword

A substantial proportion of cardiovascular disease is caused by genetic mechanisms and the total burden of inherited cardiovascular disorders exceeds that of cancer. Healthcare professionals encounter genetic cardiovascular disease in many varied clinical settings. Some inherited cardiac disorders manifest for the first time with sudden unexplained death in a young person, whereas others present with progressive symptoms or are detected incidentally. Increasingly, relatives of people with known inherited disorders are referred for counselling and screening for the same disorders. There is, therefore, a growing need for healthcare workers to develop a greater understanding of the basic principles of clinical genetics and the diverse manifestations of individual disorders.

This handbook is an excellent guide to the diagnosis and treatment of common cardiovascular disorders that should appeal not only to specialists in Inherited Cardiac Conditions, but also to less experienced readers who will almost certainly encounter patients in whom genetic factors are important.

Professor William McKenna
President of The Association of Inherited Cardiac Conditions
(www.improvement.nhs.uk/aicc/)

# Contents

# Contributors

**Rachel Butler**
Consultant/Lead-Molecular Genetics
All Wales Genetics Laboratory
Institute of Medical Genetics
University Hospital of Wales
Cardiff, UK

**Caroline Coats**
Academic Clinical Fellow
The Heart Hospital
University College London Hospitals
London, UK

**Perry Elliott**
Reader in Inherited Heart Disease/
Honorary Cardiologist
The Heart Hospital
University College London Hospitals
London, UK

**Andrew Flett**
The Heart Hospital
University College London Hospitals
London, UK

**John Gomes**
Research Fellow
Division of Medicine
Centre for Clinical Pharmacology and Therapeutics
University College London, UK

**Madeline Healey**
Specialist Registrar in Clinical Genetics
Department of Clinical Genetics
St. Michael Hospital
Bristol, UK

**Dhavendra Kumar**
Consultant in Clinical Genetics/
Lead Clinician for Cardiovascular Genetics
Institute of Medical Genetics
University Hospital of Wales
Cardiff, UK

**Pier Lambiase**
Consultant Electrophysiologist and Cardiologist
The Heart Hospital
University College London Hospitals
London, UK

**Alison Muir**
Clinical Academic Lecturer in Inherited Heart Diseases
The Heart Hospital
University College London Hospitals
London, UK

**William Newman**
Consultant/Senior Lecturer in Medical Genetics
Department of Clinical Genetics
St Marys Hospital
Manchester, UK

**Lawrence Nunn**
Research Fellow
The Heart Hospital
University College London Hospitals
London, UK

**Constantinos O'Mahony**
Research Fellow
The Heart Hospital
University College London Hospitals
London , UK

**Aaisha Opel**
Specialist Registrar in Cardiology
St Bartholomew's Hospital
London, UK

**Giovanni Quatra**
Research Fellow
The Heart Hospital
University College London Hospitals
London, UK

**Mark Rogers**

Consultant in Clinical Genetics
Institute of Medical Genetics
University Hospital of Wales
Cardiff, UK

**Graham Shortland**

Consultant Paediatrician/Lead
Metabolic Physician
Department of Child Health
University Hospital of Wales
Cardiff, UK

**Peter Thompson**

Principal Cytogeneticist
All Wales Genetics Laboratory
Institute of Medical Genetics
University Hospital of Wales
Cardiff, UK

# Abbreviations

| | |
|---|---|
| 📖 | cross reference |
| 🐁 | mouse (online reference) |
| 99mTc-DPD | 99mTc-3,3-diphosphono-1,2-propanodi-carboxylic acid |
| A | adenine |
| AAA | abdominal aortic aneurysm |
| AapoAI | apolipoprotein A-I amyloidosis |
| AApoAII | apolipoprotein A-II amyloidosis |
| ACE | angiotensin-converting enzyme |
| ACEi | angiotensin inhibitors |
| ACTC1 | cardiac actin |
| Acys | cystatin C amyloidosis |
| AD | autosomal dominant |
| ADME | absorption, distribution, metabolism, and elimination |
| AF | atrial fibrillation |
| AFD | Anderson–Fabry's disease |
| Afib | fibrinogen Aa amyloidosis |
| AGel | gelsolin |
| AHA | American Heart Association |
| ALK1 | activin-like kinase-type 1 |
| Alys | lysozyme amyloidosis |
| AMP | adenosine mono phosphate |
| APOA1 | apolipoprotein A-I |
| APOE | apolipoprotein E |
| AR | aortic regulation (cardiology) |
| AR | autosomal recessive (genetics) |
| ARMS | amplification refractory mutation system |
| ARVC | arrhythmogenic right ventricular cardiomyopathy |
| AS | Angelman syndrome |
| ASD | atrial septal defect |
| ASH | asymmetrical septal hypertrophy |
| ATP | adenosine triphosphate |
| ATP | anti-tachy pacing |
| ATTR | tranthyretin-related familial amyloidosis |
| AV | atrioventricular |
| aVF | augmented voltage unipolar left foot lead |
| aVL | augmented voltage unipolar left arm lead |

| AVM | arteriovenous malformation |
| AVSD | atrioventricular septal defect |
| BB | beta blocker |
| BHF | British Heart Foundation |
| BMD | Becker musuclar dystrophy |
| BMI | body mass index |
| BNP | brain natriuretic |
| bpm | beats per minute |
| BS | Brugada syndrome |
| BSA | body surface area |
| BWS | Beckwith–Widemann syndrome |
| C | cytosine |
| CACT | carnitine-acylcarnitine translocase |
| CAD | coronary artery disease |
| CADASIL | cerebral arteriopathy, autosomal dominant, with subcortical infarcts and leukoencephalopathy |
| CARASIL | cerebral autosomal recessive arteriopathy with subcortical infarcts and leukoencephalopathy |
| CAT | common arterial trunk |
| CAVSD | complete atrioventricular septal defect |
| CGH | comparative genomic hybridization |
| CH | chromosomal |
| CHD | congenital heart defects |
| CHD | congenital heart disease |
| CK | creatine kinase |
| CMA | Cardiomyopathy Association |
| CMR | cardiovascular magnetic resonance |
| CNS | central nervous system |
| CoA | coarctation of the aorta |
| COL3A1 | type 3 procollagen |
| COX | cytochrome c oxidase |
| CPEO | chronic progressive external ophthalmoplegia |
| CPT-1 | carnitine palmitoyl transferase 1 |
| CPT-2 | carnitine palmitoyl transferase 2 |
| CPVT | catecholaminergic polymorphic ventricular tachycardia |
| CPVT | cholaminergic polymorphic ventricular tachycardia |
| CRP | c-reactive protein |
| CRT | cardiac resynchronization therapy |
| CRT-D | cardiac resynchronization therapy with defibrillator |
| CRT-P | cardiac resynchronization therapy with pacemaker |
| CSCE | conformation-sensitive capillary electrophoresis |

| CSF | cerebrospinal fluid |
| CT | computed tomography |
| CVA | cerebro-vascular accident |
| CVM | cardiovascular malformations |
| CVS | chorionic villus sampling |
| DAD | delayed after depolarizations |
| DC | direct cardioversion |
| DCM | dilated cardiomyopathy |
| del | deletion |
| DES | desmin |
| DGGE | denaturing gradient gel electrophoresis |
| DHPLC | denaturing high-performance liquid chromatography |
| DM1 | myotonic dystrophy |
| DM1 | type 1 mytotonic dystrophy |
| DMD | Duchenne muscular dystrophy |
| DMPK | dystrophia myotonica protein kinase |
| DNA | deoxyribonucleic acid |
| DORV | double outlet right ventricle |
| dup | duplication |
| EAD | early after depolarizations |
| ECG | echocardiogram |
| ECG | electrocardiogram |
| EDMD | Emery-Dreiffus muscular dystropy |
| EDTA | EDTA blood specimen tube for molecular genetic analysis |
| EF | ejection fraction |
| ELN | elastin |
| EMG | electromyography |
| ENG | ENG |
| EPS | electrophysiological study |
| ESAC | extra structurally abnormal chromosome |
| ESC | European Society of Cardiology |
| FA | Friedreich's ataxia |
| FAP | familial amyloid polyneuropathy |
| FBN1 | fibrillin-1 |
| FDA | Food and Drug Administration |
| fDCM | familial dilated cardiomyopathy |
| FH | familial hypercholesterolaemia |
| FHD | facio-humeral dystropy |
| FHx | family history |

| | |
|---|---|
| FISH | fluorescence in situ hybridization |
| FKRP | Fukutin-related protein |
| FSHD | facioscapulohumeral muscular dystrophy |
| FTAA | familial thoracic aortic aneurysm |
| Fup | follow up |
| G | guanine |
| GA | general anaesthesia |
| Gd-DTPA | gadolinium chelate |
| GUCH | grown up congenital heart disease |
| GWAS | genome-wide association studies |
| HAMP | hepcidin antimicrobial peptide |
| HbH | haemoglobin H |
| HCM | hypertrophic cardiomyopathy |
| HD | Huntingdon's disease |
| HDL | high-density lipoprotein |
| HELLP | haemolysis, elevated liver enzymes, low platelets |
| HF | heart failure |
| HFEA | Human Fertilization and Embryo Authority |
| HHT | hemorrhagic telangiectasia |
| HLA | human leukocyte antigen |
| HLHS | hypoplastic left heart syndrome |
| HRM | high-resolution melt |
| IAA | interrupted aortic arch |
| ICC | Inherited cardiovascular condition |
| ICD | implantable cardiac defibrillators |
| ICR | imprinting control centre |
| IMD | inherited metabolic disease |
| INR | international normalized ratio |
| inv | inversion |
| IVC | inferior vena cava |
| IVF | in vitro fertilization |
| JVP | jugular venous pressure |
| KSS | Kearns–Sayre syndrome |
| LA | left atrium |
| LAD | left axis deviation |
| LAH | left anterior hemiblock |
| LBBB | left bundle branch block |
| LCAT | lecithin-cholesterol acyltransferase |
| LCHAD | long chain 3 hydroxyl-acyl-CoA dehydrogenase deficiency |
| LCSD | left cardiac sympathetic nerve denervation |

| LEOPARD | (syndrome) multiple lentigines, conduction abnormalities, ocular hypertelorism, pulmonary stenosis, abnormal genitalia, retardation of growth and deafness |
| --- | --- |
| LGE | late gadolinium enhancement |
| LGMD | limb girdle muscular dystrophy |
| LHON | Leber's hereditary optic neuropathy |
| LKAT | long-chain 3-ketoacyl-CoA thiolase deficiency |
| LMNA | lamin A/C |
| LPL | lipoprotein lipase |
| LQTS | long QT syndrome |
| LS | Leigh syndrome |
| L-TGA | congenitally corrected transposition of great arteries |
| LV | left ventricle |
| LVEF | left ventricular ejection function |
| LVH | left ventricular hypertrophy |
| LVNC | left ventricular non-compaction |
| LVOTO | left ventricular outflow tract obstruction |
| M | maternal; |
| MAD | multiple acyl-CoA dehydrogenase deficiency |
| MCAD | medium chain acyl CoA dehydrogenase deficiency |
| MD | myotonic dystrophy |
| MDT | multidisciplinary team |
| MELAS | myoclonic epilepsy, lactic acidosis with stroke |
| MERFF | myoclonus epilepsy with ragged red fibres |
| MERRF | mitochondrial encephalopathy with ragged red (muscle) fibres |
| MFM | myofibrillar myopathy |
| MI | myocardial infarction |
| MLPA | multiple ligation probe amplification |
| MNGIE | mitochondrial neurogastrointestinal encephalomyopathy |
| MPS | mucopolysaccharidoses |
| MRI | magnetic resonance imaging |
| mRNA | messenger RNA |
| MRS | magnetic resonance spectroscopy |
| MS-PCR | mutation-specific PCR |
| mtDNA | mitochondrial DNA |
| MTHFR | 5,10-methylenetetrahydrofolate reductase |
| MTOP | medical termination of pregnancy |
| MWT | maximal LV wall thickness |
| MYBPC3 | Myosin-binding protein C |
| MYOZ2 | Myozenin-2 |

| NAR | nocturnal agonal respiration |
| NARP | neurogenetic weakness with ataxia and retinitis pigmentosa |
| NHAR | non-homologous allelic recombination |
| NPV | negative predictive value |
| NS | Noonan syndrome |
| NSVT | non-sustained ventricular tachycardia |
| NTBI | non-transferrin bound iron |
| NTM | normal transmitting male |
| OFC | occipito-frontal circumference |
| OLT | orthotopic liver transplantation |
| PA | pulmonary atresia |
| PAH | pulmonary arterial hypertension |
| PAI1 | plasminogen activator inhibitor |
| PAVSD | pulmonary atresia ventricular septal defect with aorto-pulmonary collaterals |
| PCR | polymerase chain reaction |
| PDA | patent ductus arteriosus |
| PDE4D | phosphodiesterase 4D |
| PEO | progressive external ophthalmoplegia |
| PET | positron emission tomography |
| PGD | pre-implantation genetic diagnosis |
| Pgp | p-glycoprotein |
| PLAX | parasternal long-axis view |
| PND | prenatal diagnosis |
| PPCM | peripartum cardiomyopathy |
| PPM | Permanent pacemaker |
| PPV | positive predictive value |
| PS | pulmonary stenosis |
| PSAX | parasternal short-axis view |
| PWS | Prader–Willi syndrome |
| QF-PCR | quantitative fluorescent PCR |
| Qtce | Q-Tend |
| QTcp | Q-Tpeak |
| RBBB | right bundle branch block |
| RCM | restrictive cardiomyopathy |
| RNA | ribonucleic acid |
| RQ-PCR | real-time quantitative PCR |
| RV | right ventricular |
| RVOT | right ventricular outflow tract |
| S | sporadic |

| | |
|---|---|
| SADS-UK | sudden arrhythmic death syndrome |
| SAM | systolic anterior motion |
| SAP | serum amyloid P |
| SCA | spinocerebellar ataxia |
| SCARMD | severe childhood AR muscular dystrophy |
| SCD | sudden cardiac death |
| SCN5A | sodium channelopathies |
| SDH | succinate dehydrogenase |
| SLE | systemic lupus erythematosus |
| SNHL | sensorineural hearing loss |
| SNPs | single nucleotide polymorphisms |
| SPECT | single photon emission tomography |
| SQTS | short QT syndrome |
| SR | sarcoplasmic reticulum |
| SSFP GE | steady-state free procession gradient echo |
| SVAS | supra valvar aortic stenosis |
| SVT | supra ventricular tachycardia |
| T | thymine |
| T2D | diabetes type II |
| TA | tricuspid atresia |
| TAA | thoracic aortic aneurysm |
| TAAD | thoracic aortic aneurysm with dissection |
| TAPVC | total anomalous pulmonary venous connection |
| TAPVR | total anomalous pulmonary venous return |
| Tcp-e | Tpeak-end |
| TDI | tissue Doppler imaging |
| TdP | torsades de pointes |
| TDR | transmural dispersion of repolarization |
| TFP | mitochondrial trifunctional protein deficiency |
| TFR2 | transferrin receptor-2 |
| TGA | transposition of great arteries |
| TGF | transforming growth factor |
| TGFβR2 | TGFbeta receptor 2 gene |
| TIA | transient ischemic attack |
| TIMP1 | tissue inhibitor of metalloproteinase |
| TIMP3 | tissue inhibitor of metalloproteinase |
| TNN13 | Cardiac troponin I |
| TNNC1 | Cardiac troponin |
| TNNT2 | Cardiac troponin T |
| TOF | tetralogy of Fallot |

| | |
|---|---|
| TPM1 | Tropomyosin |
| TP-PCR | tandem-primer PDR |
| TSE | turbo spin echo |
| TTN | Titin |
| TTR | tranthyretin |
| TWI | T-wave inversion |
| UKGTN | UK Genetic Testing Network |
| ULSR | upper:lower segment ratio |
| UPD | uniparental disomy |
| USS | ultrasound scan |
| VCFS | velocardiofacial syndrome |
| VF | ventricular fibrillation |
| VLCAD | very long-chain acyl-CoA dehydrogenase deficiency |
| VO2 | oxygen consumption |
| VSD | ventricular septal defect |
| VT | ventricular tachycardia |
| WHO | World Health Organisation |
| WPWS | Wolff–Parkinson–White syndrome |
| XL-R | X-linked recessive |

# Chapter 1

# Introduction

# Introduction

Advances in molecular genetic technologies have resulted in increased recognition and understanding of genetic cardiovascular diseases in everyday clinical practice. In many countries, interest has been further stimulated by the publication of national guidelines for the management of families afflicted by inherited cardiac diseases that may result in premature sudden cardiac death in young people. Throughout the world multidisciplinary services for inherited cardiovascular diseases that involve cardiologists, clinical geneticists, specialist nurses and genetic counsellors are being developed. The aim of this handbook is to support this development by providing a brief practical guide to the basic principles of clinical genetics relevant to everyday cardiology practice.

In this book we use the term inherited cardiac disease to encompass a broad range of conditions that includes fetal cardiovascular disorders, congenital heart disease, cardiomyopathies, arrhythmias and disorders of blood vessels and lymphatics as well as cardiovascular disease in malformation syndromes, metabolic disorders, inherited dyslipidaemias, neuromuscular diseases, connective tissue diseases, and inherited haematological conditions. The book begins with the general principles of cardiovascular genetics and then describes the definition, aetiology, clinical presentation and treatment of specific cardiovascular diseases. Acquired conditions of the cardiovascular system (e.g. myocarditis, coronary atherosclerosis) are not covered in detail. Detailed descriptions of treatments common to familial and non-familial disease (e.g. management of heart failure) covered in other handbooks in this series will be summarized but will not be discussed in detail.

# Classification of inherited cardiovascular disease

Inherited disorders of the cardiovascular system can be grouped under the following categories:
- chromosomal conditions
- single gene or Mendelian disorders
- polygenic/multifactorial complex diseases
- mitochondrial disorders

Other modes of inheritance include genetic/genomic imprinting (📖 see Chapter 2, p. 8), genomic microdeletions/microduplications (📖 see Chapters 2 and 7) and genomic variation (📖 see Chapters 2 and 5).

A practical clinical approach to classification of inherited cardiovascular conditions is shown in Box 1.1. Details of individual category of disorders are provided in separate sections in this book.

> **Box 1.1  A practical clinical approach to classification of inherited cardiovascular conditions**
> - Congenital cardiovascular abnormalities—isolated/complex
> - Cardiovascular manifestations of multiple malformation syndromes
> - Disorders of cardiac muscle (cardiomyopathies)
> - Disorders of cardiac rhythm
> - Disorders of large- and medium-sized arteries
> - Disorders of other body systems with cardiovascular manifestations
> - Metabolic disorders with major cardiovascular manifestations

Most of the disorders listed above are primary except for some inherited multi-system disorders where cardiovascular manifestations may complicate the clinical phenotype. Victor McKusick's online database of Mendelian inheritance (🖰 http://www.nml.nih.gov/OMIM) lists several of these in different combinations.

# Chapter 2

5

# General principles of medical genetics

# DNA, genes, and the genome

## The human genome

The term human genome describes the genetic information held in human cells. The majority is encoded by a complex nuclear genome and a very small fraction by a simple mitochondrial genome. In both cases, the genetic information is encoded on deoxyribonucleic acid (DNA). Approximately 20,000 genes are encoded on human DNA; in addition, a significant proportion of the human genome consists of repetitive and non-coding DNA.

- DNA is a double-helical structure consisting of a phosphate and sugar backbone linked to nitrogenous bases; adenine (A), cytosine (C), guanine (G) and thymine (T). The specific base, sugar and phosphate comprise a nucleotide
- Each gene consists of a promoter sequence upstream of coding exons interspersed with non-coding introns (the number of exons and introns is variable) (Fig. 2.1).

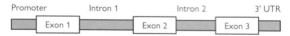

**Fig. 2.1** Gene structure.

## Gene expression

The information encoded within genes is expressed through the processes of **transcription** and **translation**. Messenger ribonucleic acid (mRNA) is synthesized from a gene sequence in the nucleus (**transcription**) and introns are spliced out. The processed mRNA sequence encodes amino acids (📖 see Table 2.1, The genetic code), which are joined to synthesise specific polypeptides in the cytoplasm to form proteins (**translation**) (Fig. 2.2).

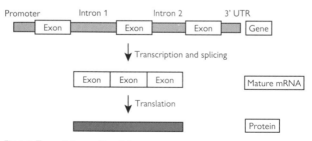

**Fig. 2.2** Transcription and translation.

## The genetic code

The synthesis of RNA and subsequently of a polypeptide is directed by the genetic code of the gene. The genetic code is a three-letter code (known as a **codon**) with four possible bases at each codon (A, T, C and G). The code specifies 20 different amino acids and is a redundant code whereby each amino acid is encoded by on average around three different codons. The genetic code also encodes termination codons (Stop) which specify that translation is complete.

**Table 2.1** The genetic code

| AAA | Lys | CAA | Gln | GAA | Glu | TAA | STOP |
|-----|-----|-----|-----|-----|-----|-----|------|
| AAG |     | CAG |     | GAG |     | TAG |      |
| AAC | Asn | CAC | His | GAC | Asp | TAC | Tyr  |
| AAT |     | CAT |     | GAT |     | TAT |      |
| ACA | Thr | CCA | Pro | GCA | Ala | TCA | Ser  |
| ACG |     | CCG |     | GCG |     | TCG |      |
| ACC |     | CCC |     | GCC |     | TCC |      |
| ACT |     | CCT |     | GCT |     | TCT |      |
| AGA | Arg | CGA | Arg | GGA | Gly | TGA | STOP |
| AGG |     | CGG |     | GGG |     | TGG | Trp  |
| AGC | Ser | CGC |     | GGC |     | TGC | Cys  |
| AGT |     | CGT |     | GGT |     | TGT |      |
| ATA | Ile | CTA | Leu | GTA | Val | TTA | Leu  |
| ATG | Met | CTG |     | GTG |     | TTG |      |
| ATC | Ile | CTC |     | GTC |     | TTC | Phe  |
| ATT |     | CTT |     | GTT |     | TTT |      |

The genetic codes of the nuclear genome are shown. The genetic code of the mitochondrial genome is very similar but differs for a small number of codons (not shown).

## Mutations and polymorphisms

Alterations of the genetic code within or nearby a gene cause **mutations** or silent **polymorphisms** depending on whether the protein encoded by the gene is significantly different from the original protein. Mutations cause a protein with altered function or reduced levels of protein to be synthesized. Polymorphisms can result in the synthesis of an identical protein (through the redundancy of the genetic code) or a protein with a tolerated amino acid change.

### Types of mutation

*1. Base substitutions*
- Nonsense (or STOP) mutations insert an early termination codon and leads to the premature truncation of the protein
- Missense mutations occur when the normal amino acid is substituted by an alternate amino acid leading to altered protein function, this may have a loss- or gain-of-function.

*2. Frameshift mutations*
- Deletions or insertions of one or several bases. The reading frame of the genetic code is disrupted. This leads to premature truncation of the protein
- Deletions or insertions of multiples of three bases. The reading frame of the genetic code is not disrupted. However, the addition or removal of amino acids may lead to altered protein function.

*3. Splice site mutations*
- The genetic code at the exon–intron boundary is altered such that correct splicing of introns does not occur in the mRNA. Splice site mutations may be located deep within introns. This may result in a truncated polypeptide and/or a polypeptide either missing or gaining amino acids.

*4. Tandem repeat expansions*
- Repetitive DNA either within or outside exons is unstable and may expand in length
- Non-coding expansions lead to disruption of gene expression or processing
- Coding trinucleotide repeat expansions are expressed (transcribed and translated) and lead to a protein with altered function.

*5. Deletions and duplications of exons and genes*
- A relatively common mutational mechanism is the deletion or duplication of single or several exons, or gene. This generally leads to protein truncation or absence of protein.

*6. Methylating or imprinting mutations*
- The expression of genes is controlled by the methylation of specific nucleotides at the DNA level. If the normal methylation pattern is disturbed, genes are switched on or off inappropriately.

### Polymorphisms
- **Synonymous polymorphisms**—alterations of the genetic code that do not result in altered protein sequence
- **Non-synonymous polymorphisms**—alterations of the genetic code that result in the insertion of a different amino acid in a protein. However, the change does not result in altered protein function.

### Unknown variants
Occasionally DNA variants are encountered where it is not clear whether the predicted change at the protein level will be deleterious. Differentiation between mutations or polymorphisms can sometimes be challenging, and may require clinical and molecular analysis of the family and functional analysis of the altered protein.

## Normal chromosomal structure

Humans have 23 pairs of chromosomes including one pair specifically assigned to male (XY) and female (XX) gender, designated the sex-chromosome pair (Fig. 2.3). The chromosomal constitution of man is complex and comprises variable amounts of euchromatin and heterochromatin visible as a characteristic banding-pattern that gives each chromosome a distinct appearance. Typically, a chromosome pair includes two homologues each comprising a short arm (p) and a long arm (q) separated by the central heterochromatin-G-C rich region—the centromere.

Chromosomal disorders result from either loss or addition of a whole chromosome (aneuploidy) or parts of chromosomes (structural). A chromosome abnormality results in major disturbance in the genomic arrangement since each chromosome or part thereof consists of thousands of genes and several non-coding polymorphic DNA sequences. The physical manifestations of chromosome disorders include growth retardation, developmental delay, and a variety of somatic abnormalities. A typical example is Down syndrome (Fig. 2.4).

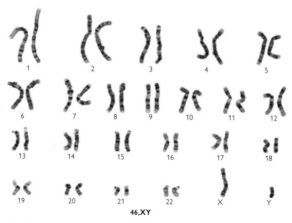

46,XY

**Fig. 2.3** Normal karyotype in a male (46,XY).

### Chromosomal disorders

Clinically significant chromosome abnormalities occur in nearly 1% of live-born births, account for about 1% of paediatric hospital admissions and are responsible for 2.5% of childhood mortality. The loss or gain of whole chromosomes is often incompatible with survival, and such abnormalities are a major cause of spontaneous abortions or miscarriages. Almost half of the spontaneous abortuses are associated with a major chromosomal abnormality, for example 45XO (Turner syndrome) or trisomy 16. It is estimated that about a quarter of all conceptions may suffer from major chromosome problems because approximately 50% of all conceptions may not be recognized as established pregnancies, and 15% of these end in a miscarriage. Essentially the major impact of chromosomal disorders occurs before birth or during early life.

Chromosomal disorders result from either loss or addition of a whole chromosome (aneuploidy) or parts of chromosomes (structural). A chromosome abnormality results in major disturbance in the genomic arrangement since each chromosome or part thereof consists of thousands of genes and several non-coding polymorphic DNA sequences. The physical manifestations of chromosome disorders include growth retardation, developmental delay, and a variety of somatic abnormalities. A typical example is Down syndrome resulting from either three copies of chromosome 21 (trisomy) (Fig. 2.4) or an addition to the long arm of chromosome 21 usually resulting from an unbalanced meiotic rearrangement of a parental chromosomal translocation between chromosomes 21 and one of the other acrocentric (centromere located at the end) chromosomes (Robertsonian translocation).

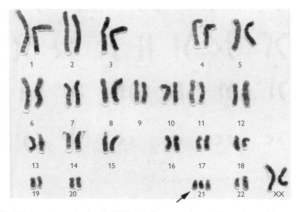

**Fig. 2.4** Karyotype of a female (XX) with Down syndrome. Note trisomy 21.

Down syndrome occurs in about 1 in 800 live births and increases in frequency with advancing maternal age. It is characterized by growth and developmental delay, often severe mental retardation, and the characteristic facial appearance recognized with upward slanting eyes. A major cause of death in these individuals is associated congenital heart defects (commonly atrioventricular septal defect and ventricular septal defect) that can complicate the clinical management in a significant proportion of Down syndrome cases. Prenatal diagnosis and antenatal assessment of the maternal risk for Down syndrome employing a variety of imaging and biochemical markers is now established clinical and public health practice in most countries.

## Mendelian inheritance

Mendelian inheritance is the classification of single gene disorders by their pattern of inheritance. 'Mendelian' refers to the work of Gregor Mendel, an Austrian monk who studied the segregation of various traits in garden peas.

Chromosomal genes are usually **bi-allelic**, i.e. there are usually two copies present. Genes found on the sex chromosomes are the exception and are **monoallelic** in males (who are XY). Mendelian inheritance patterns are determined by the location and number of copies (one or two) of the gene involved. The categories of Mendelian inheritance are **autosomal dominant**, **autosomal recessive** and **X-linked**. Mitochondrial genes are inherited in a different pattern (□ see Mitochondrial DNA, p. 16).

## Autosomal dominant inheritance

- Autosomal dominant conditions are caused by mutations in one copy of a gene pair, i.e. the conditions manifest in the heterozygous state.
- Autosomal dominant genes are located on chromosomes 1–22 (called the autosomes).
- Males and females are affected in equal proportions; in some inherited cardiovascular conditions severity may be more marked in the male
- Risk to offspring is 50% (1 in 2).
- Clinical manifestations may be variable both in distribution and severity
- Lack of clinical manifestations in a heterozygote indicates incomplete penetrance, for example autosomal dominant heypertrophic cardiomyopathy. These conditions are often seen occurring through several generations of a family e.g. long QT Syndrome (Fig. 2.5).

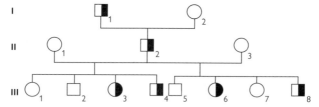

**Fig. 2.5** Pedigree illustrating autosomal dominant inheritance pattern; the affected (heterozygous) individual II.1 passed on the heterozygous mutation to four of his affected children from different marriages. Key: circle = male, square = male.

### Autosomal recessive inheritance

Autosomal recessive conditions are caused by mutations in both copies of a gene pair, i.e. they manifest in the homozygous state. Autosomal recessive conditions often appear in one generation only with no prior family history, e.g. Friedreich's ataxia (Fig. 2.6).

- Heterozygous carriers are usually asymptomatic.
- Homozygous persons are affected.
- Autosomal recessive genes are located on chromosomes 1–22.
- Male and female homozygotes are affected in equal numbers. A normal healthy sibling of a homozygous affected person carries a 2 in 3 chance to be heterozygote for the same allele.
- When both parents are carriers, the risk for affected offspring is 25%
- Consanguineous marriage (for example marrying a first cousin) may increase the chance of an autosomal recessive disorder, for example glycogen storage disease (see 📖 chapter 18).

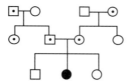

**Fig. 2.6** An autosomal recessive pedigree.

### X-linked inheritance

X-linked conditions are caused by alterations in genes found on the X chromosome. The terms **recessive** and **dominant** can be applied to X-linked conditions, although there may be some overlap. X-linked recessive disorders usually only affect males. X-linked dominant conditions affect both males and females, and are often lethal in males. The key characteristics of X-linked inheritance include:

- no male-to-male transmission
- males are always affected
- female carriers are usually healthy and apparently unaffected; mild and late manifestations are known to occur in a female heterozygote, for example Fabry disease
- risk to offspring (from a carrier mother): 50% chance for son to be affected and 50% chance for a daughter to be a carrier
- lack of family history may indicate a new mutation, but often this is misleading due to lack of adequate family history or clinical information
- x-linked conditions may appear to 'skip' a generation when they pass through an unaffected female, for example X-linked Becker muscular dystrophy or Fabry disease (Fig. 2.7)
- recurrence of an X-linked condition to an apparent non-carrier female could imply gonadal mosaicism and may carry an increased genetic risk, for example Duchenne/Becker muscular dystrophy.

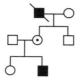

**Fig. 2.7** X-linked Fabry disease with hypertrophic cardiomyopathy.

Fig. 2.7 depicts a 30-year-old man with Fabry disease and hypertrophic cardiomyopathy. On detailed family enquiry he recalled that his grandfather had painful attacks in his extremities and died from a stroke at the age of 60 years. This may reflect Fabry disease that has passed through his mother.

## Multifactorial and polygenic inheritance

Many cardiovascular diseases are not caused by single gene disorders, but rather by a combination of genetic and environmental factors. This combination is called **multifactorial** (or **polygenic**) inheritance. The genetic factors determine the threshold for gene–environment interaction at the general population level. A lower threshold due to mutations in several genes may result in a congenital malformation (e.g. congenital heart defect) or a complex disease trait (e.g. coronary artery disease) (Fig. 2.8).

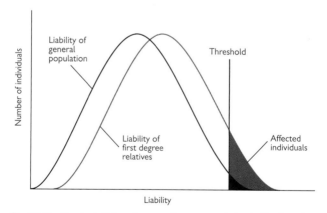

**Fig. 2.8** The Gaussian bell-shaped curve to illustrate genetic threshold, indicated by liability in the general population (shown in black). A shift to the right (in red) indicates increased liability in first degree relatives with an increased risk of recurrence. (With permission, Weatherall, 1991, Oxford University Press, UK).

The key features of multifactorial/polygenic inheritance include:
- random occurrence of clinically similar cases in the family, for example spina bifida spectrum cases (neural tube defect)
- increased likelihood of recurrence in first-degree relatives, for example parents and siblings
- increased likelihood of recurrence if the index case happens to be a female with lower incidence, for example increased risk to brother of a female with pyloric stenosis
- recurrence risks are usually small, usually around 5%; increased risk of recurrence when multiple first degree affected cases, for example higher risk to another sibling with an affected parent and sibling
- recurrence risk approximate to the square root of the incidence at birth, for example 3% recurrence risk for a congenital heart disease with a birth incidence of 1 in 1000 ($\sqrt{1}$ in 1000 = 3%; this may apply to most congenital heart diseases (2–3% recurrence risk for the next child)
- lifetime risk may be higher due to cumulative effect of several environmental factors, for example in conditions like ischaemic heart disease or hypertension, a positive family history may confer an increased risk to an individual; however, other non-genetic factors also contribute, such as smoking
- genetic factors influence, but do not determine with any certainty, the occurrence of a multifactorial/polygenic condition in an individual
- there are no reliable molecular genetic techniques to determine life-time risk; genome-wide association studies (GWAS) may help in mapping the different parts of the human genome, for example association with single nucleotide polymorphisms (SNPs), but can not be confidently used in clinical practice. A good family history is sufficient for clinical assessment, risk estimation and advising on lifestyle modifications.

### Examples of polygenic inheritance in cardiovascular conditions
- Congenital heart defects (isolated/non-syndromal)
- Atherosclerosis:
  - Ischaemic heart disease
  - Peripheral vascular disease
  - Cerebrovascular disease
- Diabetes Type II (T2D)
- Essential hypertension
- Abdominal aortic aneurysm.

## Genome-wide association studies
The explosion of genetic techniques and information in recent years has enabled large-scale studies to search for genetic variants that influence polygenic diseases. In all populations, there are areas throughout the genome where the genetic sequence varies slightly. These areas are called polymorphisms. Variation at the single nucleotide level is referred to as single-nucleotide polymorphism (SNP). Genome-wide association studies (GWAS) screen the polymorphisms present in large numbers of control and affected groups, to identify areas that confer risk for a specific condition. Most genetic variants found this way are associated with a very modest increase in risk. These variants act in combination with each other and with environmental factors consistent with multifactorial/polygenic inheritance.

# Mitochondrial inheritance

## Mitochondrial DNA

Most eukaryotes (a multicellular organism with a nucleus) possess two types of genomes—the nuclear and the mitochondrial. Mitochondrial genome is wholly contained in the mitochondrion, an intracellular organelle associated with energy generation and regulation. Mitochondrial DNA (mtDNA) codes for several proteins closely associated with oxidative phosphorylation and cellular respiration. Many nuclear genes of the respiratory enzyme chain interact with mtDNA. Apart from mutations in mtDNA, gene alterations in the respiratory enzyme complex gene system may also result in mitochondrial dysfunction manifesting with phenotypes indistinguishable from a complex multi-system mitochondrial disease.

The mtDNA genome in humans is a double-stranded circular DNA, 16.6kb in length that encodes 13 protein subunits of respiratory chain complexes, two ribosomal RNAs, and transfer RNAs. There are no intervening non-coding sequences or introns except for the D loop region that is involved in the initiation of DNA replication and transcription. Thus most mtDNA genome consists of coding sequences (Fig. 2.9). Mitochondria typically contain several copies of mtDNA and a typical human somatic cell can contain 5,000 to 10,000 copies of mtDNA representing >1% of the total DNA content of a cell. A mature oocyte may contain approximately 100,000 copies of mtDNA compared to only around 100 in a single sperm.

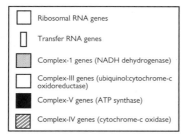

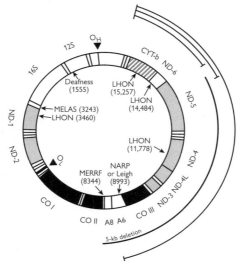

**Fig. 2.9** The circular mitochondrial genome. Note location of mtDNA mutations for major mitochondrial disorders. MELAS, myoclonic epilepsy, lactic acidosis with stroke; LHON, Leber's hereditary optic neuropathy; MERRF, mitochondrial encephalopathy with ragged red (muscle) fibres; NARP, neurological degeneration with ataxia and retinitis pigmentosa.

Reprinted from Kumar and Weatherall (eds) Genomics and Clinical Medicine. Oxford University Press, New York, 2008, Figure 6.7, page 110.

### General features of mitochondrial DNA mutations

Population studies suggest that about 1 in 400 people in the general population may have a maternally inherited pathogenic mtDNA mutation. Since mitochondria generate energy, tissues that rely on and use energy most suffer most functional disturbance. These tissues include muscle, liver, brain, heart, peripheral nerves, and endocrine glands. Different energy-dependent tissues contain varying levels of normally functioning mitochondria. The amount of mitochondria in a skeletal muscle cell may be higher compared to heart or brain.

The key features of mitochondrial inheritance include:

* mitochondrial inheritance is wholly maternal since there is virtually no paternal mtDNA present in the sperm cytoplasm. Most paternal mtDNA lies in the sperm tail that is almost completely shed at the time of fertilization during the process of penetration through the zona pellucida

* symptoms and signs of mitochondrial DNA dysfunction are extremely variable in terms of age at onset, severity and tissues/organs involved. The diagnosis of a mitochondrial disease may require a high degree to suspicion based on complex symptoms involving several systems (Table 2.2)

* some mtDNA mutations are evenly distributed (**homoplasmy**) in the same cell, tissue, or individual; for example, the presence of A1555G sequence change in an individual with sensorineural deafness or G11778A mutation in Leber's hereditary optic neuropathy (LHON)

* most mtDNA mutations are often unevenly distributed in the same cell, tissue or organ in the same individual (**heteroplasmy**). In mitochondrial disorders, because of the thousands of mitochondria in each cell, there are often variable percentages of mutant and wild-type mtDNAs between different tissues (Fig. 2.10). The different mtDNAs can vary between 0 and 100%, causing marked variation in clinical severity and the spectrum of organ involvement. In addition, the distribution of mtDNA mutations in a given tissue may also change with time (**tissue variation**), for instance falling in blood and accumulating in the non-dividing cells such as skeletal muscle

* mitochondrial function is dependent upon the wild mtDNA content that determines the specific tissue threshold (**threshold effect**). The variable mutant mtDNA load in different tissues can be judged by marked clinical variability. In some mitochondrial disorders, such as Leigh syndrome, the severity of symptoms increases sharply above a threshold mtDNA mutant load. In addition, there is preferential accumulation of mutant mtDNA in affected tissues (**selection**) to account for progressive pattern of most mitochondrial disorders, for example dilated cardiomyopathy. However, in some cell lines, for example blood, the mutant load may progressively fall.

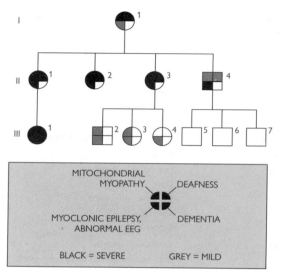

**Fig. 2.10** Pedigree of a family with mitochondrial encephalopathy with ragged-red muscle fibres (MERRF). Note segregation of different features with variable severity in the affected family members.

Adopted with permission from *Principles of Medical Genetics* by Thomas D. Gelehrter, Francis S. Collins and David Ginsburg, Williams and Wilkins, Baltimore, USA, second edition, 1998.

**Table 2.2** Multi-system involvement in mitochondrial disorders (Leonard and Schapiro 2000)

| | |
|---|---|
| Central nervous system | Developmental delay/regression |
| | Generalized seizures |
| | Ataxia |
| | Myoclonus |
| | Stroke-like episodes |
| | Encephalopathy |
| Muscle | Myopathy—weakness/fatigue/hypotonia |
| Eyes | Ptosis |
| | External ophthalmoplegia |
| | Optic atrophy |
| | Pigmentary retinopathy |
| | Cataract |
| | Sudden loss of vision |
| Ears | Sensorineural deafness |
| | Drug-induced deafness (amninoglycosides) |
| Heart | Cardiomyopathy |
| | Conduction defects |
| Pancreas | Diabetes mellitus |
| Kidney | Renal tubular dysfunction (Fanconi syndrome) |
| | Generalized aminoaciduria and glycosuria |
| Bone marrow | Sideroblastic anaemia/pancytopenia |

# Non-traditional inheritance

Preceding sections describe the most common patterns of inheritance associated with human disease. These are often referred to as *traditional patterns of inheritance*. Some human genetic diseases are caused by genetic abnormality that does not follow traditional inheritance and is assigned the term of *non-traditional inheritance*. This category includes different patterns, notably genetic/genomic imprinting, trinucleotide (triplet) repeats and disorders of genome architecture. Basic understanding of principles underlying *non-traditional inheritance* is important since transmission in some inherited cardiovascular conditions may not follow *traditional inheritance*.

## Genetic/genomic imprinting

Genetic or genomic imprinting controls gene expression without permanently altering the genetic code. Often genetic or genomic imprinting terms are used in the same context. However, genetic imprinting refers to a single gene (**specific phenotype**) whilst genomic imprinting refers to involvement of different genes dispersed through out the genome (**complex phenotype**). Genes are imprinted by the addition of a methyl group to DNA strands (to the cytosine base) which prevents gene expression. Genetic or genomic imprinting belongs to the field of **epigenetics**. Epigenetics describes the mechanisms, other than direct DNA sequence changes, that alter gene expression.

Maternal and paternal genes are usually expressed equally. However, there are certain genes that are not and instead have a parent-specific expression pattern, i.e. only one allele is active. This pattern is determined by methylation that occurs during spermatogenesis and oogenesis. Somatic cell lines also have tissue-specific imprinted genes which enable cell differentiation and function, without altering the genetic sequence. In addition to methylation abnormalities, mutations in the nearby imprinting control region (ICR) may also result in similar phenotype.

Diseases or syndromes caused by alterations in imprinted genes are called imprinting disorders. These disorders are caused by one or more of the following mechanisms:
- Deletions or mutations in the expressed copy of an imprinted gene
- Uniparental disomy (UPD) for the chromosomal homologue including an imprinted critical gene. In UPD, both homologues of a chromosome pair are inherited from one parent only. This disrupts the normal balance of expression when imprinted genes are involved. UPD results from the phenomenon of trisomic rescue where one chromosome homologue is lost during meiosis leaving two homologues belonging to one parent. UPD may be heterodisomy (different grandparental alleles) or iso-disomy (one grandparental alleles) (Fig. 2.11)
- Methylation abnormality of the main gene associated with the phenotype—hypomethylation (active) or hypermethylation (inactive)
- Mutations in the imprinting control centre gene may also result in similar phenotype.

Assisted reproductive techniques may carry an increased risk of imprinting disorders, particularly for Angelman syndrome (AS) and Beckwith–Widemann syndrome (BWS). However, due to the small numbers involved, the exact risk and mechanism is uncertain. To date, there are nine known imprinting syndromes and an estimated 200 imprinted genes described. Major examples of imprinting disorders include AS, BWS, and Prader–Willi syndrome (PWS). Congenital cardiac anomalies are not typical of these conditions, although cardiomyopathy has been reported in BWS. It is likely that some complex cardiovascular conditions may result from alterations in imprinted genes or loci, in particular those associated with ageing (apoptosis).

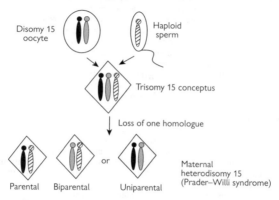

**Fig. 2.11** The origin of uniparental disomy 15 in Prader–Willi syndrome through trisomic rescue during early embryogenesis. Note different homologues (maternal heterodisomy).

Reprinted from Kumar and Elliott *Principles and Practice of Clinical Cardiovascular Genetics*. Oxford University Press, New York, 2010, Figure 3.7, page 44.

## Genetic disorders with trinucleotide repeats

Genes for few Mendelian disorders were mapped using the physical mapping approach. A search for intragenic mutations or pathogenic polymorphisms led to incidental finding of unusual presence of nucleotide clusters consistently appearing in set of three nucleotides (triplets). This set included cytosine (C) and guanine along with either adenine (A) or thymine (T). The following observations are important in understanding the pathogenic relevance of triplet repeats:

- each class of trinucleotide repeats exists in normal individuals
- a pathogenic expansion is the one that is seen in clinically symptomatic individuals.
- carriers for an X-linked disease also have an expanded allele (pre-mutation), which does not usually result in abnormal phenotype. However, it is likely that some carrier females might exhibit some manifestations as in Fragile X syndrome.

- An expanded allele in the premutation range in a male would not be associated with any clinical manifestations (normal transmitting male [NTM]), but this could further expand resulting in all daughters being carriers. However, recent studies have provided data on the existence of late-onset (~60 years) gait ataxia in NTMs.
- A normal-size CGG repeat in a normal male could undergo expansion during meiosis leading to a carrier daughter. This usually comes to light when a symptomatic grandson is confirmed to have pathogenic FRAXA expansion, formerly known as the 'Sherman paradox'.
- In some apparently normal individuals the size of the triplet repeat may fall between normal and pre-mutation ranges referred to as *intermediate allele*. The clinical significance of an expanded intermediate allele is unclear; however, this should be carefully assessed and genetic counselling offered by an experienced clinical geneticist.
- In most triplet repeat disorders, trinucleotide repeats (CAG or CTG) are present at the 5' end of the gene close to the promoter region. However, in some cases, the triplet repeat may occur at the 3' end interfering in the termination of the normal coding sequence thus leading to abnormal quantity of the gene product, for example last exon of the DM protein kinase (myotonin) gene [*DMPK*] for type 1 myotonic dystrophy (DM1).
- In some triplet repeat disorders, the expanded region can occur anywhere in the gene thus disrupting the expression of the gene.
  - In the X-linked fragile X syndrome [FRAXA], the CGG repeats are found in the 5'-untranslated region of the first exon of *FMR1*, the pathogenic gene for FRAXA.
  - In Friedreich's ataxia (FRDA), an autosomal recessive form of spinocerebellar ataxia (SCA), the expanded triplet repeat allele [GAA] occurs in the first intron of *X25*, the gene encoding frataxin.
  - In Huntington's disease (HD) and other inherited neurodegenerative disorders, the CAG triplet repeats occur within exons and encode an elongated polyglutamine tract.

**Table 2.3** Disorders with trinucleotide (triplet) repeat expansion

| Disorder | Triplet | Location | Normal size | Abnormal size range |
|----------|---------|----------|-------------|---------------------|
| FRAXA | CGG | 5'UTR | 10–50 | 200–2000 |
| Friedreich's ataxia | GAA | Intronic | 17–22 | 200–900 |
| Kennedy disease | CAG | Coding | 17–24 | 40–55 |
| SCA1 | CAG | Coding | 19–36 | 43–81 |
| Huntington's disease | CAG | Coding | 9–35 | 37–100 |
| DRPLA | CAG | Coding | 7–23 | 49–>75 |
| SCA3 | CAG | Coding | 12–36 | 67–>79 |
| SCA2 | CAG | Coding | 15–24 | 35–39 |
| SCA6 | CAG | Coding | 4–16 | 21–27 |
| SCA7 | CAG | Coding | 7–35 | 37–200 |
| SCA8 | CTG | 5'UTR | 16–37 | 100–>500 |
| Myotonic dystrophy | CTG | 3'UTR | 5–35 | 50–4000 |
| FRAXE | CCG | Promoter | 6–25 | >200 |
| FRAXF | GCC | ? | 6–29 | >500 |
| FRA16A | CCG | ? | 16–49 | 1000–2000 |

FRAX, Fragile X; UTR, untranslated region; SCA, Spinocerebellar ataxia; FRA16, Fragile 16;
DRPLA, Dentato–Rubro–Pallido–Leuysian atrophy

Few characteristics are common to trinucleotide (triplet) repeat disorders:

- inheritance pattern commonly autosomal dominant, except for Fragile X syndrome (X-linked semi-dominant) and Freidreich's ataxia (autosomal recessive)
- marked intra-familial and inter-familial clinical variation
- progressively severe clinical presentation in successive generation— a phenomenon known as *anticipation*
- four categories of triplet repeats alleles based on the size of the expansion—normal, intermediate, pre-mutation and mutation.
- some correlation with the size of the repeats. In general individuals with intermediate and pre-mutation size triplet repeats are clinically normal. However, there are few exceptions, such as in FRAXA and HD
- no detectable specific pathogenic intragenic mutations and/or pathogenic DNA polymorphism in any of the exons or introns
- abnormal triplet repeats represent unstable DNA sequences commonly at the 5' end (promoter) of the gene, and uncommonly at the intronic splice site (FA), coding sequences or exons (HD, SCA) and at the 3'end (myotonic dystrophy).

- The clinical picture predominantly in most triplet repeat disorders is neurological, but other systems may be involved including cardiovascular system (Table 2.4).

**Table 2.4** Triplets repeat disorders with cardiovascular system involvement

| Disorder | OMIM |
| --- | --- |
| Myotonic dystrophy | 160900 |
| Fragile X-FRAXA | 300624 |
| Huntington's disease | 143100 |
| Dentato–Rubro–Pallido–Leuysian atrophy (DRPLA) | 125370 |
| Spinocerebellar ataxia type 1, SCA1 | 164400 |
| Freidreich's ataxia (FRDA) | 229300 |

OMIM: Online Mendelian Inheritance in Man, Updated by Johns Hopkins University and published by NCBI, NLM (⅌ http://www.ncbi.nlm.nih.gov/omim).

## Disorders of genome architecture

Several clinically recognizable phenotypes are associated with disruption of the genome architecture. Apart from a few familial conditions, the majority of these disorders occur sporadically. Disruption in the genome is often localised to a specific chromosome region. This could be in the form of loss (**deletion**), gain (**duplication**), position change (**rearrangement, inversion**), and variation (**copy number variation**) (Fig. 2.12). Several genes are mapped to the specific critical chromosome region each contributing to the phenotype. Most of the genes have either negligible or minimal contribution to the phenotype. However, some genes are important with major contribution. The function (gene expression) in some of these genes is 'dosage dependent', correlated to the size of disruption. The term 'contiguous gene syndrome' is also used to delineate some of these conditions, as the phenotypic spectrum may have some correlation to the extent of disruption. These conditions are now classified under the broad category of 'genomic disorders' (Table 2.5). Cardiovascular manifestations often feature high within the broad phenotypic spectrum in genomic disorders.

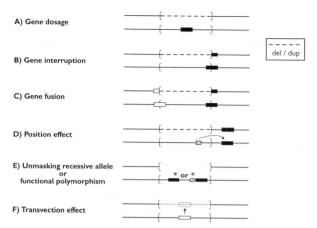

**Fig. 2.12** Different forms of genomic disruption in genomic disorders.
Reprinted from Kumar and Elliott (eds) *Principles and Practice of Clinical Cardiovascular Genetics.* Oxford University Press, New York, 2010, Figure 3.8, page 45.

The following distinctive characteristics make these conditions unique:
- phenotype is broad and varied presenting with marked clinical variation
- critical chromosome region includes several genes that are differentially expressed; expression in some of these genes is dosage dependent. The clinical picture in deleted cases is often severe but varied
- critical region is flanked with repetitive nucleotide sequences called 'low copy number repeats' or LCRs
- genomic disruption results from unequal crossing over during meiosis called 'non-homologous allelic recombination' or NHAR
- demonstration of specific disruption in the genomic architecture may help in the phenotype prediction. However, this should be used with great caution in certain clinical situations including genetic counselling and prenatal diagnosis.

**Table 2.5** Contiguous gene syndromes as genomic disorders

| Disorder [OMIM] | Inheritance | locus | Gene | Rearrangement | Size (kb) | |
|---|---|---|---|---|---|---|
| William–Beuren syndrome [194050] | AD | 7q11.23 | *ELN* | del;inv | 1600 | >320 |
| Beckwith–Wiedemann syndrome? | | 11p12 | | dup | | |
| Prader–Willi syndrome [176270] | AD | 15q11.2q13 | *SNRPN* | del | 3500 | >500 |
| Angelman syndrome [105830] | AD | 15q11.2q13 | *UBE3A* | del | 3500 | >500 |
| Dup(15)(q11.2q13) | Ch | 15q11.2q13? | | dup | 3500 | >500 |
| Triplication 15q11.2q13 | Ch | 15q11.2q13? | | trip | | >500 |
| Smith–Magenis syndrome [18290]? | 17p11.2 | | *RA13* | del | 4000 | ~250 |
| Charcot–Marie–Tooth IA | AD | 17p11.2 | *PMP22* | dup | 4000 | ~250 |
| Hereditary neuropathy pressure palsy | AD | 17p11.2 | PMP22 | del | | |
| DiGeorge/VCFS [188400] | AD | 22q11.2 | *TBX1* | del | 1500-3000 | ~225-400 |
| Male infertility [415000] | YL | Yq11.2 | *DBY* | del | 800 | |
| AZFa microdeletion | | | *USP9Y* | | | |
| AZFc microdeletion [400024] | YL | Yq11.2 | *RBMY* | del | 3500 | |

AD, autosomal dominant; Ch, chromosomal; del-deletion; dup, duplication; inv, inversion.

# Genetic laboratory techniques

# Genetic laboratory techniques

A modern genetic diagnostic laboratory includes separate sections for conventional cytogenetics, molecular cytogenetics and molecular genetics. Biochemical genetic laboratory facilities are based in selected centres. However, few tests can be requested locally to the chemical pathology laboratory. In this chapter, a brief account of molecular cytogenetics and molecular genetics is provided.

# Molecular genetics

An increasing range of molecular genetic techniques is available for the analysis of DNA. The available techniques are evolving constantly, providing improvement to the sensitivity of mutation detection and speed at which genetic conditions can be confirmed or excluded at the molecular level. The majority of molecular genetic analyses are initiated with the polymerase chain reaction (PCR), which promotes the amplification of a specific region of DNA for further molecular analysis (Fig. 3.1).

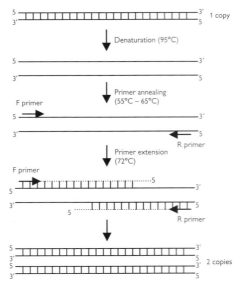

**Fig. 3.1** The polymerase chain reaction. PCR is dependent upon the design and synthesis of primers—molecules of single-stranded DNA designed to be complementary to the gene target, and Taq polymerase, a DNA replication enzyme that can tolerate being cyclically heated to 95°C. Target DNA is cyclically denatured, annealed, and extended using forward and reverse primers specific for the gene target of interest. After each round of PCR the number of copies of target DNA doubles. After 20 cycles of PCR the target DNA will have been amplified approximately a million-fold.

The type of molecular genetic analysis employed depends upon the type of mutation to be detected.

Linkage analysis of multiple affected and unaffected individuals from a single family, confirms or excludes the association of a familial genetic condition with a given chromosomal location or gene. It does not identify a familial mutation.

Gene screening describes the techniques used to detect a familial mutation, often in an index case.

Known mutation detection describes the techniques used to identify a familial mutation in at risk family members, and techniques used to detect commonly occurring mutations.

## Linkage analysis

Inherited disorders are often genetically heterogeneous being caused by mutations in several different genes, for example mutations in any of the sarcomere protein genes (*MYH7, MYBPC3, TNNT2, TNNI3, TPM1, ACTC, MYL2, MYL3*) and other genes (*LAMP2, PRKAG2* and *GLA*) are known to result in the hypertrophic cardiomyopathy (HCM) phenotype. The comprehensive gene screening of all possible genes is long, slow, and expensive. However, the inclusion or exclusion of some genes for screening can be achieved by linkage analysis dependent upon DNA samples from appropriate affected and unaffected family members being available. Subjects should be carefully assessed clinically, particularly for a late-onset or reduced penetrance genetic disorder which could be mistaken for a phenotypically similar but non-genetic cardiac muscle condition.

Polymorphic markers are regions (or single bases) of DNA which vary either in sequence or length within the normal population. The polymorphic markers are not usually associated with the pathogenesis of disease, but do show variation within the population chosen. Markers are selected that are physically closely located to the genes to be analysed. These DNA regions are amplified by PCR and typed for the polymorphic base in each familial individual. Analysis of the resulting haplotypes (the combination of alleles for each polymorphism assigned to one chromosome) determines whether the family shows linkage to the gene by identifying if every **affected family member has the same haplotype** and every **unaffected family member does not have this haplotype**.

The linkage analysis enables the exclusion and inclusion of certain candidate genes within a family and therefore promotes efficient gene screening. Fig. 3.2 illustrates linkage analysis in a large family with at least four affected individuals with Brugada syndrome. Bloods from affected and unaffected individuals were collected and their DNA was analysed for polymorphisms related to *SCN5A*, the most common sodium ion channel gene associated with Brugada syndrome. There is no consistent pattern of haplotype transmission with the disease excluding *SCN5A* as being the most likely gene associated in this family. Further linkage analysis using polymorphic markers located in close proximity to another Brugada syndrome gene (*GDPL1*) excluded this gene as well. Mutation analysis in either of these two genes is unlikely to be of any use in genetic risk estimate and accurate genetic counseling.

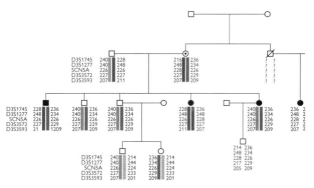

**Fig. 3.2** Linkage analysis of a Brugada family. See also colour plate section.

## Gene screening

The sequence of all exons of a gene is screened to detect various types of mutations which are often 'private' or specific to the family being analysed. Mutations are often spread throughout the gene or genes causing the inherited condition, requiring comprehensive analysis. Gene screening is therefore labour-intensive requiring the interrogation of every base of the coding sequence of a gene. Pre-screening techniques are generally quicker and cheaper but are not as sensitive as DNA sequence analysis. All methods rely upon the initial amplification of target DNA sequences by PCR.

The reporting time for gene screening is dependent upon the size of the gene(s). The detection and subsequent characterization of unknown variants extends reporting times. For genes less than 10 exons, reporting should take less than 1 month, for genes less than 10 exons, reporting should take less than 1 month, for genes less than 10 exons, reporting should take less than 1 month for genes > 10 exons reporting should take approximately 2 months.

**Table 3.1** Methods for gene screening

| Method | Types of mutation detected | Notes |
| --- | --- | --- |
| DNA sequence analysis | Missense, nonsense, frameshift, splice site, polymorphisms and unknown variants. | The gold standard for screening analysis, detecting >99% changes at the bases analysed. |
| | | Does not detect copy number changes (deletions and duplications). |
| Pre-screening analysis CSCE, HRM, DGGE, DHPLC | Missense, nonsense, frameshift, splice site, polymorphisms and unknown variants. | Pre-screening techniques that require characterization of DNA variants by sequence analysis. |
| | | <99% sensitivity for the detection of mutations, depending on the method used. |
| | | Does not detect copy number changes (deletions and duplications). |
| Copy number analysis MLPA, RQ-PCR, QF-PCR | Copy number changes such as deletions and duplications of whole exons. | Single exon deletions need verification by an independent assay. |
| | | Assays are particularly sensitive to the quality of starting DNA. |
| mRNA analysis followed by sequence or prescreening analysis | Missense, nonsense, frameshift, splice site, polymorphisms unknown variants, and copy number changes. | Relies upon the successful extraction of mRNA from the available tissue. The mRNA must be expressed within the tissue analysed. |
| | | Effective detection of splicing mutations. |

CSCE, conformation-sensitive capillary electrophoresis; HRM, high-resolution melt; DGGE, denaturing gradient gel electrophoresis; DHPLC, denaturing high-performance liquid chromatography; MLPA, multiple ligation probe amplification; RQ-PCR, real-time quantitative PCR; QF-PCR, quantitative fluorescent PCR.

### DNA sequence analysis

DNA cycle-sequence analysis is used to determine the sequence of a specific PCR product, often an exon. Within a genetic diagnostic laboratory, sequence analysis is routinely used to characterize mutations within genes and exons in patient samples. The DNA sequence of a mutation can be used to determine the impact of the DNA change at the protein level.

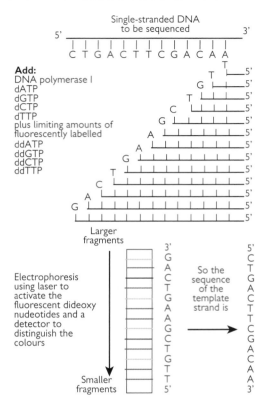

**Fig. 3.3** PCR products are denatured to create single-stranded DNA. Taq polymerase enzyme copies the single-stranded DNA template incorporating the 4 complementary nucleotides (A, C, G, and T). Limiting amounts of modified, fluorescently labelled nucleotides are also incorporated. The incorporation of modified nucleotides causes the extension of the DNA copy to halt. The process continues cyclically, like PCR, to produce different-sized DNA fragments corresponding to each position of the DNA sequence within the original PCR product. Each of the fragments has a fluorescently labelled tag corresponding to its final nucleotide of the DNA sequence. The fluorescently-labelled fragments are separated by size on an automated DNA sequencer, and the colour and size of each tagged fragment recorded to determine the DNA sequence. See also colour plate section.

DNA sequence analysis is also commonly used to detect the presence or absence of mutations in at-risk family members where the pathogenic mutation has already been identified in the index case. The at-risk family member is amplified by PCR and sequenced for the specific exon in which the mutation has been identified in the index case. Analysis of the at risk patient sample is performed alongside a normal control and the index case.

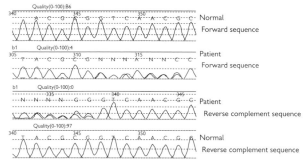

**Fig. 3.4a** DNA sequence analysis of patient and control samples for the MYBPC3 c.2545delG mutation. The MYBPC3 c.2545delG mutation is present in the patient sample but not in the normal control. The heterozygous presence of the mutation causes a frameshift within the DNA sequence resulting in the two patient alleles (one normal and one deleted) becoming superimposed upon each other.

### Pre-screening analysis

Pre-screening methods are used to detect sequence changes within DNA fragments, often exons. These methods do not determine the nature of the sequence change but provide a rapid and comparatively cheap way of determining if a change is present, requiring subsequent sequence analysis to confirm the presence of a DNA variant or mutation. Various techniques are available, often based upon the melting of paired DNA strands following PCR amplification.

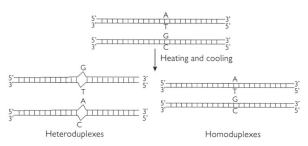

**Fig. 3.4b** Heteroduplex formation. PCR products for a specific exon are generated in a patient sample. Following PCR the sample is heated to denature double-stranded DNA and then slowly cooled to promote the formation of double-stranded DNA. If a heterozygous nucleotide change is present in the amplified DNA fragment, a heteroduplex will be formed between complementary DNA strands with differing nucleotide composition. Double-stranded fragments which have entirely complementary DNA strands form homoduplexes.

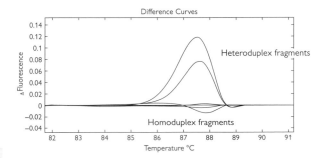

**Fig. 3.4c** High-resolution melt (HRM) analysis. Heteroduplexes and homoduplexes are melted at differing temperatures as detected by emitted fluoresence, and giving characteristic melt curves related to specific DNA variants. Heteroduplex DNA melts at lower temperatures as it comprises double-stranded DNA that is not perfectly matched. Homoduplex (normal) DNA melts at a higher temperature. Heteroduplex samples are simply identified as having different melt curves (in red). See also colour plate section.

### Copy number analysis

A significant number of pathogenic mutations result from rearrangements of DNA including gene fragments and thus disrupting the coding sequence of the gene. Rearrangements include deletions (missing gene fragments), duplications (additional gene fragments) and inversions (a gene fragment inserted in the incorrect orientation). Rearrangements can include:

- megabases (millions of base pairs) and encompass whole genes; detected by cytogenetic techniques including flourescent *in situ* hybridization (FISH) and array CGH
- single or multiple exons, or genes (hundreds to thousands of base pairs); detected by quantitative molecular methods
- single or multiple base pairs; detected by sequencing or prescreening methods.

Deletions and duplications of exons and whole genes are detected by a variety of quantitative, molecular techniques that determine copy number. MLPA is a technique that simultaneously analyses the copy number of multiple DNA fragments, it is often designed to include all the exons of a gene or genes that are known to contribute to a genetic phenotype.

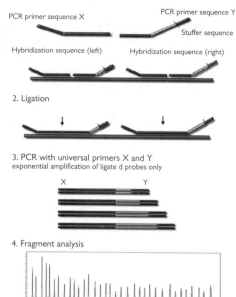

1. Denaturation and Hybridization

PCR primer sequence X

PCR primer sequence Y

Stuffer sequence

Hybridization sequence (left)     Hybridization sequence (right)

2. Ligation

3. PCR with universal primers X and Y
exponential amplification of ligate d probes only

X          Y

4. Fragment analysis

**Fig. 3.4d** Multiple ligation probe amplification (diagram courtesy of MRC Holland). Synthetic DNA probes are designed to hybridize and ligate on specific DNA fragments throughout a gene (generally one per exon). Hybridization is limited by the copy number of each gene fragment in the starting material. The ligated sequences are then amplified by PCR and separated by size. Subsequent fragment analysis includes the quantification of each PCR product, and comparison of patient samples with normal controls to determine if a deletion or duplication is present. See also colour plate section.

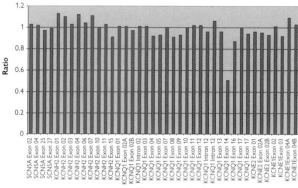

**Fig. 3.4e** 2000bp deletion of KCNQ1 exon 14. The selected exons of the *SCN5A*, *KCNH2*, *KCNQ1*, *KCNE2* and *KCNE1* genes were assayed by MLPA (mutations in these genes cause inherited arrhythmias). Results of fragment analysis have been normalized against a series of normal samples. The sample shown has two copies of each of the fragments analysed, except for KCNQ1 exon 14, for which there is only one copy. The presence of one copy of this exon was confirmed by an alternate technique, confirming it as the pathogenic mutation in this family.

### Known mutation detection

Known mutation techniques are employed when:
• a mutation has previously been detected in a family and is therefore characterized, or
• common mutations within a gene are known to cause a particular clinical presentation.

The detection of known and common mutations is generally far quicker than gene screening for 'private' mutations as only a single region of the gene needs to be analysed, and rapid techniques that detect specific mutations can be utilized.

Reporting times are generally 2 weeks for a previously characterized familial mutation or common mutation.

**Table 3.2** Molecular methods for detection of known mutations

| Method | Application | Notes |
|--------|-------------|-------|
| Real-time PCR, ARMS, MS-PCR | Detect specific mutations; nonsense, missense, splice site, small frameshifts. | Assays are designed specific for each mutation. Generally very rapid. May be multiplexed to detect several mutations simultaneously. |
| Microarray analysis | Detects specific mutations; nonsense, missense, splice site and also copy number changes. | Detects 100s of nucleotide changes simultaneously and rapidly. The development time of assays is long, and tests are therefore expensive. Few genes have sufficient common mutations for this analysis to be cost-effective. |
| Fluorescent sizing analysis, TP-PCR | Detects tandem-repeat expansions. | Repeat expansions are generally detected using PCR-based methods which are rapid. Occasionally southern blot analysis is necessary and therefore reporting times can extend to 2 months. |
| DNA sequence analysis | Detects specific mutations within a defined region; nonsense, missense, splice site, small frameshifts. | Amplification and sequence analysis of the fragment containing the known mutation only. |
| Copy number analysis; MLPA, RQ-PCR, QF-PCR | Copy number changes such as deletions and duplications of whole exons. | Assays are targeted to the known fragments containing a copy number change. Assays are particularly sensitive to the quality of starting DNA. |

ARMS, amplification refractory mutation system; MS-PCR, mutation-specific PCR; TP-PCR, tandem-primer PDR; MLPA, multiple ligation probe amplification; RQ-PCR, real-time quantitative PCR; QF-PCR, quantitative fluorescent PCR.

### ARMS analysis

The amplification refractory mutation system is commonly used for the detection of LDLR, PCSK9 and ApoE gene mutations in familial hypercholesterolaemia (FH). A PCR primer is designed to specifically amplify a common mutation and is used in conjunction with a universal return primer. The primer pairs are used in a single reaction to simultaneously amplify and interrogate a patient's DNA for multiple mutations.

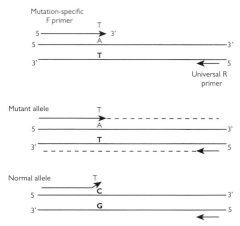

**Fig. 3.5** ARMS for a C>G mutation. A mutation-specific forward primer is designed to incorporate a thymine (T) base at the 3' end specific for a common mutation. PCR amplification proceeds when the mutant (T) base is present, however no amplification occurs when the normal (C) base is present.

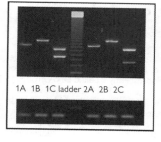
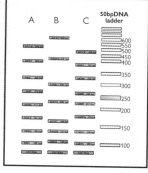

**Fig. 3.6** Multiplexed ARMS to detect 20 FH mutations (shown courtesy of Tepnel Diagnostics). Mulitple FH mutations are detected in a 3-tube assay. 2 control and any of 6–7 mutations are amplified by PCR in each reaction. Amplified products are size fractionated and compared to the 50bp DNA ladder. Sample 1: W66G mutation present; sample 2: V408M mutation present.

# Molecular cytogenetic techniques

## Fluorescence *in situ* hybridization (FISH)

### Basic principles of FISH

*In situ* hybridization detects specific nuclei acid sequences in target material fixed to a microscope slide. Fluorescence *in situ* hybridization (FISH) involves the hybridization of fluorescently labelled DNA probes to the target material. Most molecular cytogenetic FISH tests will involve the hybridization of probes to metaphase chromosomes, although interphase nuclei and solid tissue sections may also be used.

After hybridization, if the sequence corresponding to the probe is present in the target material a signal will be seen down a fluorescence microscope, if the sequence corresponding to the probe is absent from the target material no signal will be seen. Fig. 3.7 shows a 22q11 deletion detected by FISH.

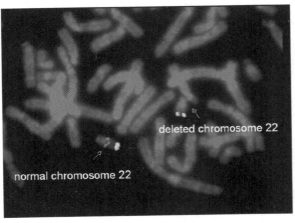

deleted chromosome 22

normal chromosome 22

**Fig. 3.7** The Vysis 22q11 region probe TUPLE1 is labelled with spectrum orange, the control probe ARSA which maps to 22q13.3 is labelled with spectrum green and DAPI has been used as a counterstain for the chromosomes. See also colour plate section.

### Types of probes

A range of types of probes are available.
- Whole chromosome paints that hybridize to the entire target chromosome.
- Repeat sequence probes that are specific for the centromeric regions of chromosomes.
- Unique sequence probes that hybridize to a sequence present in a single copy on a chromosome.

There are commercially available whole chromosome paints, centromeric probes and unique sequence probes for the common microdeletion syndromes e.g., 22q11 deletion syndrome, Williams syndrome. Probe sets are also available for screening for subtelomeric rearrangements, for the common aneuploidies found at prenatal diagnosis and for the common cytogenetic rearrangements associated with haematological malignancies. A range of fluorochromes are available for labelling of probes. This allows the simultaneous hybridization of more than one probe to the target material. Fig. 3.8 shows an insertional translocation detected by using chromosome paints labelled with different coloured fluorochromes.

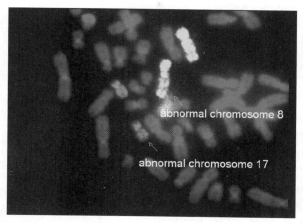

abnormal chromosome 8

abnormal chromosome 17

**Fig. 3.8** The whole chromosome 8 paint is labelled with spectrum green, the whole chromosome 17 paint is labelled with spectrum orange, and DAPI has been used as a counterstain for the chromosomes. See also colour plate section.

### Resolution of structural abnormalities
An important application of FISH is the use of chromosome paints and region specific probes such as telomeres and centromeres to characterize additional or missing chromosomal segments that cannot be identified by conventional banding techniques. This allows a more accurate delineation of structural chromosomal abnormalities and marker chromosomes detected during microscopic analysis. This subsequently allows more accurate and detailed information to be given to the referring Clinician for patient or family management.

*Microdeletion detection*

Commercially available probes are used to detect chromosomal deletions (and sometimes duplications) that are not detectable by G-banded analysis. Probes available for the more common microdeletion syndromes include:

- Angelman syndrome
- Cri du Chat syndrome
- Isolated lissencephaly sequence/Miller–Dieker syndrome
- Kallman syndrome
- Prader–Willi syndrome
- Smith–Magenis syndrome
- Williams syndrome
- Wolf–Hirschhorn syndrome
- 1p36 deletion syndrome.
- 22q11 deletion syndrome

The National Genetics Reference Laboratory Wessex provides a probe bank and key locus service for the FISH detection of the rarer microdeletion and microduplication syndromes ( http://www.ngrl.org.uk/Wessex).

*Samples for FISH analysis*

Sample requirements for FISH testing are the same as those outlined for general cytogenetic analysis (see Chapter 3, p. 50).

*FISH methodology*

Most commercially available probes are directly labelled with a fluorochrome being conjugated to a nucleotide in the probe DNA. Probes can be indirectly labelled with a hapten being conjugated to a nucleotide in the probe DNA. This is subsequently detected using fluorescently labelled reporter molecules.

- The target material is prepared on a microscope slide by conventional cytogenetic or pathology techniques.
- The probe is applied to the target material on a microscope slide and both are denatured, either at a high temperature or by using a formamide solution, and allowed to hybridize overnight. During hybridization, the denatured DNA strands of the probe will reanneal with the complementary sequences of interest on the target material.
- After hybridization there follows a series of post-hybridization washes to remove any unbound or non-specifically bound probe.
- A counterstain is added to the slide which is then analysed using fluorescent microscopy.

An example of a molecular cytogenetic report for a 22q11 deletion is given in the box.

**Example report**

- 46,XX.ish del(22)(q11.2q11.2)(TUPLE1-).
- Abnormal female chromosome complement.
- FISH studies using the Vysis 22q11 region probe TUPLE1 showed that the patient has a submicroscopic deletion of the sequences recognised by this probe.
- Conventional cytogenetic analysis showed a normal female karyotype.
- Microdeletions of chromosome 22q11 have been reported in the majority of DiGeorge syndrome and velocardiofacial syndrome cases, and in patients with non-syndromic congenital cardiac defects (Ryan et al. J Med Genet 1997; 34: 798–804). The findings are, therefore, consistent with the clinical suspicion of DiGeorge syndrome. 75% of patients with a 22q11 deletion have cardiac abnormalities.

Approximately 10% of cases have been shown to be familial; in addition, inheritance of the deletion from mildly affected or asymptomatic parents is well documented. In view of these findings, it would be advisable to carry out FISH studies on both parents to exclude the possibility that the deletion is familial. The patient herself is at a 50% risk of passing the deletion on to any offspring.

# Array comparative genomic hybridization (array CGH)

## Basic principles

Conventional chromosome analysis, which is based on G-banding, was developed in the 1970s, and is still primarily used today for routine analysis in cytogenetic laboratories. The resolution of traditional cytogenetic techniques is limited to ~5Mb at best. As a result smaller chromosomal abnormalities often remain undiagnosed. FISH does enable the identification of defined smaller genomic imbalances (~5–5000kb), but can only be applied to test for a limited number of chromosome regions simultaneously, and is unable to screen for genome-wide abnormalities. However, new technologies have recently been developed that are designed to give further information about the chromosome structure at a resolution that exceeds that of microscopic analysis.

Comparative genomic hybridization (CGH) was developed to screen the whole genome for imbalances by comparing differentially labelled test and reference samples on metaphase chromosomes.[1] However, the resolution of standard CGH is limited to around 3–10Mb. To increase the resolution substantially, microarray based comparative genomic hybridization (array CGH) was developed. Array CGH was first described in 1997,[2,3] and is based on the same principles as metaphase-CGH, except that the targets are mapped genomic clones that are spotted onto a standard glass slide instead of whole chromosomes (Fig. 3.9). Analysis of the fluorescence ratio of each target on the microarray allows the identification of copy number changes (either gains or losses). The resolution of an array is limited by the size of the insert used, and the distance between the clones, and therefore has the ability to bridge the gap between cytogenetic and molecular diagnosis. The development of the first 'whole-genome' array quickly followed.[4,5]

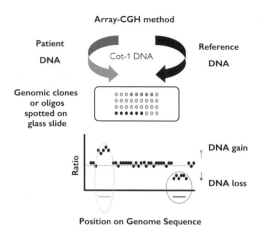

**Fig. 3.9** Laboratory process for array CGH. See also colour plate section.

Reprinted from Kumar and Elliott (eds) *Principles and Practice of Clinical Cardiovascular Genetics.*, Oxford University Press, New York, 2010; Figure 5.3, page 70.

1. Kallioniemi A, Kallioniemi OP, Sudar D, Rutovitz D, Gray JW, Waldman F, Pinkel D (1992). Comparative genomic hybridization for molecular cytogenetic analysis of solid tumours. *Science* **258**, 818–821.
2. Solinas-Toldo S, Lampel S, Stilgenbauer S, Nickolenko J, Benner A, Dohner H, Cremer T, Lichter P (1997). Matrix-based comparative genomic hybridization: biochips to screen for genomic imbalances. *Genes Chromosomes Cancer* **20**, 399–407.
3. Pinkel D, Segraves R, Sudar D, Clark S, Poole I, Kowbel D, Collins C, Kuo WL, Chen C, Zhai Y, Dairkee SH, Ljung BM, Gray JW, Alberston DG (1998). High resolution analysis of DNA copy number variation using comparative genomic hybridization to microarrays. *Nat Genet* **20**, 207–211.
4. Snijders AM, Nowak N, Segraves R, Blackwood S, Brown N, Conroy J, Hamilton G, Hindle AK, Huey B, Kimura K, Law S, Myambo K, Palmer J, Ylstra B, Yue JP, Gray JW, Jain AN, Pinkel D, Albertson DG (2001). Assembly of microarrays for genome-wide measurement of DNA copy number. *Nat Genet* **29**, 263-264.
5. Fiegler H, Carr P, Douglas EJ, Burford DC, Hunt S, Scott CE, Smith J, Vetrie D, Gorman P, Tomlinson IP, Carter NP (2003). DNA microarrays for comparative genomic hybridization based on DOP-PCR amplification of BAC and PAC clones. *Genes Chromosomes Cancer* **36**, 361–374.

# Genetic laboratory reports

Regional cytogenetics and molecular genetics laboratories will have a user manual that is available on the Internet, intranet or upon request. The user manual will detail the requirements for sending samples to the laboratory, the test repertoire of the laboratory, reporting times success rates and other reporting issues and contain useful contact numbers. The following information on cytogenetic testing has been taken from the *Regional Cytogenetics Laboratory for Wales User Manual* (with kind permission of the author, Mr. Selwyn Roberts).

### Sample requirements

Samples for genetic studies will require analysis using either molecular or cytogenetic techniques. Depending on the required test the following samples should be taken and sent to the local regional genetics laboratory. Samples should arrive within 24 hours wherever possible. As cytogenetic investigations are carried out on living cells, samples should be sent to the laboratory as soon as possible and not frozen or exposed to excessive heat.

All samples should be labelled with patient's name, date of birth, address, NHS number and other unique identifiers such as the hospital number. Each sample should be accompanied by a request form. Genetics Diagnostic Laboratory Request Forms are supplied by the laboratory to wards and clinics. Complete a form ensuring that all of the information requested on the form is provided (Fig. 3.10).

**Table 3.3**

|  | Analysis | Sample requirements |
|---|---|---|
| Cytogenetic analysis | Postnatal blood | 5ml of peripheral blood in a lithium heparin tube is required for analysis of a constitutional karyotype. For an infant, a minimum of 0.5ml is required. |
|  | Prenatal samples Amniotic fluid | 15–20ml of amniotic fluid should be taken into a sterile universal container. It is generally considered that it is safe to take 1ml of fluid for each week of gestation. |
|  | Chorionic villus | Mg should be taken and placed into medium in a sterile universal container, usually supplied by the cytogenetics laboratory. |
|  | Solid tissues and fetal material | If the infant/fetus appears fresh with no signs of maceration, cord blood or peripheral blood in lithium heparin and a sample of skin or other solid tissue should be sent. If the fetus appears slightly macerated, send a sample of fetal membranes and/or placenta. A suitable small biopsy of skin or other solid tissue should be placed in a sterile universal container, available from the cytogenetics laboratory and sent without delay. Ensure that the skin samples include the dermis and associated underlying tissue. |
|  | Haematological samples | Bone marrow aspirate samples should be taken into universal containers containing bone marrow transport medium supplied by the laboratory. Peripheral blood (5ml) should be sent in a lithium heparin tube. |
| Molecular analysis | Gene screening to identify familial mutation | 5–10ml blood in EDTA (purple top), or |
|  |  | 1–2ml blood in EDTA for neonates and newborns, or |
|  |  | 1–2cm$^2$ fresh tissue*, or |
|  |  | Paraffin fixed tissue (if no other sample is available), or |
|  |  | Guthrie cards are potential sources of DNA if no other samples are available |
|  | Predictive or confirmatory test for known familial mutation | 2–5ml blood in EDTA (purple top) |

* The laboratory should be warned in advance of the receipt of a fresh tissue sample, as these samples require immediate DNA extraction.

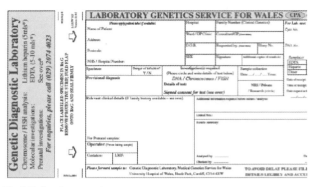

**Fig. 3.10** Sample request form.

*Known mutation tests*

Requests for predictive testing are generally only received from clinical geneticists. In the event of requests for predictive or confirmatory analyses information about the index case should also be included. The index case in whom the familial mutation has been identified should be indicated. If the index case was not previously analysed by the local genetics laboratory, a copy of the genetic report and a sample from the index patient should be arranged to be sent to the analyzing laboratory. It is preferable that the analysing laboratory confirms the presence of the previously reported familial mutation when predictive testing is performed.

Consent

If confirmation of consent is not recorded on the referral form, the laboratory will usually assume that consent has been given for testing.

For certain conditions and reasons, signed consent will be required. In particular, consent is required for predictive analyses where future disease status is predicted by a molecular analysis.

Turnaround times

*Cytogenetics*

Cytogenetic guideline reporting targets are set by the Association of Clinical Cytogenetics, *Professional Guidelines for Clinical Cytogenetics General Best Practice Guidelines* (2007).

- Prenatal diagnosis (amniotic fluid CVs and fetal blood samples).
- Rapid aneuploidy testing 95% within 3 working days.
- Karyotype result 95% within 14 calendar days.
- Postnatal diagnosis (blood and solid tissue samples).
- Rapid aneuploidy testing 95% within 3 working days.
- Urgent karyotype result 95% within 10 calendar days.
- Routine karyotype result 95% within 28 calendar days.
- Haematology/leukaemia diagnosis (bone marrow and blood samples).

- Rapid PCR/FISH testing 95% within 3 working days.
- Urgent karyotype result 95% within 14 calendar days.
- Routine karyotype result 95% within 21 calendar days.

### Molecular genetics

Molecular genetic guidelines for reporting targets were determined by Our Inheritance, Our Future. Government. White Paper on Genetics, 2003.

- Gene screening (genes >5 exons) 2–3 months.
- Common mutation analysis 20 working days/4 weeks.
- Predictive and confirmatory analysis for familial mutation 20 working days/4 weeks.
- Prenatal analysis 3 working days.

## Reporting

### Cytogenetics

Cytogenetic guidelines on reporting are set by the Association of Clinical Cytogenetics.

Cytogenetic reports should give a clear and unambiguous description of the cytogenetic results and an explanation of the clinical implications of the findings. The report of an abnormal case should include:

- karyotypic designation using ISCN nomenclature
- a clear written description of the abnormality and whether it is balanced or unbalanced
- the name of any associated syndrome
- methods used in establishing the result
- clinical interpretation to include (where appropriate):
  - whether the result is consistent with the clinical findings, and/or an indication of the expected consequences of the abnormality
  - request for follow-up of family members at risk of the same or related abnormality
  - an assessment of risk/recurrence
  - recommendation for consideration of prenatal diagnosis in future pregnancies
  - onward referral for genetic counselling.

Most reports issued by the cytogenetics laboratory will be straightforward. Clinicians should, however, be aware of the following potential reporting complications:

- an abnormal chromosome complement may only be present in a proportion of the cells in a patient (mosaicism) and may remain undetected because of its low frequency
- microdeletions will often not be detected in routine cultures. FISH testing is recommended for microdeletion syndromes (📖 see Microdeletion detection, p. 46)
- small imbalances and rearrangements may not always be detectable, because of the subtlety of the changes, or because they are submicroscopic in nature
- a fetal chromosomal rearrangement or supernumerary chromosome may be detected in prenatal diagnosis, in some case of which it may not be possible to unequivocally determine whether the fetal karyotype will cause phenotypic problems in the child

- confined placental mosaicism may be present in CVS samples, which may result in the need for further invasive testing
- trisomy correction in the placenta may result in a false negative result or undetected uniparental disomy of an imprinted chromosome in CVS samples
- false positive results, which are more common in direct preparations, QF-PCR investigations, and mosaic karyotypes, may also occur in CVS samples
- cultures initiated from placental tissue and products of conception, growth of maternal cells in the sample may give a result that is not indicative of the foetal karyotype.

### Molecular genetics

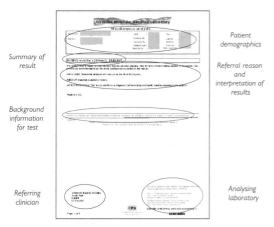

**Fig. 3.11** Molecular genetics report. See also colour plate section.

*Gene screening report outcomes*

Pathogenic mutation(s) detected (previously reported or clearly pathogenic e.g. STOP mutation)

- Confirmation of clinical diagnosis.
- Predictive testing may be offered to at-risk family members.
- Unknown variant detected (not previously reported)
  Analysis of the DNA variant is required before its pathogenicity can be established, using the following strategies
  - Search of mutation and DNA sequence databases to determine if the change has been previously seen in either affected patients or normal individuals.
  - *In silico* analysis of the DNA variant uses software to make predictions about the effect of the DNA sequence change on RNA

processing (e.g. splicing) and its resultant effect on the protein product.
- Segregation analysis explores whether the DNA variant tracks with the disease phenotype within the family. This method uses the principle of linkage analysis above. If a clinically affected individual is demonstrated not to carry the DNA variant this reduces the likelihood that the variant is the disease-causing mutation in the family. Caution must be exercised when using segregation analysis to consider the penetrance of the clinical phenotype and also whether phenocopies for the clinical phenotype may be likely.
- Some genes and variants are amenable to functional analysis to determine the nature of the DNA sequence and amino acid change within an *in vitro* system. Functional analysis is rarely available within routine diagnostic laboratories.
- Analysis of all candidate genes should be completed.

Reporting of a variant is likely to include the following phrases
- No confirmation or exclusion of clinical diagnosis.
- The DNA variant may be classified as one of the following types:
  - highly likely pathogenic
  - likely pathogenic
  - intermediate
  - unlikely pathogenic
  - non-pathogenic/polymorphic
- Further studies required to determine pathogenicity of DNA variant.
- Predictive testing will not be offered unless pathogenicity is established.
- No mutations detected.
- For many cardiac genetic conditions mutations have been described in several different genes (e.g. HoCM—*MYH7*, *MYBPC3*, *TNNT2*, *TNNI3*, *TPM1*, *ACTC*, *MYL2*, *MYL3*, *LAMP2*, *PRKAG2* and *GLA*). Therefore if a mutation is not detected in any one or a group of these genes, a diagnosis of an inherited cardiac condition can not be excluded. Even if all genes have been screened it is not possible to exclude the possibility that other genes may contribute to the clinical phenotype, or that the molecular screening technology is less than 100% sensitive.
- Alternatively, for some cardiac genetic conditions a single gene has been associated with the clinical phenotype (e.g. Fabry's—*GLA* gene). Therefore if no mutation is detected using a molecular method with approaching 100% sensitivity, the diagnosis is highly unlikely.
  - Clinical diagnosis unlikely, or, clinical diagnosis neither confirmed nor excluded.
  - (Further analysis of genes X, Y, Z recommended).
  - No predictive testing is currently available.

*Predictive analysis outcomes*

When testing an unaffected, at-risk family member for a familial pathogenic mutation:
- Familial mutation present:
  - patient at high risk of developing clinical phenotype
  - the specific risk to the patient depends upon the penetrance of the condition.

- Familial mutation absent:
  - patient at low risk of developing clinical phenotype
  - screening and/or clinical intervention may be ceased, depending upon the family structure which should be assessed by a clinical geneticist.

*Confirmatory analysis outcomes*
When testing an affected family member for a familial pathogenic mutation:
- Familial mutation present:
  - confirmation of clinical phenotype.
- Familial mutation absent:
  - exclusion of familial mutation as a cause of the patient's clinical phenotype. The relative may therefore be a phenocopy of the clinical condition within the family, or the relative may have a different mutation causing the same clinical phenotype (less likely).

# Genetic counselling

# Definition

Genetic counselling is one of the major tools for managing inherited cardiovascular conditions including single gene disorders and multifactorial conditions such as coronary artery disease (CAD) and congenital heart disease (CHD). This chapter deals with genetic counselling for cardiovascular genetic conditions that are typically transmitted in a Mendelian fashion. Typically, a genetic counsellor works within a multidisciplinary team including cardiologists, clinical geneticists, nurses, social workers, and psychologists. In some settings, families are referred directly to a clinical genetics department for genetic counselling.

### Definition

The National Society of Genetic Counsellors in the United States produced the following definition of genetic counselling which is applicable to cardiovascular genetics.

'Genetic counselling is the process of helping people understand and adapt to the medical, psychological, and familial implications of genetic contributions to disease.'

This definition is readily applicable to cardiovascular genetics and demonstrates the diversity of the genetic counsellor's role:

- education
- counselling
- working with families in dealing with psychosocial issues
- helping individuals in the family in making informed decisions.

# Role of genetic counsellors

Most referrals for genetic counselling are made when an affected individual or a close family member (consultand) seeks advice/information on an inherited condition including assessment of genetic risks, reproductive choices and genetic testing. The genetic counsellor engages with the consultand to help them to understand how their decisions fit with their values and the kind of life they want to live now and in the future. Thus genetic counselling always includes provision of information and education about the natural history of the condition in question and basic genetic information including inheritance patterns. Gaps in knowledge about the cardiovascular genetic condition and the limitations of genetic testing should also be discussed.

The expertise that genetic counsellors bring to the cardiac genetics clinic may include the following:

- understanding of the genetic basis of specific conditions
- counselling knowledge and skills
- understanding of family dynamics
- skills in working with the family while respecting the individual
- awareness that an individual's values, understanding, beliefs, and perceptions about a condition are usually built on their prior experience of the condition.

# Process of genetic counselling

Some of the key elements of the genetic counselling process are:

## Referral source

Referral for genetic counselling usually occurs in the following settings
- Primary care requesting advice on an apparently healthy but worried family member.
- Secondary care, usually cardiologist or a member of the cardiology unit
- Direct from a member of the family following a diagnosis and/or sudden cardiac death in a close relative.
- From coroner's office dealing with sudden unexplained (likely cardiac) death.
- Re-referral on a previously known family.
- Referral from another clinical genetics unit dealing with a member of the extended family.

## Confirmation of diagnosis

The following sources may need to be requested to confirm a diagnosis:
- referral letter
- medical records
- cardiology review
- death certificate
- coroner's post-mortem/outcome of inquest
- pathology reports—autopsy/specialist cardiac histopathology
- molecular genetic testing
- information from other genetic units.

## Initial contact with the consultand/family

- Introduction—role and process etc.
- Reason for referral.
- Consent for referral.
- Expectation from referral.

## Assessment/evaluation of the issues

- Appropriateness of the referral.
- Assessing immediate requirements.
- Consultand's awareness and appreciation.
- Assessment of prior genetic risks.
- Evaluation of issues pertinent to genetic counselling.
- Discussion with the clinical geneticist and/or multidisciplinary team.

## Formulation of the agenda/plan

- Prioritizing the issues and finalizing plans.
- Informing the consultand and/or family (by telephone or letter).
- Genetic clinic appointment—direct or jointly with the clinical geneticist.

## Direct appointment with the genetic counsellor

- Commonly for low-risk situation.
- Follow up appointment.
- Pre-clinic appointment.

### Discussion on consent and confidentiality issues

- Assessing level of intra-family communication and contacts.
- Informing the process and importance of consent.
- Assessing willingness to share information with other family members.
- Enquiring willingness to share information with other genetic/ cardiology units dealing with a member of the extended family.
- Assessing knowledge of current legislation on confidentiality and data-protection.

### Formal cardiac genetic clinic appointment

- Commonly joint with the consultant clinical geneticist.
- Possibly with a trainee or other career-grade geneticist on behalf of the consultant clinical geneticist.
- Usually an hour-long discussion on the nature of inherited cardiovascular condition, mode of inheritance, interpretation of the family history, specific genetic risks, likely medical implications, discussion on options, discussion on reproductive choices (if appropriate), molecular genetic testing, outcome of molecular genetic testing (stopping cardiology surveillance or continued follow-up with appropriate intervention), and agreeing on follow-up plans.

### Arranging appropriate genetic testing

- Prior information on the availability of specific molecular genetic test.
- Information on the level of sensitivity.
- Choosing the laboratory and turnaround time.
- Costs involved and agreeing with managers for payment or reimbursement.
- Recording of fully informed consent with freedom to withdraw and/or withholding results.
- Agreeing on method of result reporting—preferably at a genetic clinic appointment.

### Review of the outcome/letter

- Detailed letter on all aspects of the genetic counselling process.
- Preferably a joint letter with clinical geneticist as a co-signatory.
- Specifically to include arrangements for genetic testing, further medical consultations and follow-up.

### Review/interpretation of results

- Usually with the laboratory personnel and clinical geneticist.
- Cautionary approach to the use of technical phrases in the laboratory report.
- Care in dealing with the consultand or member of the immediate family.

### Liaison with cardiology unit/other clinical support unit

- Close links with the cardiac-genetics specialist nurse.
- Links with specialist cardiology nurses, for example heart failure or arrhythmia.
- Discussion at joint cardio-genetic multidisciplinary team meetings.

**Follow-up including dealing with members of the extended family**

- Assessing satisfaction with the genetic input.
- Questions and issues arising from the genetic clinic and/or letter.
- Review on the outcome of a negative molecular genetic test.
- Assessing the outcome of disclosure of genetic risk—both for 'high to low' or 'low to high'.
- Assessing the level and quality of appropriate medical follow-up either in primary care or secondary care.
- Dissemination of the information to other family members.
- Lifestyle and career adjustments following the genetic consultation.

# Genetic risk assessment and communication

Genetic risk assessment is usually carried out jointly with the clinical geneticist and/or genetic laboratory prior to the genetic counselling appointment. Genetic risks can be reasonably assessed by:

- pedigree analysis
- confirmation of diagnosis in the index patient (proband)
- degree of relationship to the index patient
- age and gender of the consultand
- outcome of appropriate genetic testing.

In any situation, establishing the mode of inheritance is fundamental for assessing prior genetic risk, for example 50% prior risk for being heterozygote to the healthy asymptomatic surviving sibling of a young person who died unexpectedly and with evidence of hypertrophic cardiomyopathy at post-mortem examination.

Genetic risk communication depends on whether the consultand is affected or is an unaffected relative from a family in which there is a cardiovascular genetic disease. Each consultand should receive help in appreciating the difference between inheriting the condition and developing the disease status. The types of risk may include:

- the risk of developing clinically symptomatic disease
- the risk that the condition present in the family is inherited or isolated
- the risk that a mutation will be identified in the family
- the risk of inheriting a mutation and the risk of passing on a mutation to (future) offspring
- the risk of sudden death.

It is important to highlight the following factors during risk communication:

- more than one gene causing the same condition, for example different potassium ion channel genes causing long QT syndrome
- more than one type of gene change (mutation) causing the same condition, for example the gene expression can be disrupted by either deletion, intronic splice site polymorphism, nonsense mutation or a missense mutation
- the disease-causing effect of the gene may not be 100% or incomplete penetrance
- the spectrum of symptoms and signs may not be same within a family and in different families—variability
- the natural history of the disease may be different in families and amongst the affected persons, for example no clear risks for sudden cardiac death
- perception and appreciating the risks may be different in various individuals and may be influenced by psychosocial status
- acceptance of risks may be influenced by social and cultural beliefs
- risk communication should be adjusted to person's socio-economic requirements, for example job, career and life insurance.

# Counselling for diagnostic genetic testing

This section deals only with molecular genetic testing.

If a disease-causing mutation is identified, 'predictive' gene testing can be offered to asymptomatic relatives at risk of inheriting the same mutation.

Diagnostic genetic testing for cardiovascular genetic conditions is complicated by the following factors:

- genetic heterogeneity—different mutation, alleles or genes with similar phenotype. This may be either in the same gene (allelic heterogeneity) or different genes at different loci (locus heterogeneity)
- mutations or variation of unknown or uncertain pathogenic significance
- lack of evidence for the family-specific mutation in the index case
- lack of confirmation in a clinically affected individual in the family
- mutation testing may not always be possible if the only affected family member is deceased and no tissue or genetic material (DNA) are stored.

- Genetic counselling prior to mutation detection should include a discussion about the three possible outcomes of mutation detection.

### 1. A sequence variation that is believed to be a disease-causing mutation is identified

The task of determining the pathogenicity of a sequence variation often involves consultation within a multidisciplinary team. Molecular geneticists, working together with cardiologists, clinical geneticists, and/or genetic counsellors may contribute to the assessment of the pathogenicity of a sequence change. Sequence variations are generally considered to be disease-causing if the following set of criteria can be met.

- The sequence variation is absent from a large group of control chromosomes. It is preferable for controls to be ethnically matched to the case.
- The sequence variation cosegregates with disease in the family. It may not always be possible to perform cosegregation studies because of small family size or because some affected family members may not wish to have gene testing.
- The nature of the amino acid change is significant.
- The sequence variation has been reported in other affected families, with evidence of the mutation cosegregating with disease.
- The variant is in an important functional domain of the gene (functional studies may be required to demonstrate this).

### 2. A sequence variation of unknown significance is identified

These are variations in the DNA for which there is not enough evidence to clearly categorise the variant as disease-causing, or a polymorphism, based on the criteria listed above.

When a variation of unknown significance is identified, its utility in confirming the diagnosis in a consultand with suspected disease is limited.

It **cannot be used** for predictive gene testing in at-risk relatives. The implication of identifying a sequence variation of unknown significance for first-degree relatives of all clinically affected individuals in the family is that their gene status cannot be determined and clinical screening will need to continue.

### 3. No mutation is identified

There are several explanations for this. It is possible that the disease-causing mutation in the family is present in a gene that was not tested. Alternatively, it is possible that there is a mutation in one of the genes that was tested, but the mutation detection technique employed by the laboratory missed the mutation. For example, gene sequencing is considered the 'gold standard' for mutation detection, but even gene sequencing does not detect large deletions or duplications within genes. All laboratory reports will provide information about the testing technique used and the estimated sensitivity and specificity of the technique. Many laboratories now use more than one technique for testing; MLPA, which can detect large deletions and duplications within genes not detectable by direct sequencing or gene scanning techniques, is gaining popularity as a second-tier testing technique once the primary mutation detection technique is completed and is negative.

The clinical implications of a gene-negative result, for the individual tested and the family, are the same as if a sequence variation of unknown significance was identified.

It is common practice for laboratories to report all variants found in genetic testing, whether they be disease-causing, of unknown significance or known polymorphisms (📖 see Chapter 3, Genetic laboratory techniques). It is incumbent upon both laboratory and clinical services to maintain records of all variants as knowledge of the implications of variants may change with time. Individuals attending for genetic testing should be made aware that they may be recontacted in the future if new information of clinical significance about such variations is learned.

# Predictive genetic testing

Predictive gene testing, which is also called asymptomatic gene testing, is possible only if a disease-causing mutation is known in a family. The key points in this process include:

- predictive gene testing is performed in an asymptomatic individual only; should the individual be symptomatic then this would be considered a diagnostic gene test
- the known family-specific mutation is 100% disease-causing
- the outcome of testing carries only two outcomes—the mutation is present or absent
- the risk to the individual with absent mutation is reduced to the population risk
- individuals without mutations can be reassured and no further cardiac screening is recommended
- individuals without mutations should be reassured on the negligible genetic risk to offspring
- individuals with mutations should receive further counselling on their lifetime risk for developing the cardiovascular genetic condition and will need to commence or continue targeted cardiac screening
- mutation-positive individuals should receive specific advice or information on the available prophylactic treatment such as medication or an implantable device (pacemaker or cardioverter) or both
- mutation-positive individuals may benefit from some lifestyle adjustment or modification, for example avoidance of stress and participating in competitive sports involving physical contact.

# Prenatal and pre-implantation genetic diagnosis

A number of reproductive options become available once a consultand is found to have a disease-causing mutation. These include prenatal diagnosis via chorionic villus sampling (CVS) or amniocentesis and pre-implantation genetic diagnosis.

## Prenatal diagnosis

It is important to be aware of the following basic concepts:

- CVS and amniocentesis are sample tissue from the developing placenta or fetus
- both procedures are carried out using sophisticated ultrasound imaging equipment for precise location of the fetus and placenta
- the tissue obtained is analysed for the presence of the family-specific mutation
- both procedures are associated with a risk of miscarriage. The risks generally quoted in practice are 0.5% for amniocentesis 1% for CVS. The risks may vary between centres
- CVS is most commonly performed transabdominally between 11- and 14-weeks gestation, by fine needle aspiration of chorionic cells from which DNA can be extracted and tested
- amniocentesis is commonly performed transabdominally after 15 weeks gestation by aspiration of amniotic fluid, culture of the cells suspended within the fluid, and extraction of DNA for testing. Culturing of cells can take 1–2 weeks so the result of DNA analysis can take as long as 3 weeks
- most couples undergoing above procedures do so with a view to terminating an affected fetus. However, this should not be a condition for the option of prenatal diagnosis. A couple may change the decision to terminate the affected fetus or vice versa!
- it is essential that couples considering prenatal diagnosis should be referred for formal genetic counselling and consultation with an expert in fetal medicine to assist them through the process.

## Pre-implantation genetic diagnosis

In the past 5–10 years, the use of pre-implantation genetic diagnosis (PGD) has become more widespread. Some basic concepts of this new but emerging technique include:

- PGD is the process of performing genetic analysis of an embryo for the family-specific mutation that has been identified in one of the parents
- the couple will need to undergo *in vitro* fertilization (IVF)
- the embryo is biopsied and one or two cells at the blastocyst (8 cell) stage are analysed
- testing of the cells will determine which embryos have inherited the family-specific mutation
- the embryo that does not have the mutation is transferred
- following confirmation of the pregnancy, couples are managed like any other normal pregnancy.

The European Society of Human Reproduction and Embryology PGD consortium has not reported any cases of PGD being used for cardiovascular genetic diseases except for Marfan syndrome. While the rate at which couples are using PGD to select against cardiovascular genetic conditions is currently small, the number of people requesting PGD for cardiovascular conditions is likely to increase as genetic testing for these conditions becomes more widespread. The cardiovascular genetic clinic should have as one of its responsibilities to inform the consultand about the possibility of using PGD as one of the options. Should this be the preferred choice, a referral to an IVF centre that performs PGD is recommended for detailed counselling.

Most likely users of PGD are couples:
- who have objections to termination of pregnancy
- that have had several terminations for the genetic condition present in the family in the past
- who prefer this option.

The couples need to be made aware of important limitations:
- the technique is complex and invasive
- specific permission and/or a license may be required by the PGD centre
- it may be prohibitively expensive
- the clinical pregnancy rate per embryo transfer is low with not more than 30% success rate.
- despite the best possible technique, a small false-negative risk is present
- in most cases, the resultant pregnancy is recommended to undergo CVS or amniocentesis to eliminate false negative risk.

# Genetic testing in children and adolescents

Genetic testing in children and adolescents is often challenging and requires a careful approach in dealing with complex ethical issues. In most cases it amounts to predictive genetic testing in a young child. Genetic counsellors or clinical geneticists may be involved in carrying out a diagnostic genetic test should there be reasonable clinical grounds. The genetic counsellor is responsible in facilitating and supporting the decision for carrying out a genetic test in a child or minor young person perceived to be at increased risk for an inherited cardiovascular condition.

In general the following guiding principles are used in decision making:

- the child or adolescent is confirmed to be at high prior genetic risk for developing symptoms and signs of the condition
- the family-specific mutation is absolutely confirmed to be disease-causing
- confirmation of the genetic status would allow specific and reliable long-term clinical surveillance for early detection of symptoms or signs of the condition
- specific advice or measures are known for the secondary prevention
- specific therapeutic and/or intervention devices may be used in the management following early diagnosis.

The following key factors should be kept in mind:

- wherever possible the child (10 years or older) should be included in discussion
- a parent or legal guardian has the legal right for signing the consent
- parental anxiety or concerns should not be the sole factor in the decision-making process
- children should be protected from the potential misuse of the information shared with other professionals, such as child protection, social services and educational authorities
- decision for genetic testing is in the best interest of the child or adolescent.

# Outcome of genetic counselling

The successful outcome of genetic counselling for an inherited cardiovascular disorder can be judged if the consultand and/or immediate (parents, children and siblings) family are able to:

- accept the inherited nature of the condition
- understand and appreciate the genetic risks and issues
- know and deal with their options
- make informed decisions about genetic testing
- make informed and appropriate reproductive choices
- deal with the long-term medical needs
- make appropriate lifestyle/career adjustments
- help and support members of their extended family
- working to support/help other similarly affected patients and families in the community, for example participating in patient support organizations such as British Heart Foundation (BHF), Cardiomyopathy Association (CMA) and Sudden Arrhythmic Death Syndrome (SADS-UK).

**Further reading**

Peter S. Harper *Practical Genetic Counselling*, 7th edn, Oxford University Press, New York, 2010.
Ian D. Young (2004) *Risk Calculation in Genetic Counselling*, 2nd edn. Oxford, Oxford University Press.

# Genetic testing and genetic screening

# Genetic testing and genetic screening

There are fundamental differences in genetic testing and genetic screening. However, in practice these terms are used interchangeably with often confusing interpretations.

***Genetic testing*** refers to the testing a healthy individual from a family affected with an inherited condition where the specific pathogenic genetic change, such as a chromosomal abnormality or a disease-causing change or variation in the nucleic acid sequence (gene), is already known.

Genetic testing can involve first-degree relatives (parents, siblings or children) or a family member in the extended family. The term '*cascade testing*' is commonly used when testing relatives.

It is also possible to employ conventional clinical tests (e.g., electrocardiogram for long QT syndrome, plasma cholesterol for familial hypercholesterolaemia or an echocardiogram for hypertrophic cardiomyopathy) to assess the disease risk status of an individual. However, a normal clinical screen does not rule out the possibility that an individual is carrying a genetic mutation since a number of dominantly inherited cardiovascular disorders exhibit incomplete penetrance and variable clinical expression.

***Genetic screening*** determines the genetic risk of a person belonging to a specific community or population group with a higher prevalence of a genetic condition for which a diagnostic genetic test is available. In this case, a family history is not required. It is important that there is acceptable intervention available with evidence of desired positive outcomes, for example reduced risk of developing or preventing symptoms of the condition. Examples of disorders suitable for genetic screening in particular populations include cystic fibrosis (northern Europeans), beta thalassaemia (Mediterranean people) and Tay–Sachs disease (Ashkenazi Jews).

The sole purpose of genetic screening is to offer an apparently healthy and asymptomatic individual information relevant to their own health risks, lifestyle, and the risk of having an affected child. Genetic screening inevitably has implications for other close relatives and can lead to unwanted and premature revelation of genetic risks.

# Genetic testing

## Indications

In principle, any close family member can be offered a genetic test following confirmation of the diagnosis in the index case. It is presumed that at the time of testing the person would have been healthy and asymptomatic.

Essential prerequisites prior to offering genetic testing include:
- detailed genetic counselling
- informed consent
- clinical cardiology opinion as to the clinical status any subtle changes would shift the person to the diagnostic genetic testing category as opposed to the pre-symptomatic or predictive genetic testing
- clinical genetic professional or genetic laboratory should confirm the clinical status with the cardiologist or any other relevant clinician.

The scope for genetic testing is rapidly expanding (Table 5.1). Laboratory confirmation of a molecular cytogenetic abnormality (for example 22qdeletion) or a pathogenic mutation (deletion, duplication, point mutation or a missense mutation) or a polymorphism (for example a splice site change) is the absolute requirement prior to offering genetic testing to any person with a family history of an inherited cardiovascular condition.

Clinical and laboratory methods need to be regularly reviewed in the light of new data to assess their predictive value based on sensitivity and specificity. *All genetic laboratories are required to clearly specify in the report if the pathological change is causally linked to the phenotype and pre-symptomatic or predictive genetic testing can be offered to other family members.* In case of any doubt, it is essential that the clinician or a member of the clinical team should seek confirmation from the genetic laboratory. This should be clear and unambiguous. This information is vital for genetic counselling and obtaining the informed consent.

It is also important that the genetic laboratory should be either accredited or licensed to carry out the specific genetic test. A list of accredited genetic laboratories can be found on several statutory or professional organisations, such as CPA (℘ http://www.cpa-uk.co.uk), UKGTN (℘ http://www.ukgtn.nhs.uk) and Eurogenetest (℘ http://www.eurogenetest.org). Should a gene mutation or polymorphism were found during research then this would require confirmation in an accredited genetic service laboratory.

**Table 5.1** Indications for genetic testing

| Inherited cardiovascular condition (ICC) | Clinical investigations | Genetic laboratory testing |
|---|---|---|
| Familial congenital heart disease | Clinical review, echocardiogram (ECG), karyotype and specific molecular cytogenetic abnormality (e.g., FISH for 22qdeletion) | Only applicable if a known pathogenic mutation in a specific gene, e.g. PTPN11 (Noonan syndrome), TBX1 (Velocardiofacial) and TBX5 (Holt–Oram syndrome) |
| Long QT syndrome | ECG, electrophysiological tests including epinephrine challenge | Known disease-causing mutation/polymorphism in one of the ion channel genes: SCN5A, KCNQ1, KCNE1, KCNE2, HERG etc. |
| Brugada syndrome | ECG and electrophysiological tests including azmaline/flecainide challenge | Known disease-causing mutation or polymorphism in SCN5A |
| Hypertrophic cardiomyopathy | Clinical review, ECG, echocardiogram, and cardiac magnetic resonance imaging (MRI) | Known pathogenic mutation or polymorphism in one of the cardiac sarcomere genes: MYH7, MYBPC3, Troponin C, Troponin T, Troponin I, Tropomyosin etc. |
| Arrythmogenic cardiomyopathy | Clinical review, ECG, echocardiogram and elctrophysiological tests | Known pathogenic mutation/polymorphism in one of the desmosomal genes |
| Other ICCs | Clinical review with conventional battery of cardiological investigations | Discuss with the clinical genetics team and molecular genetic laboratory for specific genes and availabilty of reliable clinical service testing |

## Essential steps in genetic testing

- Confirmation of the clinical diagnosis in the index patient.
- Verification of the family history by death certificate, post-mortem report or any other valid medical evidence.
- Confirmation of the pathogenic mutation or clinically relevant DNA polymorphism either in the index patient or any other affected family member. A copy of the report should be appended with the current medical records.
- Genetic counselling to the index patient including explicit informed consent to use the clinical and genetic laboratory information for the purpose of assessing genetic risks and carrying out genetic testing in the 'at-risk' family member seeking advice and information.

- Genetic counselling to the at-risk family member focusing on clinical aspects, inheritance pattern, genetic risks, available treatment options, scope and limitations of preventive interventions (for example, an implantable cardioverter defibrillator (ICD) or pacemaker etc.), recommended lifestyle modifications and implications on job, career, life, and medical insurance.
- Specific and unambiguous information on the genetic test including level of sensitivity, phenotype prediction and expected turnaround time.
- Fully explicit and informed consent prior to blood (or any other tissue specimen) collection.
- Record the whole process in writing for future records and share the information with the family member, referring clinician, family medical practitioner, lead of the cardiology team, and any other relevant professional.

## Establishing the clinical validity of an ICC gene mutation or DNA polymorphism

It is mandatory that any gene mutation of polymorphism should be confirmed to be pathogenic prior to consideration of its use in assessing the genetic risks to a healthy and apparently unaffected family member. There are a number of ways by which the pathogenic significance of a DNA sequence change can be established:

- Frame shift mutation, for example deletion/duplication in one of the coding exons of a gene.
- Terminating or truncating mutation, for example nonsense mutation in any of the exons towards 3' end.
- Confirmation of the pathological protein alteration resulting from a missense mutation—this could be facilitated by database search (for example Ensemble).
- Evidence to illustrate a DNA polymorphism interfering with gene function by its location (for example at 5' end) or splicing (located at one of the intronic splice junctions).
- Extensive family studies in case of a novel mutation and/or polymorphism—as many affected and unaffected. For example, finding the similar mutation or polymorphism in a healthy/unaffected family member would raise considerable doubts and thus could not be used for predictive genetic testing.
- Family linkage analysis to establish the disease-associated haplotype and correlating this with the specific gene under investigation.
- Employing RNA studies to demonstrate effect on gene-expression.
- Computer-based *in silico* analysis to work out the possible pathogenic effects.

## Genetic testing in children and young persons

Testing any child or a young person (usually under 15 years) is controversial. Apart from consent and technical difficulties, one might need to answer the core issue related to the potential health gains by carrying out a genetic test in a young family member of the family affected with an inherited disease. There are no clear answers and the final decision rests on parents and to limited extent on the child. There are a number of guidelines and suggestions for good practice. A detailed discussion on this controversial subject is beyond the scope of this section (📖 see Further reading). However, following general guidelines are likely to be helpful in dealing with request for carrying out genetic testing in a child or a young person:

- detailed genetic counselling to parents faced with the potential genetic risk to their child
- information on the ICC highlighting the available management options
- information on possible interventions including prophylactic medications and procedures to minimise clinical outcomes of having inherited the genetic abnormality
- evidence for life-long benefits of stated plan for preventive measures
- validity of informed consent keeping child's interests. Recommended age for a child to give consent for a genetic disease is agreed to be 10 years
- psych-social support to the child and parents following positive genetic testing.

## Prenatal diagnosis

The primary prevention of a genetic disease is often difficult. The practice of prenatal diagnosis (PND) is acceptable by most health practice systems and in several culturally diverse countries. Techniques of chorion villous biopsy at 11 weeks and amniocentesis at 15 weeks are established with known technical difficulties and outcomes (📖 see Further reading). This is not discussed here in detail.

Experience of PND in the secondary prevention of an inherited cardiovascular condition (ICC) is limited. This is largely due to extremely limited facilities for carrying out reliable molecular genetic diagnosis in ICC. A large majority of PND for ICC is limited to chromosome abnormality such as 22q deletion syndrome. There are several issues that pose serious challenges to the practice of PND in ICC:

- most Mendelian genetic cardiovascular diseases exhibit significant inter- and intrafamilial clinical variation
- incomplete penetrance in a number of autosomal dominant ICC
- mutational heterogeneity in large number of ICC
- clinical significance for a large number of mutations and/or DNA polymorphisms is unclear
- there is often unclear genotype–phenotype correlation of a pathogenic mutation or gene polymorphism
- the predictive value of any genetic abnormality including a chromosomal microdeletion or microduplication in PND is extremely limited and may vary from the mild to severe/lethal phenotype
- termination of an affected pregnancy is solely on the basis of detecting the genetic abnormality and **not** on the likelihood of being clinically affected
- psychosocial implications are likely as the clinical outcomes in most ICC are limited to cardiovascular morbidity and early/unexpected mortality.

## Pre-implantation genetic diagnosis

Increasing number of genetic disorders is now potentially preventable using the pre-implantation genetic diagnosis (PGD). This approach is based on employing an IVF technique of assisted reproduction and selective embryo transfer of the mutation-free embryo following the specific genetic testing in the single cell retrieved from an 8-cell stage embryo. Details of techniques are beyond the scope of this section (📖 see Further reading).

The following are a few essential prerequisites for PGD:
• confirmation of the specific genetic abnormality in the affected prospective parent, for example a chromosome abnormality such as 22q deletion or a specific gene mutation such as one of ion-channel genes in long QT syndrome
• detailed genetic counselling to focus on potential technical difficulties and limitations
• informed consent specifically for the condition and genetic abnormality under consideration
• consultation with the specialist PGD team
• explanation on genetic abnormality and genetic testing on the embryo
• discussion on the outcome of IVF including pregnancy, obstetric care, perinatal and neonatal care
• discussion on the possible need for prenatal diagnosis to reduce the risk for false-negative embryo genetic testing
• information on the legal requirement of the specific license from the statutory body such as Human Fertilization and Embryo Authority (HFEA) in the United Kingdom.

## Cascade testing

Cascade testing refers to consequential genetic testing in the extended family. This process in broadly similar to genetic testing, except that multiple family members may be involved all linked to either the index patient or the first family member in whom the diagnosis of an ICC was clinically made and confirmed by the identification of a disease-causing gene mutation or DNA polymorphism associated with one of the genes associated with ICC. It is important that all the recommended steps (📖 see Essential steps in genetic testing, pp. 79–80) are individually applied to the respective family member included in the cascade testing. Special measures might need to be applied where the cascade testing spreads to other geographic regions or even countries beyond the direct jurisdiction of the main cardiology or clinical genetic centre. Wherever possible, one of the local cardiologists or clinical geneticists should be involved to safe guard matters related to consent and confidentiality. Recently cascade testing has been introduced in Wales, UK for familial hypercholesterolemia. However, a similar approach would be applicable to any other Mendelian ICC with a confirmed pathogenic gene mutation or DNA variant.

# Genetic screening

In contrast to genetic testing, genetic screening is limited in its scope and clinical utility. This approach is directed to any person in the community or an ethnic population group with a perceived increased risk for an inherited cardiovascular disease. The person in question might not have been referred for cardiogenetic opinion. It is likely that the person in question was selected on the basis of inclusion criteria based on gender, age, body weight, smoking, alcohol consumption, and ethnic back ground. A consideration to past medical and family history is important but usually not necessarily important. The whole process may involve recording personal and medical information, carrying out a basic clinical review such as blood pressure measurement, and an electrocardiogram. It is important to record informed consent for undergoing further tests should the screening alter the lifetime risk for a specific ICC. A blood specimen or a buccal smear should be sufficient for carrying out the laboratory genetic tests.

Currently genetic screening for ICC is not routinely offered. It is often limited to collecting background information and recording basic clinical data. In most cases it is limited to checking the random blood sugar and plasma cholesterol. Carrying out an electrocardiogram in a healthy and often young person is unwanted and might lead to unnecessary further investigations. Apart from raising personal and family anxiety, this approach is controversial. Few pilot studies are underway and results of these surveys could help in designing selected population-based screening. There is no suggestion for carrying out direct mutation testing for a specific ICC.

## Limitations in genetic screening

- No specific recommendations for genetic screening in any ICC.
- Criteria for selection are unclear and not fully evidence-based.
- The process of genetic screening is not adequately validated.
- Genetic screening of children and young persons is not supported due to lack of evidence and long-term health gains.
- Clinical investigations, such as blood pressure measurement or an electrocardiogram, may lead to erroneous interpretations, irrelevant investigations, inappropriate advice and preventive measures and unpleasant outcomes.
- Most laboratory tests are **not genetic** and do not have the required sensitivity and specificity levels to warrant health surveillance.
- There are no specific recommendations for preventive or therapeutic interventions for managing the increased lifetime risk.
- Genetic screening may lead to unwanted psychological (anxiety, depression, lack of drive etc.) and socio-economic consequences (impact on job/career, difficulty in securing/improving medical and life insurance etc.).
- Health professionals may have to deal with unexpected ethical, moral and legal consequences.

## Further reading

Peter S. Harper *Practical Genetic Counselling*, 7th edn, Oxford University Press, New York, 2010.

# Chapter 6

# Congenital heart disease

# Introduction to congenital heart disease

Since most cases are now managed successfully and progress to adulthood, the prevalence of CHD in the general population has risen considerably. This rise may also reflect in an increased birth incidence due the risk of recurrence in the offspring of adults with CHD (grown up congenital heart disease or GUCH).

- Most congenital heart defects are isolated, non-syndromic and sporadic.
- The incidence of CHD is ≈7–8 per 1000 live births.
- Ventricular septal defect (VSD) is the commonest abnormality.
- CHD account for 10% of all infant deaths in Western countries and nearly half of all infant deaths attributed to congenital malformations.
- Around 15% of affected infants die in the first year, 4% of those surviving infancy dying by 16 years.
- Additional non-cardiac malformations are present in about a quarter of children with CHD.
- The presence of an associated non-cardiac malformation suggests the possibility of an underlying chromosomal abnormality or genetic multiple malformation syndrome.

# Genetics of congenital heart disease

Heritable syndromes account for approximately 7.4% of CHD, but the genetic mechanisms underlying 'sporadic' CHD are poorly understood. Approximately 12% arise from chromosomal abnormalities such as Alagille, Down, DiGeorge (22q11 deletion), Williams–Beuren, and trisomy 18, which affect cardiac developmental gene copy number. Some patients with non-syndromic 'sporadic' congenital heart disease also have 22q11 deletion. Point mutations in cardiac developmental genes (e.g. *CITED2* and *NKX2.5*) account for only a small proportion of 'sporadic' CHD.

Phenotypic heterogeneity is observed in both mouse and humans (Table 6.1). Such pleiotropy is of clinical importance in malformations such as transposition of great arteries (TGA) or tetralogy of Fallot (TOF) with substantially poorer outcomes, than for instance, an atrial septal defect (ASD).

**Table 6.1** Phenotypic heterogeneity in patients with congenital heart disease resulting from non-synonymous mutations in single genes and certain chromosomal disorders

| Gene | Cardiac phenotypes |
| --- | --- |
| CFC1 | TGA, ASD, AVSD, VSD, PDA, L-atrial isomerism, DORV, heterotaxy |
| CITED2 | TOF, ASD, VSD, TAPVR, TGA |
| CRELD1 | AVSD, heterotaxy |
| GATA4 | TOF, AVSD, AS, PS, dextrocardia |
| LEFTY A | HLHS, AVSD, dextrocardia, heterotaxy |
| TBX5 | ASD, VSD, AVSD, HLHS, TOF, CAT, TA, DORV, TAPVR |
| TBX20 | ASD, VSD, valve defects |
| JAG1 | ASD, AVSD, VSD, TOF, PA, PDA, PS, CAT |
| NKX2-5 | ASD, VSD, TOF, DORV, L-TGA, IAA, HLHS, PAVSD |
| NOTCH1 | AS, TOF, VSD |
| PROSIT240 | TGA, VSD, coarctation of aorta |
| PTPN11 | PS, PDA, ASD |
| ZIC3 | Situs inversus, TAPVR, HLHS, VSD, TGA, DORV, PS |
| 22q11del | IAA, VSD, CAT, PAVSD, TOF |
| Trisomy 21 | AVSD, VSD, TOF |

AS, aortic srenosis; ASD, atrial septal defect; APUS, absent pulmonary valve syndrome; AVSD, atrio-ventricular septal defect; BAV, bicuspid aortic valve; CA, coarctation of aorta; CAT, common arterial trunk; DORV, double outlet right ventricle; HCM, hypertrophic cardiomyopathy; HLHS, hypoplastic left heart syndrome; IVC, inferior vena cava; IAA, interrupted aortic arch; L-TGA, congenitally corrected transposition of great arteries; PA, pulmonary atresia; PAVSD, pulmonary atresia ventricular septal defect with aorto-pulmonary collaterals; PDA, patant ductus arteriosus; PPAS, peripheral pulmonary artery stenosis; RAA, right aortic arch; TA, tricuspid atresia; TGA, transposition of great arteris; TOF, tetralogy of Fallot; TAPVR, total anomalous pulmonary venous return.

# General aspects of CHD management

The management of CHD requires integrated and appropriately resourced multidisciplinary care. The multidisciplinary team (MDT) should include the following:

- Fetal/neonatal cardiology: fetal/neonatal diagnosis, leading the management plan, advising parents, and supervising the cardiology aspects of management.
- Surgical intervention: provided at the tertiary/supraregional paediatric cardiothoracic surgery unit.
- Paediatric cardiology: monitoring the general paediatric aspects of care, growth and development progress, parental support and guidance in accordance to the needs of the child.
- Clinical genetics: assessment and diagnosis of the underlying genetic condition including multiple malformation syndrome, genetic counselling, clinical and genetic surveillance of close family members, supporting and advising on reproductive choices, participating in the management of high-risk pregnancy including prenatal diagnosis.
- GUCH service: usually an adult cardiologist with special interest in congenital heart diseases; main role in the delivery and supervision of MDT management of a known case of complex or syndromic form of CHD progressing to adult age group (15–16 years) (☐ see Further reading).

Further reading

Goodship J. and Wren, C *Congenital cardiovascular malformations*, in Kumar and Elliott (eds), *Principles and practice of clinical cardiovascular Genetics*, Oxford university Press, New York, 2010.

# The genetic consultation in CHD

Whilst the major concern for parents of children with a CHD is the well-being of their child the questions that dominate the genetic consultation are 'Why did it happen?' and 'Will it happen again?' This is addressed by taking the family history, documenting maternal health and exposures in pregnancy and assessing whether the child has an isolated CHD or additional abnormalities.

## Family history

A three-generation family history should always be recorded before giving recurrence risks. In addition to providing more accurate information this may identify a family that is large enough to map and identify a causative gene.

The incidence of CHD is higher in monozygotic twins. As it is not uncommon for one of a twin pregnancy to be lost before term one should ask specifically if a first trimester obstetric ultrasound was performed and how many embryos were seen: the family is unlikely to volunteer this information as they will not be aware of its importance.

### Maternal history

Maternal illness increases the risk of CHD. Specifically:

- rubella is rare in countries with vaccination programmes but should still be considered
- untreated phenylketonuria is associated with a greater than sixfold increase in CHD risk, including TOF, ventricular septal defect (VSD), patent ductus arteriosus (PDA) and single ventricle. Strict dietary control before conception and in the first seven weeks of gestation reduces this risk
- diabetes mellitus increases the risk of laterality disturbance, transposition of the great arteries, atrioventricular septal defect, VSD, hypoplastic left heart, outflow tract defects and PDA. Good glycemic control before conception and during pregnancy decreases the risk but may be difficult to achieve
- epilepsy increases the risk of congenital malformations including CHD, possibly due a direct teratogenic effect of anticonvulsant therapy or an indirect effect of perturbed folate metabolism.

CHD is also a feature of fetal alcohol syndrome, thalidomide embryopathy and isoretinoin embryopathy.

## Examining the child

CHD often occurs in combination with other malformations or dysmorphic features which provide clues to a chromosomal or syndromic diagnosis. Such a diagnosis has implications for the management of the child (e.g. risk of learning, hearing or visual impairment) and family (e.g. recurrence risk). Specific features to note include:

- height, weight and head circumference
- developmental milestones

- limb abnormalities (polydactyly (pre- or post-axial); abnormalities of the thumb/radial ray)
- quality of speech and speech development (e.g. velopharyngeal insufficiency is common in children with chromosome 22q11 deletion).

If there are multiple congenital malformations, dysmorphic features, pre-and postnatal retardation of growth, unexplained developmental delay or any combination of these features in association with CHD, chromosome analysis should be requested unless the pattern is that of a recognizable Mendelian syndrome.

# Genetic investigations in CHD

## Cytogenetics

Standard cytogenetic analysis to examine the karyotype for a major aneuploidy or a structural abnormality is helpful. This may be combined with FISH for 22q deletion in a case with complex CHD, particularly with an outlet abnormality. Other specific FISH examination should be requested in particular CHDs (e.g. 7q deletion in supravalvular aortic stenosis: Williams–Beuren syndrome). It is important to discuss the case with the cytogenetic laboratory or clinical geneticist prior to blood specimen collection.

## Molecular genetics

Mutation analysis in certain genes associated with some complex CHDs and multiple malformation syndromes is now possible (Table 6.2). An up-to-date list of approved and accredited molecular genetic laboratories can be found in online resources, for example UK Genetic Testing Network (UKGTN), European genetic testing network (Eurogentest) and North American Genetic testing network (GeneTests). A discussion with the clinical geneticist and the laboratory is important for specimen collection and complete information on sensitivity and specificity of the mutation analysis. Whilst identification of an underlying mutation may not be helpful in making the diagnosis, it may help in advising the long-term prognosis and providing options for prenatal or pre-implantation genetic diagnosis.

**Table 6.2** Genetic laboratory investigation in congenital heart disease
CHD/syndrome gene/chromosomal abnormality investigation

| Total anomalous venous drainage | 22qdup | Karyotype; FISH |
|---|---|---|
| Atrio-ventrcular septal defect | Trisomy 13,18 21; 3p25del | Karyotype; FISH |
| Transposition of great arteries | 22q11del | FISH |
| Truncus arteriosus | NKX2.6; 22q11del | Mutation testing/FISH |
| Tetralogy of Fallot | 22q11del | FISH |
| Interruption of the aorta | 22q11del | FISH |
| Coarctation of the aorta | 45X; 22qdel | Karyotype; FISH |
| Supra valvular aortic stenosis | Elastin/7q microdeletion | Mutation testing/FISH |
| Left hypoplastic heart syndrome | 1p36del; 11qdel; 2211qdel | Karyotype; FISH |

# Genetic counselling

Most referrals for genetic counselling include complex congenital heart defects or a multiple malformation syndrome with a significant cardiovascular phenotype. Preparation and conduct of genetic counselling, usually by an expert genetic counsellor, normally follow the conventionally agreed principles and practice of genetic counselling (📖 see Chapter 4, Genetic counselling). The aim is to provide information on CHD or malformation disorder, factual information on possible causes specifically highlighting the genetic factors, recurrence risks in future childbearing, reproductive options and available management options.

In most cases discussion is focussed on multifactorial/polygenic inheritance. For discussion related to chromosomal, Mendelian or mitochondrial inheritance see respective chapters in this book. Most consultees appreciate a detailed explanation on the role of many genes with a small combined effect leading to congenital heart defect similar to many other single or even complex congenital anomalies. The outcome of genetic counselling is generally positive supported by explanation, low recurrence risks (see Table 6.3) and reassurance through available reproductive and management options.

Recurrence risk for most CHDs are between 2–3% except for two consecutive affected siblings. These are derived from family studies and are therefore empiric. Recurrence risk to a first-degree relative, sibling or offspring, is approximately equal to the square root of the birth incidence in the general population. For example, an incidence of 1 per 1000 live birth for VSD will reflect in a recurrence risk estimate of approximately 3%. Empiric recurrence risk estimates are available for both unspecified (Table 6.3) and specific CHDs (Table 6.4). These are for guidance only. It is important to consider individual factors in calculating the recurrence risks.

**Table 6.3** Recurrence risks (%) for first degree relatives in unspecified congenital heart disease (adapted from Harper, 2003)

| | |
|---|---|
| Population incidence | 0.5 |
| Sib of isolated case | 2–3 |
| Half-sib or other second degree relatives | 1–2 |
| Offspring of isolated case: | |
|   Father | 2–3 |
|   Mother | 5–6 |
| Two affected sibs/sib-parent | 10 |
| More than 2 affected first-degree relatives | 50 (approx.) |

**Table 6.4** Genetic risks in congenital heart disease: all percent (adapted from Harper, 2003)

| Defect | 1 affected sib | Father affected | Mother affected |
|---|---|---|---|
| Ventricular septal defect 3 | 2.5 | | 9.5 (provisional) |
| Atrial septal defect | 2.5 | 1.5 | 6 |
| Patent ductus arteriosus 3 | 2 | | 4 |
| Fallot's tetraology | 2.5 | 1.5 | 2.5 |
| Arteriovenous canal defect | 2.5 | 1 | 14 (provisional) |
| Pulmonary stenosis | 2 | 2 | 6.5 |
| Aortic stenosis | 2 | 5 | 18 (provisional) |
| Transposition of great vessels | 1.5 | | |
| Hypoplastic left heart syndrome | 3 | | |
| Pulmonary atresia | 1 | | |
| Common truncus | 1 | | |
| Tricuspid atresia | 1 | | |
| Ebsteins' anomaly | 1 | | |

# Total anomalous pulmonary venous connection

In total anomalous pulmonary venous connection (TAPVC) all four pulmonary veins fail to connect with the left atrium and instead join the systemic venous system. The connection is variable in position and in degree of obstruction:

- supracardiac: to the innominate vein or superior vena cava
- infradiaphragmatic: to the hepatic or portal vein; this is most likely to be obstructed.
- intracardiac: to the coronary sinus or right atrium.
- associated with ASD: with flow from the right to the left atrium.

Infants with TAPVC present with a combination of cyanosis and heart failure. Surgical repair entails reconnection of the pulmonary veins to the left atrium. The long-term outlook for survivors of surgery is very good although in some infants there is recurrent and progressive pulmonary vein stenosis. Medium-term mortality ranges from 8–35%, being significantly better if total anomalous pulmonary venous connection is an isolated malformation.

Most cases of TAPVC are sporadic but a few families with multiple affected individuals in more than one generation are reported. TAPVC is associated with cat-eye syndrome, which is caused by an additional marker chromosome derived from chromosome 22. Formation of the marker chromosome is mediated by interchromosomal recombination between inverted low copy repeats on chromosome 22. Thus the marker comprises two centromeres with satellites (ribosomal RNA genes) with two copies of the proximal region of the long arm of chromosome 22 between them. Usually this is a mosaic chromosome abnormality, that is, the marker is present in only a proportion of cells, such that affected individuals have four copies (tetrasomy) of the genes on proximal chromosome 22q11 in a proportion of their cells.

# Complete atrioventricular septal defect

Complete atrioventricular septal defect (CAVSD) is a major malformation of the lower part of the atrial septum, the inlet part of the ventricular septum and the atrioventricular valve(s). There is a common atrioventricular valve in place of the mitral and tricuspid valves. The common valve usually has five leaflets and is often regurgitant. CAVSD is present in around 30 per 100,000 live births. The majority of infants present with heart failure or an incidental murmur. Some infants with a relatively high pulmonary resistance remain well with no murmur or heart failure, in which case the defect may be inoperable when the diagnosis is made. Without treatment, the natural history is premature death from heart failure in infancy or from irreversible pulmonary vascular disease (Eisenmenger's syndrome) in later childhood or early adult life. Surgical repair involves patch closure of the VSD, division of the common atrioventricular valve into left and right atrioventricular valves and patch closure of the ASD. In most cases post-operative atrioventricular valve function is good although reoperation for atrioventricular valve regurgitation is sometimes necessary.

Sixty per cent of CAVSD cases have Down syndrome (CAVSD accounts for almost half of the CVMs seen in Down syndrome). CAVSD is also associated with trisomies 13 and 18, chromosomal deletions (e.g. chromosome 3p25 deletion), Smith–Lemli–Opitz syndrome and Ellis–van Creveld syndrome. Isolated CAVSD is usually sporadic, but a few families with incomplete penetrance have been reported.

# Tetralogy of Fallot

Key features (see also Fig. 6.1):
- subaortic ventricular septal defect
- anterior displacement of the aorta
- complex right ventricular outflow obstruction.

TOF is the commonest type of cyanotic heart disease in infancy, occurring in around 30 per 100,000 live births. Most diagnoses are made in infancy after recognition of cyanosis or a heart murmur. Management depends on the severity of the outflow obstruction. Excessive or increasing cyanosis, or hypercyanotic 'spells', are managed by an early palliative aorto-pulmonary shunt, which increases the pulmonary artery flow. Definitive repair comprises closure of the ventricular septal defect and relief of the pulmonary outflow obstruction. The median age at repair in many units is around one year with a surgical mortality of 1%. Pulmonary regurgitation is a late complication after surgery that may require further surgery in adult life.

Tetralogy of Fallot is usually an isolated malformation but can be associated with other CVMs such as anomalous pulmonary venous connection, atrioventricular septal defect. It is present in 15% of children with 22q11 deletion and this deletion is present in around 5–10% of infants with TOF. TOF also occurs in around 5% of children with trisomy 21 and trisomy 21 accounts for around 5% of infants with TOF. It is also associated with trisomies 13 and 18 and a number of multiple malformation syndromes.

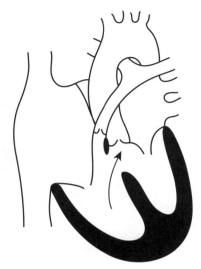

**Fig. 6.1** Tetralogy of Fallot. Note overriding of the aorta and pulmonary stenosis; presence of ventricular septal defect creates a right–left shunt.

Reprinted with permission from *Principles and Practice of Clinical Cardiovascular Genetics*. Oxford University Press, New York, 2010; Chapter 9, pp. 139–149.

# Hypoplastic left heart syndrome (HLHS)

Key features (see also Fig. 6.2):
- imperforate aortic valve
- underdeveloped left ventricle
- hypoplastic or atretic mitral valve.

Pulmonary venous return enters the right atrium from the left atrium and the only outlet from the heart is through the pulmonary artery. The systemic circulation is duct-dependent. The aortic arch is hypoplastic and the ascending aorta is very small, acting simply as a conduit for flow into the coronary arteries.

The natural prevalence is around 20 per 100,000 live births but is reduced by antenatal diagnosis and termination of pregnancy. The median age at diagnosis is about 2 days in those diagnosed postnatally.

Immediate treatment is with a prostaglandin infusion. Previously, infants were often allowed to die because of the poor results of intervention, but radical palliative surgery (the Norwood operation and variants that connect the right ventricle to a reconstructed aorta) can be performed. Actuarial 4-year survival for infants undergoing a Norwood operation is reported at 44%.

HLHS is usually a sporadic malformation but there is a familial association with other left sided malformations (e.g. bicuspid aortic valve and coarctation of the aorta). HLHS is associated with chromosomal syndromes (Turner syndrome, 45,X); 1p36 microdeletion and Jacobsen syndrome (11q23-qter deletion); and non-chromosomal syndromes such as Rubenstein–Taybi syndrome.

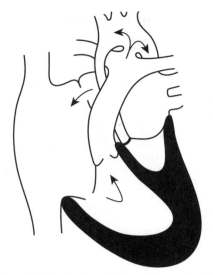

**Fig. 6.2** Left hypoplastic heart syndrome. Note marked narrowing of the left ventricular space.

Reprinted with permission from *Principles and Practice of Clinical Cardiovascular Genetics*. Oxford University Press, New York, 2010; Chapter 9, pp. 139–149.

# Transposition of the great arteries

This is the commonest cyanotic congenital heart disease presenting in newborn infants, occurring in around 30 per 100,000 live births. In 'simple' transposition the main abnormality is ventriculo-arterial discordance (the aorta arises from the right ventricle and the pulmonary artery from the left ventricle) (Fig. 6.3). Separate pulmonary and systemic circulations are incompatible with life and early after birth some cross-flow between the circulations is maintained by patency of the duct and the foramen ovale. Most infants present in the first few days of life with cyanosis. On recognition of cyanosis, infants are started on prostaglandin infusion to maintain ductal patency and undergo balloon atrial septostomy. Early repair with an arterial switch operation has a surgical mortality of less than 5%. TGA is rarely found in association with genetic syndromes but is one of malformations with highest relative risk in offspring of diabetic mothers.

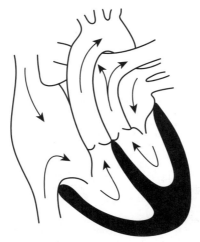

**Fig. 6.3** Transposition of the great arteries. Note aorta arising from the right ventricle and pulmonary artery from the left ventricle.

Reprinted with permission from *Principles and Practice of Clinical Cardiovascular Genetics.* Oxford University Press, New York, 2010; Chapter 9, pp. 139–149.

# Truncus arteriosus

Truncus arteriosus, or common arterial trunk, is a major malformation of the outflow of the heart occurring in around 10 per 100,000 live births.[1] It results from failure of septation of the ventricular outlets and the proximal arterial segment of the arterial tube (Figs 6.4a and b) to produce a single outlet valve overriding a subarterial ventricular septal defect. Both left and right ventricular outflow occurs through the valve into a common trunk which then separates into aorta and pulmonary arteries. The mode of connection of the pulmonary arteries to the trunk is variable. The truncal valve is usually tricuspid or quadricuspid and may be stenosed and/or regurgitant. There is often a right aortic arch and sometimes interruption of the aortic arch. Early primary repair involves patching the ventricular septal defect to the right of the truncal valve and removing the pulmonary arteries from the common trunk to leave the left ventricle connected to the aorta via the truncal valve (neoaortic valve) and placement of a conduit from the right ventricle to the pulmonary arteries to complete a biventricular repair. Results are good but later conduit replacement is inevitable.

About 10% of infants with chromosome 22q11 deletion have truncus and 30–40% of cases of truncus arteriosus occur in the context of 22q11 deletion. Truncus is also associated with maternal diabetes. A recessive pedigree has been reported that was found to have an *NKX2.6* mutation.

1. Hoffman J (1987) Incidence mortality and natural history. In: Anderson RH, Mc Cartney FJ, Shinebourne EA, Tynun M, eds. *Pediatric Cardiology*, Churchill Livingstone, London.

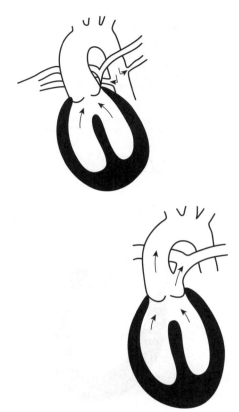

**Fig. 6.4** Truncus arteriosus—single trunk of the aorta arising from both right and left ventricle. There is subarterial ventricular septal defect; pulmonary artery may arise from the right ventricle (a) or direct from the aorta (b).

Reprinted with permission from *Principles and Practice of Clinical Cardiovascular Genetics.* Oxford University Press, New York, 2010; Chapter 9, pp. 139–149.

# Supravalvar aortic stenosis

Supravalvar aortic stenosis (SVAS) is a rare malformation characterized by stenosis of the ascending aorta at the sinotubular junction (Fig. 6.5) sometimes associated with stenosis of other systemic arteries and pulmonary arteries, and abnormalities of the aortic valve. Other malformations (mitral valve abnormalities, coarctation of the aorta, ventricular septal defect) are reported.

SVAS occurs in the context of Williams–Beuren syndrome in 50% of cases. When it occurs as an isolated malformation it can be familial, segregating as a dominant trait due to mutations in the elastin gene (ELN).

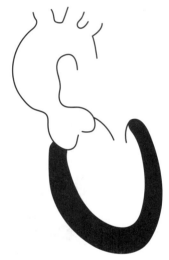

**Fig. 6.5** Supravalular aortic stenosis. Note narrowing of the proximal aorta just above the aortic valve.

Reprinted with permission from *Principles and Practice of Clinical Cardiovascular Genetics.* Oxford University Press, New York, 2010; Chapter 9, pp. 139–149.

# Coarctation of the aorta

Coarctation of the aorta (CoA) can present from prenatal to adult life but most are diagnosed in infancy. There is narrowing of the distal aortic arch adjacent to the ductus (Fig. 6.6). It is often accompanied by hypoplasia of the proximal aorta and sometimes of the aortic arch. About 40% of affected infants have an associated cardiac malformation; the commonest being VSD or bicuspid aortic valve; aortic valve stenosis, mitral valve abnormalitied and more complex cardiac malformations are also common. CoA It is the commonest cause of heart failure or cardiovascular collapse in the newborn. Infants can present with a murmur, heart failure or failure to thrive or hypertension beyond infancy. The surgical mortality of CoA repair is low and the overall outcome depends on the associated malformations. CoA is associated with Turner syndrome (45,X).

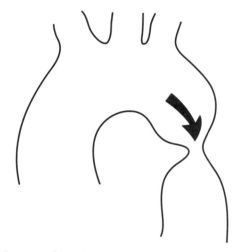

**Fig. 6.6** Coarctation of the aorta.

Reprinted with permission from *Principles and Practice of Clinical Cardiovascular Genetics*. Oxford University Press, New York, 2010; Chapter 9, pp. 139–149.

# Interruption of the aortic arch

In interruption of the aortic arch (IAA) a portion of the aorta fails to develop and the descending aorta is entirely supplied via the ductus. The interruption may be distal to the left subclavian artery (type A) or between the left carotid and the left subclavian arteries (type B) ([] Fig. 6.7). Interruption of the aortic arch is always associated with a major cardiac abnormality such as VSD, aortopulmonary window, truncus arteriosus, or other complex malformations.

As the lower half of the body has an entirely duct-dependent circulation, closure of the duct can result in haemodynamic collapse and death within hours. 50% go home without recognition of the problem, but present with heart failure or death before 6 weeks of age. Treatment is by primary repair of the aortic arch and additional procedures depending on associated abnormalities. Life expectancy is reduced due to residual or recurrent arch obstruction. 50% of cases of IAA type B occur in the context of chromosome 22q11 deletion and 15% of infants with 22q11 deletion have IAA.

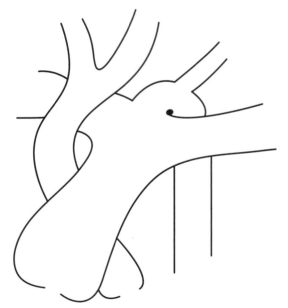

**Fig. 6.7** Interruption of the aortic arch. Note descending aorta is supplied directly by the ductus.

Reprinted with permission from *Principles and Practice of Clinical Cardiovascular Genetics.* Oxford University Press, New York, 2010; Chapter 9, pp. 139–149.

# Prenatal diagnosis

Most parents with one affected child with a CHD may contemplate another child. An increasing number of prospective parents at risk for having another affected child are attracted to the availability for prenatal diagnosis. However, this choice is commonly guided by their instinctive feeling of 'to know before birth' than 'to wait till the child is born'. Genetic counsellors should ensure that this parental decision was made with the help of all available information including recurrence risk applicable to their specific circumstances. Whilst most clinical genetics units have a dedicated prenatal diagnosis team, it is important to offer the opportunity to consult a fetal medicine team. This multidisciplinary team approach is acknowledged as the good practice in prenatal diagnosis.

Prenatal diagnosis for CHD commonly includes one or more of the following:

- anomaly ultrasound examination at 18 weeks gestation to include heart, brain, kidneys, and skeletal system. In addition, measurements for growth and other body parameters can also be recorded
- fetal echocardiography usually following the anomaly ultrasound examination. In some cases, this could be carried as early as 12 weeks when the four-chamber view of the heart is possible. Serial scans are carried out in most cases till 18 weeks gestation
- conventional and molecular cytogenetics
- targeted molecular genetic testing.

# Management of congenital heart disease

The management of congenital heart disease requires an integrated adequately resourced multidisciplinary care. The MDT should include the following led by a dedicated clinician representing the specific area of management.

• Fetal/neonatal cardiology: fetal/neonatal diagnosis, leading the management plan, advising parents and supervising the cardiology aspects of management.

• Surgical intervention: usually provided at the tertiary/supraregional paediatric cardiothoracic surgery unit equipped and fully resourced in dealing with any form of complex single or multiple congenital cardiovascular malformations. A number of surgical techniques are employed by specialised paediatric cardiothoracic surgical units. These are beyond the scope and remit of this book and the reader is recommended to refer to other resources, preferably a discussion with a member of the surgical unit.

• Paediatric follow-up: monitoring the general pediatric aspects of care, growth and development progress, parental support and guidance in accordance to the needs of the child.

• Clinical genetics support: assessment and diagnosis of the underlying genetic condition including multiple malformation syndrome, genetic counselling, clinical and genetic surveillance of close family members, supporting and advising on reproductive choices, participating in the management of high-risk pregnancy including prenatal diagnosis.

• GUCH: usually an adult cardiologist with special interest in congenital heart diseases, main role in the delivery and supervision of MDT management of a known case of complex or syndromic form of CHD progressing to adult age group (15–16 years). This aspect of care is not generally available due to lack of adequate resources. The working group of the British Cardiovascular Society on GUCH has made several recommendations (📖 see Further reading).

## Further reading

Kumar and Elliott (eds). *Principles and Practice of Clinical Cardiovascular Genetics*, Oxford University Press, New York, 2010.

British Cardiovascular Society Working group on Grown Up Congenital Heart disease (GUCH).

# Cardiovascular manifestations in chromosomal disorders

# Introduction

Chromosomal conditions are associated with congenital heart disease (☐ see Chapter 6, Congenital heart disease for specific defects), cardio-myopathies and arrhythmias. It is uncommon to encounter a functional disturbance alone in association with a chromosome aberration. This section summarizes cardiac anomalies that may co-exist with other anomalies in recognizable multiple malformation chromosomal syndromes. It is important to note that some of these multiple malformation syndromes may also present without a detectable chromosome aberration. Causation of most congenital heart disease is multifactorial/polygenic. Congenital heart diseases are associated with chromosome abnormalities where disruption in few selected genes in the specific chromosome region may be aetiologically important (Table 7.1). However, a small proportion may be due to mutations in single genes, also referred to as Mendelian malformation syndromes.

Chromosome abnormalities are broadly classified as being **numerical** (45, 47, 48 etc.) or **structural** (microdeletion, microduplication, ring chromosome, inversion and iso-chromosome) (☐ see also Chapter 2, General principles of medical genetics). Any variation from the normal human chromosome diploid number (46, XX or 46, XY) is referred to as *aneuploidy* (*a*—abnormal, *neu*—number, *ploidy*—chromosome). Conversely, any structural variation with normal diploid number is referred to as being structural. In both instances, there is a large genomic disruption resulting in a spectrum of malformations or functional disturbance that is often recognizable as a **multiple malformation syndrome**.

Overall around 30% of all children with a chromosome abnormality have CHD. Some chromosome abnormalities (for example trisomy 18) are associated with a very high rate of CHD. Some chromosome deletions or duplications also have a strong association with a *specific* congenital heart defect (for example duplication of chromosome 21 in Down syndrome and AVSD).

**Table 7.1** The spectrum of chromosome abnormalities with cardiovascular malformations

| Cardiovascular malformation | Chromosome abnormality |
|---|---|
| Atrial septal defect | Paternal disomy 14; maternal disomy 16; microdeletion—1p36; 5q35; 6p25; 9q34; 15q24–q26 |
| Atrio-ventricular septal defect | Maternal disomy 16; 8p23 microdeletion |
| Cardiomyopathy | Ch.14 paternal disomy; microdeletion—1p36; 5q35; 17q25 |
| Coarctation/interrupted aorta | Mosaic chromosome 16; maternal disomy 16; 6p25 microdeletion; 22q11 microdeletion; 22q11.2 microduplication; 45X Turner |
| Cardiac situs inversus/dextrocardia | 6p27 microdeletion |
| Duplicated/right aortic arch | 12p13 microdeletion; 22q11 microdeletion |
| Double outlet right ventricle | 8p23 microdeletion |
| Fallot's tetralogy | Microdeletion 5q11.2; 9q34; 22q11 & 22q11.2 microduplication |
| Hypoplastic left heart syndrome | Microduplication 22q11.2; microdeletion 1p36, 8p23, 11q26, 15q24–q26; 20q11 |
| Patent ductus arteriosus | Maternal disomy 2; paternal disomy 6; paternal disomy 14; microdeletion—5q35; 6p25; 9q34 |
| Pulmonary stenosis | Microdeletion 5q35; 9p13; 20qdel |
| Ventricular septal defect | Mosaic trisomy 10; paternal disomy 10; maternal disomy 16; microdeletion—1p36; 1q44–qter; 4q35; 5q35; 6p25; 9q34; 17q25; 19p13; 22q11 |
| Unspecified congenital cardiac anomaly | Submicroscopic microdeletion—9q34; 10p15; 11q25; 18q23; 20q11 |

# Trisomy 21 (Down syndrome)

Trisomy 21 is the most common aneuploidy syndrome with an estimated birth prevalence of 1 in 600 to 800 live births. The majority of cases of Down syndrome are caused by free trisomy 21 and in these cases there is no need to karyotype parents. In 5% of cases the additional chromosome 21 is due to an unbalanced translocation, classically but not invariably a Robertsonian translocation, in which two acrocentric chromosomes have fused at the centromere or within the short arm. In these cases parental karyotyping should be arranged because a parent carrying a balanced Robertsonian translocation involving chromosome 21 is at risk of future recurrence of Down syndrome.

## Major clinical features

- Mild to moderate muscular hypotonia.
- Flat facial profile with upslanting palpebral fissures, brachycephaly and small round ears.
- Short neck with redundant nuchal skin.
- Atlanto-axial instability (1 in 5).
- Single palmar (simian) crease (just under half of affected children).
- Most frequent extracardiac congenital malformation is duodenal atresia.
- Cardiovascular anomaly (80%) may be present including atrioventricular septal defect (AVSD) in 47% and ventricular septal defect (VSD) in about a quarter of cases. Other cardiovascular anomalies include tetralogy of fallot (TOF), atrial septal defect (ASD) and isolated mitral cleft. In addition, mitral valve prolapse and aortic regurgitation in adult life are more common in Down syndrome than in the general population.
- Seizures of minor or major nature affect 1 in 4 individuals, often of adult onset.
- Medical complications of hypothyroidism and coeliac disease may occur in later age.
- Depression and early onset of memory loss (similar to Alzheimer's disease) may affect adults with Down syndrome.

# Trisomy 18 (Edwards syndrome)

Trisomy 18 is the second most common autosomal aneuploidy after Down syndrome with a birth incidence of around 1 in 3000. Median survival of those born alive is three days with no babies living longer than a year though the cardiac problem was rarely implicated as the cause of death.

Major clinical features
- Finger clenching with second and fifth overlapping third and fourth.
- Babies are small for gestational age.
- Dysmorphic appearance: prominent occiput, low-set ears, micrognathia, small palpebral fissures and a short sternum.
- CHD in about 87% cases: VSD, AVSD, hypoplastic left heart (HLH), double outlet right ventricle (DORV), TOF, subvalvar pulmonary stenosis, transposition of the great arteries (TGA) and coarctation of the aorta (COA).
- Extracardiac malformations, commonly gastrointestinal (e.g. umbilical hernia, omphalocele) and urogenital systems (horseshoe kidney, hydronephrosis, polycystic kidneys).

# Trisomy 13 (Patau syndrome)

The most common aneuploidy syndrome (1 in 5,000 live births). The median survival may range from four days to just under six months. Most cases of Patau syndrome have straightforward trisomy 13. In these cases there is no need to karyotype parents. In others the additional chromosome 13 is due to an unbalanced translocation, classically though not invariably a Robertsonian translocation. In these cases parental karyotyping should be arranged because a parent carrying a balanced Robertsonian translocation involving chromosome 13 is at risk of future recurrence of Patau syndrome.

**Major clinical features**
- Midline cleft lip and/or cleft palate (often bilateral).
- Postaxial polydactyly.
- Structural brain abnormalities—absent septum pellucidum, absent corpus callosum and holoprosencephaly.
- Cardiovascular malformations (CVM) may include VSD, ASD, AVSD, TOF, DORV, pulmonary stenosis (PS) and left isomerism.
- Scalp defects.
- Other midline congenital malformations.

# Turner syndrome

Incidence is approximately 1/2000 girls. A karyotype of 45,X is seen in approximately 50% of cases; others have various structural abnormalities of the X chromosome including isochromosomes comprising 2 copies of Xq(iXq), deletions and mosaicism.

## Major clinical features

- Redundant nuchal skin or neck webbing with a low posterior hairline.
- Oedema of the dorsum of hands and feet in the perinatal period that resolves later.
- Deep-set, hyperconvex nails.
- Broad chest with wide-spaced nipples.
- CHD (around 50%)—most common coarctation of aorta/interrupted aortic arch; aortic valve abnormalities are commonly seen with 45X karyotype.
- Structural renal malformations, for example horseshoe kidney (60%).
- Growth retardation—usually proportionately short.
- Delayed or failure to develop secondary sexual characteristics.
- Infertility and premature ovarian failure in almost all girls with a 45,X karyotype.
- Intelligence is within the normal range in most cases.

It is important to note that above clinical features can be milder or even absent if there is mosaicism with a normal cell line. Girls with mosaicism can have normal secondary sexual development and fertility followed by premature ovarian failure.

# Cat-eye syndrome

Caused by tetrasomy for 22q11.2. The additional piece of chromosome, made up of 2 copies of material from chromosome 22, is identifiable on a standard karyotype as an extra piece of chromosome (a marker extra structurally abnormal or ESAC chromosome). As the marker chromosome is unstable, it is often lost from some cells, leading to the mosaic karyotype in some cases.

## Major clinical features

- Coloboma of the iris (60%) giving the 'cat-eye' look—may be unilateral or bilateral and can extend to involve the choroid and retina.
- Pre-auricular pits and tags (87%), in addition, the pinna can be malformed or even absent, with or without associated atresia of the external auditory meatus.
- Mild to moderate growth and developmental delay (50%).
- Urogenital abnormalities—horseshoe kidneys, unilateral renal hypoplasia, imperforate anus with a fistula and cryptorchidism in males (around 30%).
- Congenital heart defects (around 30%) including anomalous pulmonary venous drainage (19%), Fallot's tetralogy, coarctation/interrupted aortic arch and hypoplastic left heart syndrome.

# Mosaic aneuploidies

Any chromosome abnormality can occur as numerical (mosaic aneuploidy) or structural. Mosaic structural chromosome changes may be somatic indicating a specific clonal origin. This phenomenon is well known in relation to oncology where it is somatic in most cases confined to specific tissues, such as lymphocytes in lymphocytic leukaemias. A number of aneuploidies are lethal resulting in first trimester miscarriage (e.g. trisomy 16, one of the most common chromosome abnormalities present in aborted conceptuses). Such a chromosome abnormality in the mosaic form may be compatible to survival and delivered as a live born infant. There are examples of live born mosaic trisomy 16. It is likely that a number of congenital anomalies might co-exist with a mosaic aneuploidy including cardiovascular malformation.

# Microduplication syndromes

A microduplication syndrome is a partial aneuploidy with normal diploid number of chromosomes. There are several examples known each with a broad spectrum of clinical features. It is likely that in some cases the physical abnormalities are subtle and may remain undiagnosed. Occasionally, a microduplication may manifest following the phenomenon of genetic imprinting if it happened to be on either the paternal or maternal haploid chromosomes. In such a situation there is additional material belonging to one parental chromosome described as *uniparental disomy* (🕮 see Chapter 2, General principles of medical genetics). However, in most cases, the duplicated segment includes several dosage sensitive genes. The clinical spectrum may include several minor and major congenital anomalies. Cardiovascular malformations (CVMs) are often noted. Different types of CVMs may be associated with a specific microduplication syndrome. For example, 22q11.2 microduplication (Cat-eye syndrome) is known to present with Fallot's tetralogy and hypoplastic left heart syndrome. A discussion with the cytogeneticist or clinical geneticist is recommended to establish causal relationship of CVM with the specific duplicated chromosome segment (🕮 see also Further reading).

# Microdeletion syndromes

Most microdeletion syndromes represent haploinsufficiency of dosage-sensitive genes. Several genes may be lost within the deleted chromosome segment. The term 'contiguous gene syndrome' is used to describe most microdeletion syndromes. The variation in the clinical picture often correlates with the loss of gene functions. This may also be brought about by loss of gene function dependent upon the 'parent of origin'. Loss of a 'tumour-suppressor gene' within the deleted segment amounts to 'one-hit' and may lead to tumorigenesis in the event of the 'second-hit', whether inherited or acquired. Fig. 7.1 illustrates chromosomes commonly encountered microdeletion syndromes. A brief account of some of these syndromes that are likely to present in a clinical genetic or paediatric cardiology practice is given here (📖 see Further reading.)

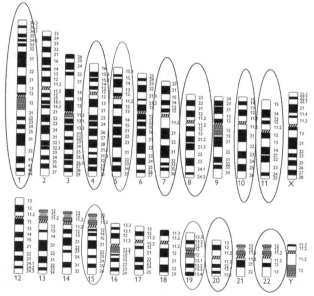

**Fig. 7.1** Microdeletion syndromes with cardiovascular manifestations.

## 1p36 deletion syndrome

Deletion of chromosome 1p36 is among those microdeletion syndromes that have been more recently identified. Its incidence has been estimated to be as high as 1 in 5000. Deletions vary in size—some are cytogenetically visible but the majority are only identified with a specific FISH test; around 25% of deletions may be cytogenetically visible. The clinical spectrum is wide.

### Major clinical features

- developmental delay, muscular hypotonia and seizures
- characteristic facial appearance, with deep-set eyes, straight eyebrows and a broad nasal bridge
- cardiovascular anomalies common and include structural congenital heart defects (70%) and non-compaction cardiomyopathy (around 20%). Septal defects (VSD, ASD) are most frequent, but a significant proportion of children are also born with PDA, TOF and valve abnormalities. Ebstein anomaly and other tricuspid valve defects are also described.

## 4p deletion syndrome (Wolf–Hirschhorn syndrome)

The phenotype of Wolf–Hirschhorn syndrome was descibed long before its association with microdeletion of the short arm of chromosome 4. Prevalence is around 1 in 50,000. The terminal 4p deletion may be visible on a standard karyotype in 58% of cases, but specific FISH testing should be requested if this diagnosis is suspected and chromosomes are normal. Submicroscopic deletions account for the remaining 42% of cases. About 85% of cases occur *de novo*. Parental karyotypes should be checked to ensure that balanced translocations involving 4p16.3 are not missed as a cause.

### Major clinical features

- Microcephaly and pre- and postnatal growth retardation.
- Dysmorphic facial appearance with broad and prominent nasal bridge giving rise to comparison with the appearance of a 'Greek Helmet'. This and the arched eyebrows, sometimes associated with ptosis, make up the characteristic facial appearance.
- Congenital heart disease is seen in around 45%, most often septal defects (ASD and VSD).
- Seizures and moderate to severe development delay in around 50%.
- Cleft palate, talipes and hypospadias are common.

## 5p deletion syndrome (Cri du Chat syndrome)

The incidence of this microdeletion syndrome is 1/50,000 in newborn infants. The cause of cri du chat syndrome is a microdeletion of chromosome 5p. Some larger deletions are detected on a standard karyotype, however if the diagnosis is strongly suspected and the karyotype appears normal, FISH testing should be requested. In 85% of cases there is a *de novo* deletion of 5p and 15% of cases are the unbalanced product of a parental balanced translocation. The latter will have a risk of recurrence in future pregnancies, so genetic counselling, and karyotyping, for parents is important.

## Major clinical features

- Pre- and postnatal growth retardation.
- Microcephaly.
- A 'cat-like' cry in infancy (from which the syndrome takes its name) and developmental delay.
- Characteristic facial appearance—round face, hypertelorism, high nasal bridge, micrognathia.
- Talipes, congenital hip dislocation and inguinal herniae.
- Premature greying of the hair in adulthood.
- Congenital heart disease is present in around 15 and 20% of patients; septal defects (mostly VSD and some ASD) in around 40%, patent ductus arteriosus (PDA) (40%) and up to 10% may have either TOF or pulmonary stenosis.

## 7q11 deletion syndrome or Williams syndrome

Around 90% of Williams cases have a deletion of chromosome 7q11.23 that is identified on a standard FISH test. The genetic basis of supravalvar aortic stenosis was elucidated through investigation of a family in which non-syndromic SVAS segregated with a balanced chromosome transloca- tion. One breakpoint of this reciprocal translocation disrupted the elastin gene at chromosome 7q11.23, a locus that had already shown to be linked to SVAS in two unrelated families with autosomal dominant SVAS. Point mutations in *ELN* have since been found in autosomal dominant SVAS and *ELN* maps to the Williams syndrome critical region, confirming that this is the gene responsible for CHD in Williams syndrome. Patients who lack one functional copy of *ELN* typically have stenotic lesions of the outflow tract but the range of cardiac phenotypes includes a normal cardiovas- cular system to a persistent truncus arteriosus. Point mutations in ELN may account for about one-third SVAS patients.

## Major clinical features

- Pre/postnatal growth delay leading to proportionate short stature.
- Hypercalcaemia in infancy.
- Characteristic facies with stellate irides, periorbital fullness and prominent lips.
- Cardiac malformations are common and include supravalvar aortic stenosis (around 70%) and peripheral pulmonary artery stenosis (around 30%); arterial stenosis may affect other organs (e.g. kidneys). Supravalvar aortic stenosis accounts for <1% of all CHD, but a high proportion of the cardiac defects found in patients with Williams syndrome.
- Developmental delay in most cases with a happy and friendly social behaviour often referred to as 'cocktail party' manner.

## 8p23 microdeletion syndrome

Major cardiovascular manifestations associated with the syndrome of 8p23 microdeletion include conotruncal lesions, atrial septal defects, atrio- ventricular canal defects and pulmonary valve stenosis. The critical region is approximately 5cM in size and harbours a number of genes including zinc finger transcription factor GATA-4. Evidence suggests that deficiency of *GATA-4* may contribute to the phenotype of patients with monosomy of 8p23.1. Other transcription factor genes critical for cardiovascular development include *TBX1, TBX3, TBX5* and *NKX-2.5.*

## 10p15 deletion syndrome

Increasing number of 22q deletion negative cases with clinical features of 22q deletion syndrome are reported to have a microdeletion of chromosome 10p15.

### Major clinical features

- Prominent forehead with frontal bossing.
- Abnormal external ears with down-slanting palpebral fissures.
- Small mandible with or without cleft palate.
- Variable degree of myopia.
- Cardiac anomalies similar to 22q microdeletion cases.
- Cryptorchid/undescended testes.
- Syndactyly of 2/3 toes.
- Muscular hypotonia and learning difficulties with developmental delay.

## 11q23-qter deletion (Jacobsen syndrome)

Terminal deletion of the long arm of chromosome 11 is an uncommon chromosome abnormality affecting fewer than 1 in 100,000 children. Jacobsen syndrome is the eponymous name given to terminal 11q deletions In most cases of Jacobsen syndrome a cytogenetically visible 11q deletion is identified. This can be *de novo* or it can be the unbalanced product of a balanced parental translocation.

The clinical phenotype includes congenital malformations affecting the CVS, thrombocytopenia and abnormal leukocyte function, craniosynostosis, renal tract, central nervous system (CNS) and eye malformations and facial dysmorphism. Reviews have described and compared the physical characteristics of over 100 individuals with partial monosomy for 11q.

### Major clinical features

- Metopic synostosis causing trigonocephaly (50%) compared to 20% of all individuals with isolated craniosynostosis.
- Unusual type of thrombocytopenia (Paris–Trousseau thrombocytopenia) in around 90% of patients.
- Around 50% patients may have a distinctive congenital heart anomaly—HLH accounts for around 13% in Jacobsen syndrome compared to only 1.5% of all cases of CHD; an additional 11% have mitral stenosis, probably as part of the HLH spectrum.

## 15q24-26 deletion syndrome

This is similar to cases with a ring chromosome 15 with *de novo* deletions of the distal part of 15q (q26.3, q26.2 and/or q26.1). Depending on the size of the deletion, these patients may be missing one copy of the insulin-like growth factor receptor gene (*IGF1R*) and some do have features suggestive of Russell–Silver syndrome. In some cases, clinical features may be similar to Fryns syndrome, Prader–Willi and Angelman syndromes.

**Major clinical features**

- Growth and developmental delay
- Microcephaly
- Triangular face with hypertelorism, high arched palate, abnormal ears and micrognathia
- Brachydactyly
- Congenital cardiac malformations—atrial septal defect, aortic stenosis and hypoplastic left heart
- Urogenital abnormalities

### 19p13 deletion syndrome

Multiple congenital anomalies occur in the microdeletion 19p13 syndrome.

**Major clinical features**

- Prenatal onset of growth retardation including microcephaly
- Dysmorphic facies—hypertelorism, flat nose, micrognathia, low-set ears, down-turned corners of the mouth
- High arched palate
- Umbilical hernia
- Non-specific sensorineural deafness
- Punched-out lesions of the retina
- Red cell abnormalities
- Complex heart defects
- Ligamentous laxity
- Learning difficulties with social and communication problems

### 20p deletion syndrome (Alagille syndrome)

Alagille syndrome (Arterio-hepatic dysplasia) is a variable familial condition characterized with neonatal jaundice, congenital cardiac and skeletal abnormalities. Some cases have been shown to have a deletion of the short arm of chromosome 20. The critical gene is *JAG1* located within the deleted chromosomal segment and codes for Jagged-1 protein. A patient with TOF and a butterfly vertebra, but no other features of Alagille syndrome was found to have a deletion of 20p12 encompassing the *JAG1* gene. Another patient with pulmonary stenosis, and a family history of this condition, was also found to have a mutation in this gene although there were no other features of Alagille syndrome. In one study, 61 individuals with features of Alagille syndrome had *JAG1* mutations and in 5 cases mosaicism was present. The possibility of mosaicism (around 8%) can complicate genetic counselling, as these individuals can be very mildly affected. An affected girl with a microdeletion of 20p is reported whose mother had mosaicism for this deletion and was phenotypically normal. Genetic counselling is also complicated by the finding of mutations in relatives, approximately half of whom may not meet the clinical criteria for Alagille syndrome.

Major clinical features

- Intrahepatic cholestasis due to a paucity of intrahepatic bile ducts (occasionally extrahepatic as well) resulting in prolonged neonatal jaundice (91%), although a quarter may develop jaundice later in infancy.
- Characteristic facies—prominent forehead with deep-set eyes and long nose with a flattened tip.
- The mandible may gradually become prominent.
- Cardiac lesions (85%) are predominantly peripheral pulmonary stenosis but might include pulmonary valve stenosis, partial anomalous venous drainage or atrial and ventricular septal defects.
- Ocular lesions may include anterior chamber defect (particularly posterior embryotoxon), pigmentary retinopathy (88%) and optic disc drusen bilaterally (80%) (95% of cases may have unilaterally).
- Other anomalies may include oligodontia, oral xanthomas and cutaneous xanthomas.
- Skeletal changes consist of hemi- or butterfly vertebrae (87%), shortening of the distal phalanges, radius or ulna, bilateral radio-ulnar synostosis and features of caudal regression.
- Short stature is common (50%) and there is occasional developmental delay with learning difficulties (16%).

A thorough clinical review supported by relevant radiological and cardi-olgical investigations should be carried out in a suspected case of Alagille syndrome. This should be supported by cytogenetic analysis, specifically to exclude 20p12 microdeletion using molecular cytogenetic methods including FISH. Molecular genetic testing for mutations in the *Jagged1* gene is recommended in a cytogenetically negative case and may be positive in about two-third of cases.

### 22q11 deletion syndrome (DiGeorge syndrome; velocardiofacial syndrome)

The deletion is rarely visible on routine karyotype hence a specific test should be requested when the diagnosis is considered, either FISH on chromosome spreads or a DNA-based test depending on your diagnostic laboratory. Around 90% of deletions are *de novo*, 10% are familial, so genetic counselling is recommended. Clinical presentation in an affected parent or sibling can be mild. Parental karyotyping should always be performed. The principle of investigating the relatively small genomic region shared in common by CHD patients with microdeletion syndromes to find a gene or genes that are involved in cardiogenesis is well-illustrated by research that identified TBX1. There are two lines of evidence that TBX1, a cardiac transcription factor within the 22q11 deleted region is a major player in the cardiac phenotype. Since *TBX1* was first proposed as the gene responsible for the cardiac phenotype in 22q11.2 deletion, point mutations in this gene have been found in human subjects with conotruncal heart lesions. However, TBX1 mutations do not seem to be a common cause of isolated conotruncal CVM. Transgenic studies on mice provide good evidence supporting *TBX1* gene associated with cardiac anomalies in VCFS or Di George syndrome.

The phenotype associated with chromosome 22q11 deletion is highly variable.

**Major clinical features**
- Congenital heart disease (75%)—of these 14% have VSDs, 14% have interruption of the aortic arch, 10% have pulmonary atresia (with or without VSD) and 17% have TOF. A further 9% have truncus arteriosus.
- Cleft palate, often involving the soft palate (submucous cleft palate) presenting with velopharyngeal insufficiency.
- Neonatal hypocalcaemia with tetany.
- Variable immunodeficiency due to T-cell quantitative and qualitative abnormalities.
- Growth retardation and developmental delay in most cases.
- Communication difficulties due to speech and language delay.
- Structural renal tract anomalies.
- Increased risk of psychiatric disorder (schizophrenia) in both childhood and adult life.

Although the association between the deletion and a phenotype was first detected through investigation of children with DiGeorge syndrome it rapidly became apparent that the same deletion was present in children with velocardiofacial syndrome (VCFS) and conotruncal anomaly face syndrome. The term '22q11 deletion syndrome' is more useful than the eponyms 'DiGeorge' and 'VCFS' because there is such marked phenotypic variation. Within a single family one can find individuals who have never presented to medical attention, individuals with velopharyngeal insufficiency and learning difficulties and also individuals with hypocalcaemia, low T-cell counts and CHD (DiGeorge syndrome) all resulting from the same deletion. Overall, a high proportion of all children with 22q11 deletion have serious CHD that is likely to require surgical correction or palliation.

# Genetic counselling

Parents and close family members of a child with a chromosome abnormality complicated with multiple malformations should be referred to the medical genetics service for genetic counselling. It is likely the child or the family was known to the specialist paediatric cardiology unit for medical and/or or surgical care ( see Management). The purpose of the medical genetic consultation would be multifold including explanation of chromosome abnormality, delineation of the phenotype, assessment of recurrence risk estimates, long-term outcome or prognosis and availability of the reproductive options including prenatal diagnosis ( see Prenatal diagnosis).

The format of approach and conduct of the genetic counselling should normally follow the commonly adopted *non-judgemental and non-directive* principle (see Chapter 4, Genetic counselling). The emphasis should always be providing parents and close family members clear and concise information focusing on recurrence risk estimates and reproductive options for any future child-bearing. In most cases, recurrence risks are small, limited to around 1% in a live newborn child. However, this could be higher if this was confirmed to be related to a parental balanced chromosome rearrangement (*autosome–autosome* translocation or *autosome–sex chromosome* translocation) or structural abnormality (*para/pericentric inversion*). In such a situation, recurrence risk estimate is based upon chromosomes involved, specific chromosome segments involved, history of a previous child born with multiple anomalies, history of recurrent miscarriages or fetal wastage, and evidence from the literature of live-born cases surviving through the childhood. In most cases, probability of a live-born child with an unbalanced chromosome complement is small, limited to not more than 5%. However, this estimate may vary subject to the availability of specialist fetal/perinatal and neonatal multidisciplinary care.

# Prenatal diagnosis

Prenatal diagnosis of a chromosome abnormality likely to be complicated with a single or complex cardiovascular malformation is increasingly chosen as one of the options by parents with a previously affected pregnancy. In some cases, the spectrum of congenital anomalies is extended to involve other body systems. The request for prenatal diagnosis could generate from either a discussion with the fetal medicine team or may result following genetic counselling (📖 see Genetic counselling). Parents are offered the opportunity to make an informed decision for prenatal diagnosis with an understanding for the option of medical termination of pregnancy (MTOP) in the event of the pregnancy confirmed to be affected. However, the decision for MTOP should not be a condition and parents should be allowed to change their mind reflecting altered view and/or personal circumstances.

As far as possible, the pregnancy is managed in a specialist fetal medicine unit supported by the specialist prenatal diagnosis team from the medical genetics service. Discussion prior to the consent should include aspects of techniques of chorion villous biopsy (CVB) (minimum at 11 weeks) or amniocentesis (minimum at 15 weeks) for fetal chromosome analysis (📖 see Chapter 4, Genetic counselling). Information on the technique and risks involved for miscarriage is implicitly explained. It is important to clarify that the decision for MTOP would be based solely on the finding of abnormal chromosome constitution and **not** on actual cardiovascular anomaly with or without associated other structural abnormality. This approach allows performing MTOP as early as 13–14 weeks gestation. However, in some cases, parents may choose to defer MTOP till confirmation of a cardiovascular anomaly by a detailed anomaly ultrasound examination including fetal echocardiography around 20-week gestation. This approach would delay carrying out performing MTOP to around 22-week gestation. Whenever possible, parents may be offered an opportunity to make contact with other parents with experience of having undergone prenatal diagnosis in similar circumstances.

# Management

The management of a pregnancy affected with an abnormal chromosome constitution complicating a cardiovascular anomaly and/or other structural anomalies should be assigned to the multidisciplinary team equipped with specialists in fetal medicine, fetal cardiology, neonatal/paediatric cardiothoracic surgery, clinical genetics, specialist neonatal care and long-term support extending to the first few years of life. The pregnancy should be closely monitored throughout and arrangements for childbirth made in the unit with facilities for immediate specialist neonatal care including cardiothoracic surgical intervention. This approach may offer a high level of assurance to parents and as well as the obstetric and midwifery units. In most cases, the immediate outcome in terms of survival may be significantly improved. However, the long-term survival and quality of life may depend on other associated anomalies, physical growth and neurodevelopment complicating the chromosome abnormality.

### Further reading

Brewer C., *et al.* (1998). A chromosomal deletion map of human malformations. *Am J Hum Genet* **63**: 1153–1159.

Jones K (ed). *Smith's Recognizable patterns of human malformation*, 5th edn. Saunders, Philadelphia, PA. (2007).

Schinzel A. (2001) *Schinzel's Catalogue of unbalanced Chromosome Aberrations in Man*, 2nd edn. De Gruyter, Berlin. (2001).

# Cardiomyopathies

# Classification

Classifications of heart muscle disease are complex and have inevitable limitations due to overlap between categories, progressive disease processes and continuing expansion of knowledge of these diseases. The oldest definition of cardiomyopathy dates from 1957 when the cardiomyopathies were defined as 'subacute or chronic disorders of heart muscle of unknown or obscure aetiology'. A Task Force was set up by the World Health Organisation (WHO) and the International Society and Federation of Cardiology to establish a consensus on definition and nomenclature and the first was published in 1980, then updated in 1995.

Expert panels of the American Heart Association (AHA) and European Society of Cardiology (ESC) have published new classifications in 2006 and 2008, respectively. These have significant similarities in that they both exclude ischaemic heart disease and valvular disease but also have important differences. The AHA classification includes channelopathies as cardiomyopathies while the ESC classification is based on specific morphological and functional phenotypes that are further classified into familial and non-familial disease.

## American Heart Association Classification 2006 (see Table 8.1)

### Definition

'Cardiomyopathies are a heterogeneous group of diseases that usually (but not invariably) exhibit inappropriate ventricular hypertrophy or dilatation and are due to a variety of causes that frequently are genetic. Cardiomyopathies either are confined to the heart or are part of generalized systemic disorders, often leading to cardiovascular death or progressive heart failure-related disability.'

Cardiomyopathies are classified into two major groups based on organ involvement:

- *primary cardiomyopathies* are confined to heart muscle
- *secondary cardiomyopathies* show cardiac involvement as part of a large number and variety of generalized systemic or multi-organ disorders.

**Table 8.1** AHA classification for cardiomyopathies

| | | |
|---|---|---|
| Primary cardiomyopathies | Genetic | Hypertropic cardiomyopathy (HCM)/arrhythmogenic right ventricular cardiomyopathy (ARVC)/left ventricular non compaction (LVNC)/conduction defects/mitochondrial myopathies/ion channel disorders |
| | Mixed | Dilated cardiomyopathy (DCM)/restrictive |
| | Acquired | Inflammatory/Takotsubo/peripartum/tachycardia induced/infants of IDDM mothers |
| Secondary cardiomyopathies | Infiltrative | Amyloidosis, Gauchers, Hurler's, Hunter's |
| | Storage | Fabry's, glycogen storage disease, Niemann–Pick disease, haemochromatosis |
| | Toxicity | Drugs, heavy metals |
| | Endomyocardial | Endomyocardial fibrosis, Loeffler's endocarditis |
| | Inflammatory | Sarcoidosis |
| | Endocrine | Diabetes, hyperthyroidism, hypothyroidism, hyperparathyroidism, phaeochromocytoma, acromegaly |
| | Cardiofacial | Noonan's, lentiginosis |
| | Neuromuscular | Friedreich's ataxia, Duchenne–Becker muscular dystrophy, myotonic dystrophy |
| | Nutritional | Beriberi, scurvy, selenium |
| | Autoimmune | Systemic lupus erythematosus, dermatomyositis, scleroderma |
| | Consequence of cancer therapy | Anthracyclines, radiation, cyclophosphamide, |

**European Society of Cardiology Classification 2008
(see Table 8.2)**

*Definition*

A cardiomyopathy is 'a myocardial disorder in which the heart muscle is structurally and functionally abnormal, in the absence of coronary artery disease, hypertension, valvular disease and congenital heart disease sufficient to cause the observed myocardial abnormality'.

They are grouped into specific morphological and functional phenotypes and each phenotype is then subclassified into familial and non-familial forms. The non-familial forms are then subclassified into idiopathic and acquired cardiomyopathies in which the ventricular dysfunction is a complication of the disorder rather than an intrinsic feature of the disease.

**Table 8.2** ESC classification for cardiomyopathies

| Cardiomyopathies | HCM | Familial/genetic | Unidentified gene defect |
|---|---|---|---|
| | DCM | | Disease subtype |
| | ARVC | | |
| | restrictive cardiomyopathy (RCM) | Non-familial/ non-genetic | Idiopathic |
| | Unclassified | | Disease subtype |

**Table 8.3** Examples of genetic and non-genetic causes for cardiomyopathy

| | HCM | DCM | ARVC | RCM | Unclassified |
|---|---|---|---|---|---|
| Familial | Familial, unknown gene | Familial, unknown gene | Familial, unknown gene | Familial, unknown gene | Left ventricular non-compaction |
| | Sarcomeric protein mutations | Sarcomeric protein mutations (see HCM) | Intercalated disc protein mutations | Sarcomeric protein | • Barth syndrome |
| | • β myosin heavy chain | Z-band | • Plakoglobin | • Troponin I (RCM +/- HCM) | • Lamin A/C |
| | • Cardiac myosin binding protein C | • Muscle LIM protein | • Desmoplakin | • Essential light chain of myosin | • ZASP |
| | • Cardiac troponin I | • TCAP | • Plakophilin 2 | | • α-dystrobrevin |
| | • Troponin-T | Cytoskeletal genes | • Desmoglein 2 | Familial amyloidosis | |
| | • α-tropomyosin | • Dystrophin | • Desmocollin 2 | • Transthyretin (RCM + neuropathy) | |
| | • Essential myosin light chain | • Desmin | Cardiac ryanodine receptor (RyR2) | • Apolipoprotein (RCM + nephropathy) | |
| | • Regulatory myosin light chain | • Metavinculin | | | |
| | • Cardiac actin | • Sarcoglycan complex | Transforming growth factor-β3 (TGFβ3) | Desminopathy | |
| | • α-myosin heavy chain | • CRYAB | | Pseuxanthoma elasticum | |
| | • Titin | • Epicardin | | Haemochromatosis | |
| | • Troponin C | Nuclear membrane | | Anderson—Fabry disease | |
| | • Muscle LIM protein | • Lamin A/C | | Glycogen storage disease | |
| | Glycogen storage disease (eg Pompe; PRKAG2, Forbes', Danon) | • Emerin | | | |

(Continued)

Table 8.3 (Contd.)

| HCM | DCM | ARVC | RCM | Unclassified |
|---|---|---|---|---|
| Lysosomal storage diseases (eg, Anderson—Fabry, Hurler's) | Mildly dilated CM | | | |
| Disorders of fatty acid metabolism | Intercalated disc protein mutations (see ARVC) | | | |
| Carnitine deficiency | Mitochondrial cytopathy | | | |
| Phosphorylase B kinase deficiency | | | | |
| Mitochondrial cytopathies | | | | |
| Syndromic HCM | | | | |
| • Noonan's syndrome | | | | |
| • LEOPARD syndrome | | | | |
| • Friedreich's ataxia | | | | |
| • Beckwith—Wiedermann syndrome | | | | |
| • Swyer's syndrome | | | | |
| Other | | | | |
| • Phospholamban promoter | | | | |
| • Familial amyloid | | | | |

| | HCM | DCM | ARVC | RCM | Unclassified |
|---|---|---|---|---|---|
| Non-familial | Obesity | Myocarditis (infective/toxic/immune) | Inflammation | Amyloid (AL/prealbumin) | Tako Tsubo cardiomyopathy |
| | Infants of diabetic mothers | Kawasaki disease | | Scleroderma | |
| | Athletic training | Eosinophilic (Churg Strauss syndrome) | | Endomyocardial fibrosis | |
| | Amyloid (AL/prealbumin) | Viral persistence | | • Hypereosinophilic syndrome | |
| | | Drugs | | • Idiopathic | |
| | | Pregnancy | | • Chromosomal cause | |
| | | Endocrine | | • Drugs (serotonin, methysergide, ergotamine, mercurial agents, busulfan) | |
| | | Nutritional—thiamine, carnitine, selenium, hypophosphataemia, hypocalcaemia | | Carcinoid heart disease | |
| | | Alcohol | | Metastatic cancers | |
| | | Tachycardiomyopathy | | Radiation | |
| | | | | Drugs (anthracyclines) | |

ARVC, arrhythmogenic right ventricular cardiomyopathy; DCM, dilated cardiomyopathy; HCM, hypertrophic cardiomyopathy; RCM, restrictive cardiomyopathy.

# Hypertrophic cardiomyopathy (HCM): definition and diagnosis

## Definition
Left ventricular hypertrophy in the absence of loading conditions to account for the observed degree of hypertrophy.

The prevalence of HCM in the general population is approximately one in 500 adults.

Approximately 50% of adults with HCM have mutations in genes encoding sarcomeric proteins.

HCM also occurs in association with systemic diseases capable of mimicking the sarcomeric cardiac phenotype (see Table 8.4).

Histologically, most cases of HCM are characterized by a triad of disorganization ('disarray') of cardiac myocytes and myofibrils, myocardial fibrosis, and small vessel disease.

## Assessment of cardiac morphology
- Maximal wall thickness of ≥15mm is classically used as a diagnostic criterion, but milder hypertrophy is compatible with HCM.
- The hypertrophy is typically asymmetric and involves the anterior ventricular septum.
- The left ventricular cavity is small and measure of global systolic function (ejection fraction) are usually normal.
- Left ventricular outflow tract obstruction is seen in ~30% of patients but is not pathognomonic of HCM (can also occur in elderly patients with angulated aortas and sigmoid septums).
- Hypertrophied papillary muscles often cause mid left ventricular cavity obstruction.

## Assessment of loading conditions
- Co-existent conditions that cause hypertrophy (e.g. obesity, athletic training, and systemic hypertension) can make the diagnosis of HCM problematic. (📖 Athletic heart p. 170).
- HCM in other family members or a DNA-based diagnosis may help clear diagnostic dilemmas.

## Further reading
Hughes S.E. (2004) The pathology of hypertrophic cardiomyopathy. *Histopathology* **44**: 412–427.
Maron B.J., *et al.* (2003) American College of Cardiology/European Society of Cardiology Clinical Expert Consensus Document on Hypertrophic Cardiomyopathy: A report of the American College of Cardiology Foundation Task Force on Clinical Expert Consensus Documents and the European Society of Cardiology Committee for Practice Guidelines. *Eur Heart J* **24**: 1965–1991.

**Table 8.4** Causes of hypertrophic cardiomyopathy

| Causes of hypertrophic cardiomyopathy |
| --- |
| Sarcomere protein gene mutations |
| Anderson-Fabry disease |
| Glycogen storage diseases |
| Respiratory chain diseases |
| Fatty acid metabolism |
| Friedreich's ataxia |
| Amyloid |
| Noonan's syndrome |

# Clinical family screening for HCM

HCM is usually inherited as an autosomal dominant trait with incomplete penetrance and variable expression. Probands should be informed of the familial nature of the disease and the genetic risk to other family members. All individuals undergoing screening should be counselled appropriately ( see Genetic counselling Chapter 4).

## Screening protocol

- Screening consists of history, clinical examination, electrocardiography, and two-dimensional echocardiography.
- Electrocardiographic changes usually precede the development of hypertrophy.
- Screening should be more intensive during adolescence and early adulthood since the development of hypertrophy is associated with body growth:
  - <12 years: systematic screening not recommended unless there is a sinister family history
  - 12–18 years: screening every 6–12 months
  - >18 years: ongoing screening every 3–5 years as disease expression can occur in middle age and beyond.
- Echocardiographic or electrocardiographic abnormalities without an alternative diagnosis have a high probability of being the expression of the same gene mutation affecting the proband.
- For the clinical diagnosis of HCM to be established in a first-degree relative one of the following requirements needs to be satisfied (see Table 8.5):
  - One major criterion, or
  - Two minor echocardiographic criteria, or
  - One minor echocardiographic plus 2 minor ECG criteria.

## Further reading

McKenna W.J., et al. (1997) Experience from clinical genetics in hypertrophic cardiomyopathy: proposal for new diagnostic criteria in adult members of affected families. *Heart* **77**: 130–132.

**Table 8.5** Screening criteria for HCM in first-degree relatives

|  | **Major criteria** | **Minor criteria** |
|---|---|---|
| Echocardiography | Left ventricular (LV) wall thickness >13mm in the anterior septum or posterior wall or >15mm in the posterior septum or lateral free wall | LV wall thickness >12mm in the anterior septum or posterior wall or >14mm in the posterior septum or lateral free wall |
|  | Severe SAM with septal contact | Moderate systolic anterior motion (SAM) with no septal contact |
|  |  | Redundant mitral valve (MV) leaflets |
| Electrocardiography | Left ventricular hypertrophy (LVH) and repolarization changes (Romhilt and Estes) | Complete bundle branch block (BBB) or (minor) interventricular conduction defect (in LV leads) |
|  | Abnormal Q (>40ms or >25% R wave) in at least 2 leads from II, III, aVF (in absence of left anterior hemiblock), V1–V4; or I, aVl, V5–V6 | Deep S V2 (>25mm) |
|  | T-wave inversion in leads I and aVL (>3mm) (with QRS-T wave axis difference >30°), V3–V6 (>3mm) or II and III and aVF (>5mm) | Minor repolarization changes in LV leads |

Modified from McKenna *et al. Heart* 1997; **77**: 130–132.

# HCM caused by sarcomeric protein gene mutations

- The first mutation was discovered in 1990 in the β-myosin heavy chain. Subsequently many hundreds of mutations have been identified in over a dozen genes.
- Collectively the known causal genes and their mutations account for approximately 50% of all HCM cases.
- They are generally inherited as an autosomal dominant trait.
- The majority of HCM mutations are missense mutations.
- Individuals carrying identical sarcomeric gene mutations have marked phenotypic variability.
- Modifier genes probably enhance or protect against effects of the mutation.
- Approximately 5% of patients will have more than one genetic defect (on the same or on two different genes).
- Genetic testing of all genes has to be complete in all patients even if a first genetic defect has been found.

## Genes for thin filament proteins
- 10–15% of cases.

### Cardiac troponin T (TNNT2)
- Located on chromosome 1q23.
- 27 mutations found to date to cause HCM.
- Show milder hypertrophy but higher proportion of arrhythmias and sudden cardiac death.
- Functional studies suggest that increased calcium sensitivity of cardiac muscle contraction is involved in the pathogenesis.

### Cardiac troponin I (TNNI3)
- Located on chromosome 19q13.
- 26 mutations identified to date.
- Relative prevalence 3–5%.
- Calcium sensitizing effect on cardiac muscle contractions observed with enhanced systolic function and impaired diastolic function.

### Cardiac troponin C (TNNC1)
- Located on chromosome 3p21.
- Rare mutation identified in late onset disease phenotype.
- Decrease in myofilament calcium sensitivity.

### alpha tropomysin (TPM1)
- Located on chromosome 12q22.
- 11 missense mutations found to cause HCM.
- Relative prevalence 3–5%.
- Heterogeneous phenotype of intermediate severity.
- Calcium sensitizing effect on cardiac muscle contraction.

### Cardiac actin (ACTC1)

- Located on chromosome 15q14.
- Seven missense mutations found to date.
- Rare cause with relative prevalence 1.5%.
- Decreased thermal stability of actin monomer and impaired filament formation.

## Mutations in genes for thick filament proteins

### β-Myosin (MyH7)

- Gene (*MYH7*) located on chromosome 14q12.
- At least 167 mutations identified to date in both exon and intron.
- Relative frequency 35–50% (one of commonest causes HCM).
- Some specific mutations identified with more malignant phenotype with early onset, 100% penetrance and a high incidence of premature sudden death.
- Other variants associated with near normal life expectancy.

### Essential myosin light chain (MYL3)

- Located on chromosome 3p21.
- Four missense mutations identified to date.
- Relative frequency <1%.
- Associated with a benign prognosis and low mortality rate.
- Very subtle increase in myofilament calcium sensitivity reported.

### Myosin-binding protein C (MYBPC3)

- Located on chromosome 11p11.
- At least 134 mutations identified to date in both exon and intron.
- One of the most common causes of familial HCM.
- Associated with later onset, less hypertrophy, lower penetrance and a better prognosis compared with mutations in MYH7 or cTNT.
- Delayed onset may pose risk of sudden death in individuals previously considered unaffected, therefore lifelong periodic screening necessary.

## Mutations in genes for titin and Z-disc proteins

### Titin (TTN)

- Located on chromosome 2q31.
- Two missense mutations identified to date.
- Infrequent cause of familial HCM (<1%).
- Has role in determining passive muscle stiffness and myofilament calcium sensitivity.

### Z-disc proteins

- Several mutations identified in the T-cap gene (*TCAP*) and in the MLP gene (*CSRP3*).
- All rare causes of familial HCM (<1%).

### Myozenin-2 (MYOZ2)

- A missense mutation identified in a large family.
- Characterized by early-onset symptoms, pronounced hypertrophy and cardiac arrhythmias.

# HCM pathophysiology

### Molecular biology and genetics

The pathophysiological link between genetic mutation and LV hypertrophy appears to be mediated by functional abnormalities induced by specific mutations in sarcomeric proteins. However, studies of individual myocyte function show both increased and decreased force and velocity of contraction and do not predict the clinical phenotype. There is evidence of impaired cardiac energetics at an early stage with reduced adenosine triphosphate (ATP) production and impairment of calcium-ATP homeostasis.

### Diastolic dysfunction

A hallmark feature of HCM is diastolic dysfunction. Myocyte disarray, hypertrophy, fibrosis, and abnormal calcium handling all contribute to impaired LV relaxation and increased LV filling pressures. Pressure-volume relations during LV filling can differ from those seen in other causes of LVH and indicate increased diastolic ventricular interaction in HCM.

### Left ventricular outflow tract obstruction (LVOTO)

The mechanism of LVOTO is multifactorial with abnormal flow vectors and pushing and drag forces involved. Systolic anterior motion (SAM) is exacerbated by malposition of the mitral valve, papillary muscles and elongated leaflets (Fig. 8.1). The timing and duration of mitral–septal contact correlates with the degree of LVOTO and LV ejection time.

### Myocardial ischaemia

Angina-like chest pain occurs in HCM due to increased myocardial oxygen demand and possibly compression of epicardial vessels due to LV hypertrophy. Positron emission tomography (PET) and magnetic resonance imaging (MRI) studies have demonstrated impaired micro vascular flow in patients with HCM and histological studies confirm medial thickening, enlargement of the endothelial cells and luminal narrowing of small arteries and arterioles.

### Systolic dysfunction

Progression to systolic dysfunction occurs in 5–10% of patients with HCM and is associated with ventricular wall thinning, LV dilatation and irreversible heart failure. This so-called 'end-stage' phase has a poor prognosis and mortality rate of 11% per year.

### Abnormal vascular responses

A paradoxical vasodilator response to orthostatic stress is seen in some patients with HCM and may explain syncope and abnormal blood pressure responses associated with more severe disease. The mechanism for inappropriate vasodilatation may be baroreceptor activation or secondary to myocardial ischaemia. Propranolol and paroxetine can improve vascular response to exercise.

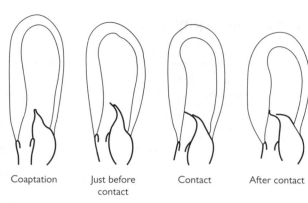

Coaptation        Just before        Contact        After contact
                  contact

**Fig. 8.1** Systolic anterior motion of the mitral valve causing LVOTO. Reproduced with permission from Sherrid MV *et al.* An echo cardigraphic study of the fluid mechanics of obstruction in hypertrophic cardiomyopathy. *J Am Coll Cardiol*, 1993 Sep, 22(3):816–25, with permission form Elsevier.

# Echocardiography in HCM

There are few if any pathognomonic echo features of HCM as many abnormalities are also seen in other conditions associated with left ventricular hypertrophy (such as hypertension, amyloid and valve disease).

## Distribution of hypertrophy

Hypertrophy predominantly affects the LV but in 20% there is right ventricular (RV) involvement as well. The extent and distribution of hypertrophy is identified by a series of parasternal short axis images (Fig. 8.2). Common patterns are described:

- asymmetrical septal hypertrophy (ASH) which is defined as a septal to posterior wall thickness ratio of 1.5 to 1
- concentric hypertrophy
- apical hypertrophy
- localized basal septal hypertrophy (overlaps with that commonly seen in elderly and hypertensive patients).

## Systolic and diastolic function

LV cavity is typically small and non-dilated. Systolic function is usually normal or 'supranormal' with vigorous contraction and ejection fraction typically >60%. Diastolic function is commonly impaired due to a thick non-compliant ventricle. Diastolic dysfunction should be graded using MV inflow and pulmonary venous Doppler patterns together with mitral annular tissue Doppler velocities (Fig. 8.3).

## Left ventricular outflow obstruction

Characterizing obstruction requires careful assessment of the mitral valve. M-mode echocardiography is useful to demonstrate systolic anterior motion (SAM) of the anterior mitral valve leaflet and premature closure (fluttering) of the aortic valve.

Mitral regurgitation due to SAM is typically an eccentric jet directed posteriorly, unless there is co-existing MV pathology. MV leaflets are often elongated and papillary muscles hypertrophied. Look for an echo-bright 'impact lesion' at the point of mitral-septal contact and turbulent blood flow in the outflow tract.

LVOT gradient should be measured at rest in the apical long axis and 5-chamber view. CW Doppler of LV outflow typically shows a dagger shape representing late peaking systolic obstruction (Fig. 8.4). A provokable gradient may be detected using Valsalva manoeuvre, nitrates or exercise stress. An mid-cavity gradient can often be seen using Doppler.

## Left atrium

Left atrial size is often increased in patients with HCM and is associated with diastolic dysfunction, LVOTO, poor exercise capacity, atrial fibrillation and an overall worse prognosis. LA volume is more reproducible that diameter measured in a single view.

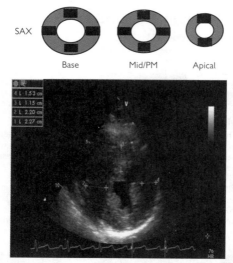

**Fig. 8.2** Serial short-axis views of the left ventricle at the level of the mitral valve, papillary muscles and apex, demonstrating the segments of myocardial wall measured routinely in patients with HCM. Reproduced with permission from L.K. Williams, M.P. Frenneaux, and R.P. Steeds. Echocardiography in hypertrophic cardiomyopathy. *European Journal of Echocardiography*, (2009) 10, iii9–iii14.

| | Normal | Mild | Moderate | Severe |
|---|---|---|---|---|
| | | ↓ Relaxation | ↓ Relaxation<br>↓ Compliance<br>↑ LVEDP | ↓ Relaxation<br>↓ Compliance<br>↑↑ LVEDP |
| | | Abnormal relaxation | Pseude-Normal | Restrictive filling |
| LV inflow Doppler | | | | |
| E/A ratio | 1–2 | <1 | 1–2 | <2 |
| IVRT (ms) | 50–100 | >100 | 50–100 | >50 |
| Dt (ms) | 150–200 | >200 | 150–200 | >150 |
| Pulmonary venous Doppler | | | | |
| PV$_S$>PV$_D$<br>PVa (m/s)<br>a$_{aur}$–A$_{aur}$ (ms) | PV$_S$>PV$_D$<br><0.35<br><20 | PV$_S$>PV$_D$<br><0.35<br><20 | PV$_S$<PV$_D$<br>≥0.35<br>≥20 | PV$_S$<<PVD<br>≥0.35<br>≥20 |
| Mitral annular tissue Doppler | | | | |
| E$_m$/A$_m$ | 1–2 | <1 | <1 | <<1 |
| E/E$_m$ (septum)<br>E/E$_m$ (lateral) | <8<br><10 | -<br>- | >15<br>>10 | -<br>- |

**Fig. 8.3** Left ventricular diastolic function. BSE guidelines adapted from Rakowski, H. *JASE* 1996.

# Tissue Doppler imaging in HCM

### Pre-clinical detection of HCM

Reduced myocardial tissue Doppler velocities are seen in patients with HCM even before the development of LVH. Therefore tissue Doppler imaging (TDI) might be used to detect pre-clinical disease in gene carriers (Figs. 8.3 and 8.5) although other conditions such as coronary artery disease, hypertension and diabetes mellitus also alter tissue Doppler velocities. The age at which velocities become abnormal is not clear.

### Distinguishing athletes

TDI may help separate physiological hypertrophy seen in athletes from that seen in HCM or hypertension. Combing TDI variables with wall thickness and flow propagation velocities provides the most sensitive and specific evaluation.

### Monitoring treatment

TDI has been used to monitor response to alcohol septal ablation and various drug treatments where improvements in diastolic velocities parallel a reduction in filling pressures, outflow gradient and an increase in exercise capacity.

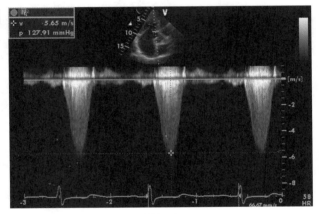

**Fig. 8.4** Typical dagger appearance of LV outflow velocity.

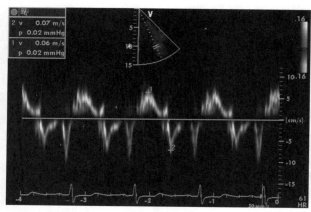

**Fig. 8.5** Tissue Doppler imaging in HCM.

# Stress echocardiography in HCM

Assessment of sub-aortic gradients with exercise echocardiography should be a routine part of evaluation of patients with HCM. Whilst LV outflow gradients are detected in only 25% patients at rest, they are evident in up to 70% of patients during exercise. These patients often report exertional dyspnoea or pre-syncope and are candidates for medical or surgical treatment. When LVOT obstruction is severe the gradient may become holosystolic and can be difficult to distinguish from MR.

## LV function

Stress echocardiography is useful in detecting systolic dysfunction in patients with HCM and a normal resting left ventricular ejection function.

## Exercise TDI

Augmentation of LV longitudinal function during exercise is blunted in patients with HCM, suggesting these patients have abnormal longitudinal functional reserve.

# Cardiovascular magnetic resonance imaging in HCM

Cardiovascular magnetic resonance (CMR) is a valuable tool in the assessment of the patient with HCM. Combining multiple techniques in one scan allows for a sophisticated evaluation of LV/RV cardiac function, hypertrophy, morphology, flow, velocities, perfusion, and fibrosis.

Clinical uses of CMR in HCM include detecting early disease expression, characterizing established disease and distinguishing phenocopies.

**Early disease**

- The first signs of phenotypic expression in HCM may be difficult to detect with imaging.
- 2D echocardiography has several limitations in this regard. It is reliant on adequate acoustic windows and the fixed probe on the chest wall necessitates oblique cross-sectioning in short axis of the LV.
- Hypertrophy in HCM can be confined to relatively small regions of the LV chamber that may be obscured or have inadequate border definition on echo. When HCM is suspected and the ECG is abnormal with a normal echo, CMR may pick up missed hypertrophy (5% of cases in some series).
- Several minor cardiac morphological abnormalities have been associated with early disease expression—for example crypts (also described as clefts or recesses), particularly of basal inferior wall. Their significance remains unclear and the presence of a few may be part of the normal spectrum.

**Apical involvement**

- Echo views of the apex are technically challenging due to near field artefact. In patients suspected to have apical variant HCM, (particularly negative T waves anteriorly) CMR may elucidate missed hypertrophy.
- Small apical aneurysms are clearly demonstrated on CMR.
- Apical cavity obliteration, thrombus, and LV non-compaction can be identified.

**Contrast-enhanced CMR**

- Gadolinium chelate (Gd-DTPA) contrast agents identify focal areas of fibrosis.
- Gd-DTPA is exclusively extracellular and accumulates in areas of scar making the area brighter on MRI—a phenomenon called late gadolinium enhancement (LGE).
- LGE is common in HCM, occurring in up to 70% of patients.
- LGE is correlated with clinical risk markers for sudden death, non-sustained ventricular tachycardia (NSVT), atrial fibrillation (AF) and progression to heart failure.

## Obstruction

- Left ventricular outflow tract is readily assessed by rest and stress echocardiography.
- CMR can be useful when there are complicating factors such as multilevel obstruction, RV outflow obstruction, aortic membranes or poor echo windows.

## Phenocopies

- Other conditions may present with LVH and cause diagnostic difficulty.
- Examples include storage disorders such as Anderson–Fabry's disease (AFD), amyloid and athletes heart.
- CMR, at least in the early stages, may help refine the differential diagnosis, pointing to specific etiologies.
- Typically AFD patients have basal infero-lateral LGE in the early stages but this may be absent.
- Cardiac amyloidosis produces subendocardial LGE affecting all four chambers diffusely and a characteristic dark blood pool.

## Progressive disease

- The natural history of HCM over time occasionally progresses to include wall thinning, cavity size increase and a reduction in ejection fraction and heart failure.
- This process is often associated with extensive LGE on contrast CMR (Fig. 8.6).
- CMR in this scenario can demonstrate thrombus formation on early contrast images.

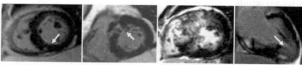

Subtle LGE of the RV insertion points - A frequent finding in HCM

Septal LGE

Extensive LGE of the septum associated with progressive disease

Apical LGE sometimes associated with apical aneurysm

**Fig. 8.6** Short axis sections on cardiac magnetic resonance imaging.

# HCM symptom management (drugs)

No pharmacological treatment has been shown to alter prognosis in HCM. It is current practice to initiate drug therapy when symptoms develop or if LVOTO is present.

### Beta-blockers

Major actions:
- slow heart rate
- prolong diastole and reduce ventricular filling pressures
- reduce exercise induced outflow obstruction
- suppress arrhythmias
- lessen myocardial ischaemia.

High doses are often required to be effective in HCM though problems with fatigue, insomnia, impotence and bradycardia may limit their use.

### Calcium channel blockers

- When beta-blockers are poorly tolerated or contraindicated, verapamil is a suitable alternative providing good symptom relief and improved exercise duration.
- It is often more effective in patients without obstruction where chest pain is the main symptom.
- Use with caution in those with obstruction where its vasodilatory effect may exacerbate outflow tract gradient.
- Adverse effects include hypotension, atrio ventricular (AV) block and heart failure.

### Disopyramide

- This Class 1a anti-arrhythmic agent may be used with beta-blockers or verapamil when a residual gradient and symptoms persist.
- A dose response effect is seen.
- Anticholinergic side effects and QT prolongation may limit the maximal dose to below 600mg/day.
- The observed benefit is not always long-lasting and symptoms may recur as early as 12 months after starting therapy.

### Angiotensin-converting enzyme (ACE) inhibitors and angiotensin II receptor blockers

- As HCM progresses a subgroup (5–10%) will develop systolic heart failure.
- In the absence of LVOTO, treatment with ACE inhibitors, angiotension II receptor blockers and diuretics is usually implemented although the prognostic benefits of these interventions are not known.
- Some patients will develop restrictive physiology when diuretics are the mainstay of treatment and negative inotropic agents must be used with caution.

### Anticoagulation

- Atrial fibrillation (AF) is the most common arrhythmia in HCM and is usually poorly tolerated due to a stiff poorly compliant ventricle.
- Anticoagulation with warfarin is recommended in all those with paroxysmal or chronic AF.

- Aspirin is often initiated in the presence of left atrial (LA) enlargement alone.

## Endocarditis prophylaxis

- The incidence of endocarditis in HCM is usually confined to those with LVOTO or concomitant MV disease.
- Current NICE guidelines do not recommend antibiotic prophylaxis routinely in HCM and instead encourage maintenance of good oral health.

## Further reading

National Institute for Health and Clinical Excellence (2008) *Prophylaxis Against Infective Endocarditis in Adults and Children Undergoing Interventional Procedures.* London: National Institute for Health and Clinical Excellence.

# Treatment of left ventricular outflow tract obstruction

Patients with symptomatic LVOTO refractory to medical treatment are considered for more invasive management. The mechanism and site of obstruction must be taken into consideration when planning intervention. Whilst surgery is considered the gold standard, the decision must take into account available expertise and patient co-morbidities.

### Surgery

Ventricular septal myectomy (Morrow procedure) is considered the gold standard to treat refractory symptoms and LVOTO. Surgery is performed via an aortotomy—a rectangular trough is created in the basal septum by making two parallel incisions, which are then connected proximally below the aortic valve and extended distally to beyond the point of mitral–septal contact and subaortic obstruction (Fig. 8.7). The procedure significantly improves symptoms in 70%, reduces risk of sudden death and delays progression of heart failure, such that long-term survival after myectomy equates with non-obstructive HCM (Fig. 8.8). In specialist centres surgical mortality is <1% with the major complications being complete heart block and ventricular septal defect. In cases of mid-cavity obstruction the myectomy can be extended to allow mobilization of the papillary muscles. Mitral valve replacement can also relieve obstruction but is reserved for those with inherent mitral valve abnormalities as operative complications are higher. Re-do myectomy is uncommon.

### Dual chamber (DDD) pacing

Dual chamber (DDD) pacing with a short AV delay is an option for reducing symptoms related to LVOTO and has been subject to randomized controlled trials. The mechanism is presumed due to altered electrical activation of the interventricular septum. A clinical response does not always correlate with reduction in LVOT gradient. Results are most favourable in the elderly population who often have localized basal septal hypertrophy, however a significant placebo effect is recognized. The deleterious effects of long-term DDD pacing in HCM is not known.

### Alcohol septal ablation

Percutaneous alcohol septal ablation involves careful injection of alcohol into one of the septal branches of the left anterior descending artery to produce a localized area of necrosis. This results in thinning of the basal septum, widening of the outflow tract and a gradual elimination of obstruction over 3–6 months. Complications include extensive myocardial infarction and AV block. Myocardial contrast echocardiography is recommended prior to injection to ensure the correct area is targeted.

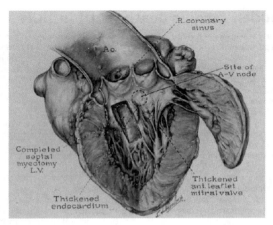

**Fig. 8.7** The Morrow Procedure. Reproduced with permission from Morrow AG et al. (1975). Operative treatment in hypertrophic subaortic stenosis. Techniques and the results of pre and postoperative assessments in 83 patients. *Circulation* 1975; **52**, 88–102.

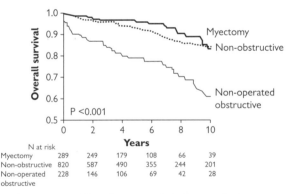

**Fig. 8.8** Long term survival from all cause mortality in 3 groups of patients with HCM. Reproduced from Ommen SR et al. (2005). Long-Term Effects of Surgical Septal Myectomy on survival in patients with obstructive Hypertrophic Cardiomyopathy. *J Am Coll Cardiol*, 2005, **46**, 470–476, with permission from Elsevier.

# Sudden cardiac death (SCD) in HCM

- Early studies from tertiary referral centres with highly selected patients reported annual mortality rates of up to 6% but contemporary studies have shown survival rates similar to that of the general population of the same age and sex.
- Susceptibility to SCD varies substantially between individuals.
- SCD can occur at any age with a peak in incidence during late adolescence and young adulthood.
- SCD is caused primarily by ventricular arrhythmias caused by:
  - myocardial hypertrophy which causes dispersion of repolarization and refractoriness making the myocardium vulnerable to triggered arrhythmias
  - disarray and fibrosis which create areas of conduction block predisposing to re-entry arrhythmias
  - abnormal ion fluxes during repolarization of cardiomyocyte cell membranes cause after-depolarizations and triggered activity
  - additional modifiers may induce ventricular arrhythmias:
    — myocardial ischaemia caused by intimal and medial smooth muscle cell hyperplasia of the small intramural coronary arteries
    — left ventricular outflow tract obstruction
    — diastolic dysfunction
    — abnormal autonomic function.
- Each patient should be risk stratified for SCD, and reassessed temporally.

# Management of the risk of SCD in HCM

### Lifestyle modifications for the prevention of SCD

- SCD has been associated with intense competitive exercise.
- International guidelines suggest that athletes with HCM should be advised against participation in competitive sports.

### Secondary prevention of SCD

- Survivors of cardiac arrest have a high annual mortality rate (~5%).
- International guidelines support the use of internal cardioverter defibrillator (ICDs) for secondary prevention.
- Treatment with anti-arrhythmics is not reliable in preventing SCD.

### Primary prevention of SCD

The current approach to risk stratification for SCD relies on an assessment of a small number of routinely collected clinical parameters. International guidelines rank these risk factors into 'major' and 'possible'.

#### *Major risk factors*

- Ventricular arrhythmias:
  - non-sustained ventricular tachycardia (NSVT) defined as 3 or more ventricular complexes at a rate of ≥120 beats per minute is associated with SCD especially in young patients
  - in patients ≤30 years of age, NSVT is associated with a fourfold increase in the relative risk of SCD
  - the duration, frequency or rate of NSVT does not influence its predictive accuracy
  - NSVT becomes more common in patients >30 years of age but the relative risk for SCD decreases
  - ventricular ectopy and ventricular couplets are present in ~80%, and ~40% of patients respectively but have no prognostic value.
- Family history of SCD secondary to HCM:
  - pedigree analysis should be undertaken in every patient
  - pedigree analysis is often limited by lack of accurate information
  - post-mortem reports and death certificates should be sought
  - a single SCD in a large family with multiple affected members is probably less predictive than a single SCD in a small family with only two or three affected members.
- Maximal wall thickness ≥30mm:
  - maximal wall thickness ≥30mm is associated 2–4-fold increase in the relative risk of SCD but the majority of patients with SCD have a maximal wall thickness <30mm
  - the extent of hypertrophy is also associated with SCD
  - suboptimal echocardiographic images may limit accurate assessment of hypertrophy, and alternative modalities such as cardiac MRI may be required.
- Unexplained syncope:
  - unexplained syncope with one or more episodes within the previous 12 months is associated with SCD
  - unexplained syncope on exertion, especially in children and adolescents, is particularly worrisome.

- Abnormal blood pressure response to exercise:
  - failure of systolic blood pressure to rise by more than 20–30 mm Hg from baseline is associated with SCD in patients <40 years of age
  - probably related to abnormal autonomic responses
  - children and young adolescents normally have a flat blood pressure response to exercise limiting the use of this parameter in this group.

### Possible risk factors

Other clinical parameters have been proposed as markers of risk but the data are either preliminary or inconclusive:
- atrial fibrillation
- late gadolinium enhancement
- competitive sports
- left ventricular outflow tract obstruction ≥30mmHg.

### Global risk burden approach

In the setting of primary prevention, there is little evidence to suggest that any one risk factor is more predictive of SCD than another (🕮 Table 8.6). However, the aggregation of these risk factors in an individual patient is thought to reflect the severity of the underlying myocardial disease and thus the risk for SCD.
- Patients with ≥2 risk factors have a 72% six-year survival with a 4% to 5% annual risk of SCD and are thus candidates for ICD implantation.
- Patients without any major risk factors for SCD do not require aggressive primary prevention as the mortality rate is <1%/year.
- Patients with a single risk factor constitute about 25% of HCM patients with a six year survival rate of 93%. However, 5% of SCD occurs in patients with a single risk factor and it is challenging to identify those with a single risk factor who are at greatest risk for SCD. The presence of 'possible' risk factors may favour implantation of an ICD.

## Further reading

Elliott P.M., et al. (2000) Sudden death in hypertrophic cardiomyopathy: identification of high risk patients. *J Am Coll Cardiol* **36**: 2212–2218.

Maron B.J., et al. (2003) American College of Cardiology/European Society of Cardiology Clinical Expert Consensus Document on Hypertrophic Cardiomyopathy: A report of the American College of Cardiology Foundation Task Force on Clinical Expert Consensus Documents and the European Society of Cardiology Committee for Practice Guidelines. *Eur Heart J* **24**: 1965–1991.

**Table 8.6** Clinical parameters associated with SCD (modified from ACC/ESC Guidelines, *EHJ* 2003; **24**: 1965–1991, and Frenneaux M.P. *Heart* 2004; **90**: 570–575.)

| Major clinical parameter | PPV % | NPV % |
| --- | --- | --- |
| Non-sustained ventricular arrhythmias | 25 | 85 |
| Family history of SCD | 28 | 88 |
| Unexplained syncope | 25 | 86 |
| Maximal LV wall thickness ≥30mm | 13 | 95 |
| Abnormal blood pressure response to exercise | 15 | >95 |

PPV, positive predictive value; NPV, negative predictive value.

# Management of atrial arrhythmias in HCM

Atrial fibrillation affects about a quarter of HCM patients, with an incidence of 2% per annum.
- Risk factors:
  - left atrial dilation (a consequence of diastolic dysfunction, left ventricular outflow tract obstruction and SAM-related mitral regurgitation)
  - increasing age.
- Complications:
  - deteriorating function, especially with left ventricular outflow tract obstruction
  - increased risk of death from heart failure
  - increased risk of stroke.

## Anticoagulation
- Systemic embolization in the presence of atrial fibrillation has an incidence of 2.5% per year.
- Left atrial dilation increases the risk of embolization even further.
- Warfarin anticoagulation is the cornerstone of treatment.
- Some investigators promote the use of either aspirin or warfarin in patients with significantly enlarged atria, even in the absence of atrial fibrillation.

## Rhythm control
Restoration of sinus rhythm is almost always attempted in view of the symptomatic improvement experienced by most patients.
- Direct current shock cardioversion:
  - more in recent onset atrial fibrillation
  - transoesophageal examination should be considered in patients with severely enlarged left atria as left atrial appendage clots form despite adequate anticoagulation
  - class III anti-arrhythmics can be used to help maintain sinus rhythm post electrical cardioversion.
- Pulmonary vein isolation:
  - used in cases that are refractory to DC shock cardioversion or anti-arrhytmics
  - most patients require multiple procedures
  - anti-arrhythmics are frequently required post ablation
  - more successful for paroxysmal atrial fibrillation.

## Rate control
- AV blocking agents can be used to control the ventricular rate.
- Digoxin should be avoided:
  - poor efficacy
  - can exacerbate the severity of left ventricular outflow tract obstruction.

- In drug-resistant cases with permanent atrial fibrillation, AV nodal ablation with right ventricular pacing (or biventricular pacing if the systolic function is impaired) has been used.

## Further reading

Olivotto I., Maron B.J., Cecchi F. (2001) Clinical significance of atrial fibrillation in hypertrophic cardiomyopathy. *Curr. Cardiol Rep.* **3**: 141–146.

# Differentiation of HCM from hypertensive heart disease

### The heart in hypertension

- LVH is initially a compensatory process representing an adaptation to increased ventricular wall stress. The prevalence of LVH in a general population sample ranges from 3–5% but to >50% of those >70years.
- Non-haemodynamic factors also play a role in determining which hypertensive patients develop LVH and to what extent. These factors include age, sex, race, body mass index (BMI), diabetes and dietary salt intake.
- The compensatory increase in LV mass eventually is no longer beneficial and becomes a pre-clinical disease and an independent risk factor for congestive cardiac failure, ischaemic heart disease, arrhythmia, sudden death and stroke.
- As well as concentric LVH, left atrial dilatation, diastolic dysfunction with impaired relaxation and reduced chamber compliance are recognized.
- The prevalence of diastolic dysfunction in hypertensive patients depends on the method of measurement and may be as high as 72%, even in the absence of concentric remodelling.

### Hypertensive heart disease vs hypertrophic cardiomyopathy

- Hypertension typically produces concentric remodelling of the left ventricle as opposed to asymmetric septal hypertrophy.
- Moderate to severe hypertrophy (≥15mm) is rare in white people with mild to moderate hypertension.
- The presence of a family history of cardiac hypertrophy in a non-hypertensive relative or a positive gene test increases the likelihood of hypertrophic cardiomyopathy as opposed to hypertensive heart disease.
- The diagnosis of HCM in black patients with hypertension is more difficult since hypertrophy is not rare in hypertensive black patients.
- SAM of the mitral valve is a recognized but rare finding in hypertensive heart disease (<1%).
- In hypertension, treatment with anti-hypertensive agents can result in regression of LVH accompanied by diminished ventricular arrhythmia, improved diastolic dysfunction, preservation of systolic function and resolution of microvascular ischaemia.

# Common diagnostic dilemmas—racial variants

- The differentiation between a hypertrophic cardiomyopathy phenotype and normal heart is influenced by the race of the subject.
- Published data comparing cardiomyopathy patients and controls according to ethnicity is lacking.
- The presence of a family history of LVH in a normotensive relative would point to a diagnosis of hypertrophic cardiomyopathy.
- The upper limits of LV wall thickness used to discriminate physiological LVH from HCM are established in Caucasian athletes.
- In 1998 in a healthy, middle-aged, biracial population ECG abnormalities were found in 8% black subjects compared to 5% white subjects.
- Two studies published in 2008 compared black and white athletes:
  - 18% black athletes exhibited LVH compared to just 4% white athletes
  - 3% black athletes had LVH ≥15mm compared to 0% of white athletes
  - in elite American football players, ECG abnormalities were present in 30% black players compared with 13% white players and 15% of other race players
  - black race was an independent predictor of ECG abnormalities
  - ECG abnormalities most commonly included increased precordial voltages and repolarization abnormalities.

Criteria to differentiate physiological from physiological hypertrophy are not available but this is an important area requiring further investigation to help identify those at risk as well as preventing false positive results preventing participation in sports for normal individuals.

# Athletic heart

## Athletes

Differentiation between pathological and physiological hypertrophy is clinically important and increasingly required by governing bodies prior to sports participation. No single test is sensitive or specific and careful assessment, often with a three-month period of detraining, is needed to distinguish the athlete from the patient with hypertrophic cardiomyopathy. The major differences are shown in Table 8.7.

**Table 8.7** Major differences between the athlete and the patient with hypertrophic cardiomyopathy

| Athlete's heart | Hypertrophic cardiomyopathy |
|---|---|
| History of athletic training | Family history of HCM or SCD |
| Asymptomatic | Palpitations, syncope, |
| ECG: LVH, sinus bradycardia | ECG: Q waves, ST depression, deep T wave inversion |
| Peak VO$_2$ >100% predicted | Low aerobic capacity |
| MWT < = 13mm | MWT > = 13mm |
| LV cavity size increased | Small LV cavity size |
| Normal diastolic function | Diastolic dysfunction |
| Normal longitudinal function | Abnormal TDI indices |

SCD, sudden cardiac death; LVH, left ventricular hypertrophy; VO$_2$, oxygen consumption; MWT, maximal LV wall thickness; TDI, tissue Doppler imaging.

## Obesity

Hypertension, obstructive sleep apnoea and coronary artery disease contribute to left ventricular hypertrophy associated with obesity. There is some evidence that an independent 'obesity cardiomyopathy' exists where concentric LVH occurs independent of systemic disease. Waist circumference, BMI and duration of obesity are risk factors and pathogenesis involves insulin resistance, adipokines, lipotoxicity, microvascular changes, inflammation and sympathetic and renin–angiotension system activation. Pre-clinical disease may be detected by echocardiography with early diastolic and TDI abnormalities. Weight loss is effective and associated with reverse LV remodelling.

# Friedreich's ataxia

Friedreich's ataxia (FRDA) is a neurodegenerative disease that primarily affects the nervous system and the heart.

## Incidence
- 1:36,000–1:50,000.
- Most common inherited ataxia in individuals of Western European origin.
- Also found in people of North African and Middle Eastern origin but not reported in other ethnic groups.

## Aetiology
- Inherited as an autosomal recessive trait.
- Caused by an unstable GAA repeat expansion in intron 1 of the FRDA gene on chromosome 9.
- ~96% patients homozygous for this repeat.
- Remaining patients compound heterozygotes with the GAA expansion in one allele and an inactivating mutation in the coding region of the other allele.
- This gene encodes the mitochondrial matrix protein frataxin, which is involved in cellular iron homeostasis and is essential for survival.
- In FRDA frataxin levels are significantly reduced resulting in multiple enzyme deficits, increased mitochondrial iron accumulation and susceptibility to oxidative damage.

## Clinical features
- Progressive limb and gait ataxia.
- Loss of deep tendon reflexes.
- Extensor plantar responses.
- Loss of position and vibration sense in lower limbs.
- Dysarthria.
- Age of onset and age at which patients become wheelchair bound is inversely correlated with the length of the GAA repeat expansion
- Hypertrophic cardiomyopathy.
- Diabetes mellitus (due to a combination of insulin resistance and inadequate insulin response).

## Cardiac features
- Hypertrophic cardiomyopathy detected by echocardiography is present in most patients but is often asymptomatic.
- Increasing age at diagnosis of FRDA is associated with decreased risk of cardiomegaly.

### ECG
- Abnormalities detected in approximately 90% patients.
- Commonest finding inferolateral repolarization abnormalities.
- Development of Q waves has an unfavourable prognostic value with regard to the evolution towards LV dilatation and impaired function.
- Patients typically complain of palpitations, exertional dyspnoea or angina.

*Echocardiography*
- Hypertrophy characterized by either concentric or asymmetrical hypertrophy with preserved systolic function.
- Hypertrophy is usually mild and obstruction uncommon.

## Management
- A variety of therapeutic strategies are under development.
- Antioxidants, coenzyme Q10, vitamin E.
- Idebenone has been reported to decrease the cardiac hypertrophy in patients, but large-scale studies are required to confirm this.
- Coenzyme Q10 given in combination with vitamin E has produced a prolonged improvement in cardiac and skeletal muscle bio-energetics.
- Other novel therapeutic approaches emerging include:
  - erythropoeitin—to increase frataxin expression
  - pioglitazone—stimulates mitochondrial function
  - deferiprone—oral iron chelator
  - gene therapy and protein replacement.

# Cardiac amyloidosis

Cardiac amyloidosis refers to a group of disorders characterized by extracellular deposition of insoluble fibrils derived from aggregation of misfolded, normally soluble proteins. There are several forms of cardiac amyloidosis, each with its unique features and management strategy. They may be acquired or hereditary and are classified according to the precursor protein.

Regardless of the precursor protein, amyloidosis type is virtually indistinguishable with light microscopy. All forms show an amorphous proteinaceous substance that demonstrates apple green birefringence under polarized light when stained with Congo red.

## AL amyloidosis
- Previously known as primary amyloidosis.
- Most commonly diagnosed form of amyloidosis.
- Occurs equally in men and women, usually >50 years.
- AL fibrils derived from monoclonal immunoglobulin light chains.
- Any B-cell dyscrasia (including myeloma, lymphoma, macroglobulinaemia) can cause, but >80% due to subtle and otherwise 'benign' gammopathies.
- Multi-organ infiltration typical.
- Heart affected in up to 90% cases.
- 50% patients present with symptoms of heart failure.

### Clinical features
- Rapidly progressive signs and symptoms.
- Median survival 15 months.
- **Symptoms:** dyspnoea, chest discomfort, weight loss, syncope.
- **Signs:** peripheral oedema, elevated jugular venous pressure (JVP), ascites, periorbital purpura and easy bruising, macroglossia (10–20%), carpal tunnel syndrome, (postural) hypotension, hepatomegaly, autonomic/sensory neuropathy, proteinuria, nephritic syndrome, pleural effusions.
- Classical features commonly present in later stages of the disease.

### Electrocardiogram
- Low voltage ECG (QRS amplitude 10≤mV in all limb leads or ≤1mV in all precordial leads) in 46%.
- Pseudo-infarct pattern (Q waves with no infarct on echo) in 47%.
- Combination of the above seen in 25% patients.
- Atrial arrhythmias (most commonly AF) 10–15%.
- Extreme axis deviation.

### Echocardiogram
- Images should be interpreted in context of clinical picture.
- Most commonly biventricular thickening and increased LV mass.
- Increased echogenicity of the myocardium with a granular or 'sparkling' appearance (low sensitivity).
- Systolic function normal until the more severe stages of the disease with a potential disproportionate reduction of longitudinal function.

- Diastolic dysfunction is the hallmark of this disease
  - abnormal mitral inflow patterns,
  - reduced diastolic velocities on tissue Doppler
  - abnormal strain and strain rate imaging patterns
- Bi-atrial enlargement 27–50%
- Thickening of valve leaflets
- Thickening intra-atrial septum in a minority
- Pericardial effusion

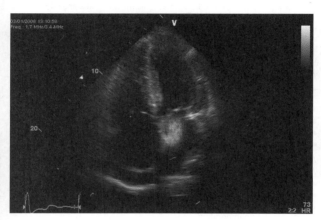

**Fig. 8.9** Image of echo of amyloidosis.

### Magnetic resonance imaging

- Global sub-endocardial late gadolinium enhancement 60–70%.
- Likely to represent interstitial expansion from amyloid infiltration.
- Abnormal myocardial and blood-pool gadolinium kinetics with atypically dark appearance of the blood pool.
- Reflects similar myocardial and blood T1 values attributable to high myocardial uptake and fast blood pool washout.

### Cardiac catheterization

- Right-sided heart catheterization enables accurate haemodynamic assessment.
- Pressure tracings reveal a dip and plateau or square root sign indicative of restrictive physiology.
- Coronary angiogram is usually normal.

### Cardiac biomarkers

- Troponin increased due to myonecrosis and small vessel ischaemia secondary to amyloid deposition.
- Brain natriuretic (BNP) levels increased due to diastolic dysfunction.
- Both correlate to disease severity and prognosis.

### Tissue diagnosis
- Apple-green birefringence when stained with Congo red when viewed under a polarizing microscope.
- Fine needle aspiration of abdominal fat positive in >70% patients.
- Endomyocardial biopsy is virtually 100% sensitive due to the wide deposition of AL amyloid throughout the heart.

### Tissue diagnosis
- I123-labelled serum amyloid P (SAP) specifically binds with all types of fibril (via a calcium-mediated mechanism). SAP scans provide information on the presence and distribution of amyloid deposits in the body, but cannot image the beating heart.
- 99mTc-3,3-diphosphono-1,2-propanodi-carboxylic acid (99mTc-DPD) scintigraphy can detect amyloid deposition in the myocardium in tranthyretin TTR but not in AL amyloidosis.

### Other investigations
- Serum immunoglobulin free light chains assay can quantify the aberrant circulatory protein precursor (85–98% sensitivity) and can be serially monitored to assess disease progression and response to therapy.
- Serum and urine immunofixation.
- Urine electrophoresis.
- Bone marrow biopsy.

### Management and -rognosis
*Management of cardiac-related symptoms*
- Mainstay of treatment of heart failure is diuretic therapy.
- Meticulous attention to fluid balance and daily weights.
- High incidence of thromboembolism associated with AF therefore anticoagulation imperative.
- Beta blockers poorly tolerated due to bradycardia/hypotension.
- Vasoactive drugs should be used with caution due to risk of profound hypotension.
- Both digoxin and calcium blockers bind to amyloid fibrils and can result in digoxin toxicity at therapeutic doses or profound hypotension with calcium blockers.
- Sudden death is common with most deaths due to electromechanical dissociation.
- Pacemakers should be used in those who fulfill conventional implantation indications.
- Implantable cardioverter defibrillators have not been shown to prolong survival.

*Treatment of the underlying disease*
- Therapy aimed at stopping the production of the paraprotein responsible for the formation of amyloid.
  - Oral chemotherapy (melphalan and prednisolone).
  - High-dose chemotherapy coupled with peripheral autologous stem cell rescue (contraindicated if congestive heart failure, syncope, arrhythmias, renal failure, poor functional status or involvement of >2 visceral organs).
- Heart transplantation not generally accepted due to poor long-term survival secondary to disease recurrence in the allograft.

## Other forms of acquired amyloidosis

### AA amyloidosis

- A complication of chronic inflammatory conditions such as rheumatoid arthritis, familial Mediterranean fever, chronic infections, inflammatory bowel disease.
- Accumulation of the acute-phase response, serum amyloid A.
- Renal disease is the most common feature (proteinuria and renal failure).
- Cardiac involvement typically is clinically insignificant.
- Treatment of the underlying process can reverse the disease.
- New biological agents that inhibit tumour necrosis factor and interleukin-1 potently suppress acute phase response.
- Colchicine prevents AA amyloidosis in familial Mediterranean fever.

### Senile systemic amyloidosis

- An age-related disease due to deposition of fibrils derived from normal wild-type transthyretin.
- Large male predominance.
- Rare <60 years.
- Almost always slowly progressive with median survival 75 months.
- Invariably presents as congestive heart failure as it has major predilection for the heart.
- Bifasicular block on ECG common, with progression to complete AV block not infrequent, requiring pacemaker implantation.
- Biventricular pacing should be strongly considered in these patients as they may deteriorate with pacing due to ventricular dyssynchrony.
- Carpal tunnel syndrome is a common clinical feature.
- Exclusion of a plasma cell dyscrasia is mandatory.
- Screening should be performed to exclude a mutant transthyretin.
- No specific treatment.
- Death is usually due to congestive heart failure or arrhythmias.

### Isolated atrial amyloidosis

- Unclear if any clinical significance.
- Commonly seen at post-mortem in elderly patients.
- Amyloid fibril originates from atrial natriuretic peptide.
- Non-systemic deposition isolated to the atria.
- More common in females and in the presence of atrial fibrillation or valvular disease.

### Haemodialysis-related amyloidosis

- Due to the deposition of accumulated β2 microglobulin from long-standing uraemia.
- Clinical effect of cardiac deposition minimal.
- Predominant symptoms due to joint involvement.
- Renal transplantation normalizes β2 microglobulin concentration and improves joint pain.

### TTR-related familial amyloidosis

- Tranthyretin (TTR)-related familial amyloidosis (ATTR) is the most frequent form of hereditary systemic amyloidosis.
- TTR is a single polypeptide chain of 127 amino acid residues encoded by a single gene on chromosome 18 with 4 exons.
- TTR is a tetrameric plasma transport protein for thyroid hormone and retinol-binding protein/vitamin A synthesized in the liver.
- ATTR is inherited as an autosomal dominant trait with variable penetrance.
- The majority of TTR mutations are a single nucleotide substitutions.
- Over 80 different amyloidogenic mutations reported (many in single individuals or families).
- Most ATTR carriers are heterozygous for a pathogenic mutation and express both normal and variant TTR.

#### Geography
- Some TTR mutations are found in extended kindreds in particular geographic locations.
- The most common is Val30Met, which leads to 'type I familial amyloid polyneuropathy' (FAP) in Portugal, Sweden and in Japan.
- Val122Ile is present in 4% of African-Americans.
- Thr60Ala is the most common cause of ATTR in the UK and Ireland.

#### Clinical
- Phenotypic heterogeneity linked to the type of TTR mutation, geographic cluster and endemic or non-endemic distribution.
- In classic endemic TTR Val30Met type of FAP, sensorimotor polyneuropathy is common. The neuropathy usually starts at 30–35 years of age with small-fibre dysfunction in the lower limbs. Motor function is usually only affected at an advanced stage.
- Autonomic neuropathy occurs relatively early, resulting in severe orthostatic hypotension, bowel disturbance, erectile dysfunction, urinary retention, and incontinence.
- In Japanese and Portuguese patients with the non-endemic, 'late-onset' Val30Met TTR mutation, autonomic dysfunction is milder, and sensory loss and cardiomyopathy are more common. Swedish patients have age at onset in mid-50s, with much slower disease progression.

Other neurological features of ATTR include include:
- carpal tunnel syndrome
- vocal hoarseness (recurrent laryngeal nerve palsy)
- scalloped pupil deformity
- vitreous opacities
- stroke, seizures, hydrocephalus, spastic paralysis, spinal cord infarction
- renal involvement is generally **not** a feature of ATTR.

#### Cardiac
- Patients with the Val30Met mutation from endemic clusters tend to have less severe heart involvement in comparison non-endemic areas or other mutations.
- In endemic areas of Portugal and Japan, conduction disturbances are the single most frequent form of cardiac involvement, whereas

congestive heart failure due to amyloidotic cardiomyopathy is a rare, age-related manifestation.
- Patients in non-endemic areas are more prone to develop severe cardiac amyloidosis.

*Diagnostic examinations*
📖 see AL amyloid.

### Specific treatments
*Orthotopic liver transplantation*
- As the liver is mainly responsible for transthyretin production, orthotopic liver transplantation (OLT) decreases circulating mutant TTR in the serum and stabilizes symptoms.
- Long-term survival after OLT is 77% at 5 years.
- Factors influencing outcome include:
  - continued production of variant transthyretin in the choroid plexus, which occurs with some TTR mutations
  - mutation
  - duration of neurological symptoms
  - nutritional status
  - oculoleptomeningeal amyloidosis.
- Prophylactic pre-operative pacemaker implantation is often performed in patients with evidence of cardiac autonomic involvement.

*Combined heart–liver transplantation*
- Patients with amyloidotic cardiomyopathy have an increased perioperative morbidity and mortality.
- Cardiovascular complications account for about two-fifths of deaths after OLT (almost half of which of which occur within the first 3 months).
- Progression of cardiomyopathy even after successful OLT has been observed even in patients whose cardiac involvement was only mild up to the time of transplantation.
- It is currently thought that wild-type TTR deposition can increase dramatically in the presence of a pre-existing template of amyloid in the heart.
- No more than 30 reports of combined heart–liver transplant available in the literature.

### Other forms of hereditary amyloidosis
*Apolipoprotein A-I amyloidosis (AApoAI)*
- Apolipoprotein A-I is the main constituent of high-density lipoprotein particles.
- About half of apolipoprotein AI is synthesized in the liver and the other half in the small intestine.
- ApoAI gene is located on chromosome 11.
- Twelve different ApoAI gene mutations (mostly single nucleotide substitutions) associated with deposition of apolipoprotein A-I amyloid.
- All forms of apolipoprotein A-I amyloidosis are inherited as autosomal dominant traits.
- Clinical onset varies from the third decade of life to advanced age.

- The kidney is the most frequently affected organ, and death is usually caused by renal failure.
- Other sites of involvement include liver, spleen, and occasionally the heart.
- In rare cases, cardiac involvement can lead to massive hypertrophy.

*Apolipoprotein A-II amyloidosis (AApoAII)*
- Apolipoprotein AII, is predominantly synthesized by the liver and the intestines.
- Point mutations in the apoAII gene cause autosomal dominant amyloidosis.
- Clinically, characterized by early adult onset of progressive renal failure.

*Lysozyme amyloidosis (ALys)*
- Lysozyme is a ubiquitous bacteriolytic enzyme present in external secretions and in leukocytes, macrophages, gastrointestinal cells and hepatocytes.
- Four different lysozyme gene mutations (Trp64Arg Ile56Thr, Asp67His, Phe57Ile) cause an autosomal dominant non-neuropathic form of hereditary amyloidosis.
- Gastrointestinal involvement has been seen in nearly all reported cases of lysozyme amyloidosis, varying from mild abdominal discomfort to severe malabsorption syndrome.
- Megaloblastic anemia due to acid folic deficiency secondary to amyloid deposition in the small intestine described.
- Renal manifestations are frequent.
- Other clinical manifestations include sicca syndrome, bone marrow infiltration and heart involvement.

*Gelsolin (AGel)*
- Gelsolin amyloidosis relatively common in Finland.
- Caused by a mutation (Asp187Asn) in plasma gelsolin, an actin-modulating protein.
- Main clinical manifestations are corneal lattice dystrophy, cranial neuropathy, and cutis laxa.
- Peripheral and autonomic neuropathy, and cardiac or renal involvement can also occur.

*Fibrinogen Aα amyloidosis (AFib)*
Fibrinogen amyloidosis (AFib) is an autosomal dominant disease with low penetrance, caused by point mutations in the fibrinogen A alpha chain gene (about six amyloidogenic mutations in the fibrinogen Aα-chain have been identified, the most common being Glu526Val. Kidneys are the main site of amyloid deposition. Cardiac involvement has yet to be reported.

*Cystatin C amyloidosis (ACys)*
This disease, documented in a seven-generation pedigree in north-west Iceland (hereditary cerebral haemorrhage with amyloidosis, Icelandic type, HCHWA-I) is a rare, fatal, autosomal dominant condition, directly linked

to a Leu68Gln mutation in the cystatin C protein sequence, a cysteine protease inhibitor. Mutant cystatin C forms amyloid in brain arteries and arterioles, and to a lesser degree in tissues outside the central nervous system such as the skin, lymph nodes, testis, spleen, submandibular salivary glands, and adrenal cortex.

# Noonan syndrome

Noonan syndrome (NS) is a phenotypically heterogeneous clinical disorder characterized by certain recognizable physical abnormalities, most commonly facial dysmorphia, short stature and cardiac abnormalities.

## Incidence
- 1:1,000–1:2,500 live births.
- One of the most common syndromes.

## Aetiology
- May occur sporadically (50%) or in a pattern consistent with autosomal dominant inheritance.
- Predominance of maternal transmission.
- Mutations in five known genes have been demonstrated and together account for 60–80% of cases: *PTPN11, KRAS, SOS1, NF1* and *RAF1*.
- Genes are all-important in the pathway of growth hormone action.

### PTPN11
- Located on chromosome 12.
- Encodes the protein tyrosine phosphatase.
- Mutations result in a gain of function and are reported in 59% familial NS and 37% sporadic.

### KRAS
- Encodes for K-Ras protein.
- Mutations lead to gain in function.
- Mutations found in <5% NS cases.

### SOS1
- Located on chromosome 2.
- Encodes a protein component of the RAS–ERK cascade.
- Mutations found in 20% NS cases.
- Possible to diagnose NS clinically in the absence of positive genetic findings.

## Clinical features

### Facial features
- Shows considerable change with age and is most striking in the neonatal period but often very subtle in adulthood.
- Broad, high forehead.
- Hypertelorism.
- Low-set, posteriorly rotated ears.
- Short neck with excess nuchal skin.
- Ptosis.

### Other physical features
- **Growth:** feeding difficulties, failure to thrive (60%), puberty delayed by average 2 years, average adult height below 3rd centile.
- **Chest deformities:** pectus carinatum superiorly, pectus excavatum inferiorly (70–95%), increasing inter-nipple distance, thoracic scoliosis (15%).
- Joint hyperextensibility 50%.

- Cubitus valgus 50%.
- Talipes equinovarum 12%.
- Undescended testes at birth 77% ± reduced fertility in adult males.
- Urinary tract malformation 10%.
- Bleeding diatheses 55% due to factor deficiencies, thrombocytopenia, platelet function defects.
- Lymphatic vessel dysplasia 20%.
- Ophthalmic: 60% due to strabismus, refractive errors or amblyopia.
- Hearing loss 15–40% usually due to otitis media.
- Hepatosplenomegaly unrelated to cardiac failure 26–51%.
- Mental retardation 15–35% (usually mild).

### Cardiac abnormalities

- Pulmonary valve stenosis with dysplastic features 50–62%.
- Hypertrophic cardiomyopathy 20%.
- Atrial septal defects 6–10%.
- Ventricular septal defects 5%.
- Persistent ductus arteriosus 3%.
- Rarer—AV canal defects/coarctation of aorta.

### Hypertrophic cardiomyopathy in Noonan's syndrome

- More common in PTPN11 mutation negative subjects.
- Reported to have a strong association with RAF-1 mutations.
- Arrhythmia and sudden cardiac death less common than in non-syndromic HCM.
- Mortality high in children with progressive heart failure (25% mortality).
- Outflow tract obstruction described.

## Diagnosis

- Clinical + scoring system based on phenotypic characteristics.

## Differential diagnoses

- Turner syndrome.
- Cardio-facio-cutaneous syndrome.
- Costello syndrome.
- Neurofibromatosis type 1.
- LEOPARD syndrome (multiple lentigines, conduction abnormalities, ocular hypertelorism, pulmonary stenosis, abnormal genitalia, retardation of growth and deafness).

## Management

- Majority of children grow up and function normally.
- Periodic cardiac evaluation with ECG, echocardiogram, ambulatory ECG monitoring.
- Growth hormone is effective in improving adult height in children with NS and is safe for subjects with cardiovascular involvement.

# Dilated cardiomyopathy (DCM)

DCM is characterized by impaired function and dilatation of the left or both ventricles in the absence of coronary artery disease and/or abnormal loading conditions to cause the observed myocardial abnormality.

DCM is defined as familial (fDCM) when one or more blood relatives of the proband are affected by DCM or sudden cardiac death at a young Age (<35years). Other causes of DCM are shown in Table 8.8.

Dilated cardiomyopathy is among the most common causes of heart failure in the young and a major reason for cardiac transplantation. The exact prevalence of DCM in the general population is unknown. The prevalence ranges from 14.0/100,000 population in Japan to 36.4/100,000 population in the USA.

The true incidence of inherited or familial DCM is not known. In the absence of a non-genetic cause of DCM, approximately 20–50% of the apparently 'idiopathic' cases have evidence of familial disease.

## Assessment of cardiac morphology and function

For the diagnosis of DCM the following 2 criteria need to be met:
- Left ventricular systolic impairment.
- Ejection fraction of the left ventricle <0.45 and/or fractional shortening <25%.
- Left ventricular dilatation:
  - left ventricular end-diastolic diameter >117% of the age and body surface area corrected value
  - the Henry equation, $(45 \cdot 3(\text{body surface area})^{1/3} - 0 \cdot 03(\text{age}) - 7 \cdot 2)$ is used to calculate the predicted left ventricular end-diastolic diameter, corrected for age and body surface area
  - the degree of left ventricular enlargement required for the diagnosis reflects the cautious approach of the current guidelines (117% corresponds to +2 SD of the predicted normal limit +5%).

## Assessment of loading conditions

Systemic hypertension, significant valvular and pericardial disease, coronary artery disease should be excluded.

## Further reading

Richardson P., et al. (1996) Report of the 1995 World Health Organization/International Society and Federation of Cardiology Task Force on the Definition and Classification of cardiomyopathies. *Circulation* **93**: 841–942.

Taylor M.R., Carniel E. and Mestroni L. (2006) Cardiomyopathy, familial dilated. *Orphanet. J Rare. Dis.* **1**: 27.

**Table 8.8** Non-familial causes of DCM

| | |
|---|---|
| Chemotherapy | Anthracyclines, Trastuzumab, tyrosine kinase inhibitors |
| Radiotherapy | Mantle radiotherapy |
| Nutritional | Selenium and thiamine deficiency |
| Toxins | Ethanol, cocaine |
| Iron overload | Thalassaemia, haemochromatosis |
| Inflammatory | Sarcoid, autoimmune disorders, vasculitis, giant cell myocarditis |
| Infections | Viral, bacterial infections, Chaga's disease |
| Endocrine disorders | Hypo/hyperthyroidism, Cushing's/Addison's syndrome, phaeochromocytoma |
| Post partum | DCM that develops during the last month of pregnancy or within 5 months of delivery in previously healthy women |
| Tachycardia induced DCM | Incessant atrial or ventricular tachycardia cause DCM which reverses once the tachycardia is controlled. |
| Idiopathic | No cause found after appropriate investigations |

Modified from Elliott P. et al. (2008) *Eur Heart J* **29**: 2, 270–276.

# Histological findings in DCM

- Cardiac mass is increased indicating hypertrophy, but because of the dilatation ventricular wall thickness is normal.
- Mural thrombi are frequently present in the left ventricle and atria.
- Mild focal scarring of the mitral and tricuspid leaflets and secondary dilatation of their annuli are common.
- The epicardial and intramural coronary arteries are normal.
- Microscopic features include:
  - hypertrophy and degeneration of myocytes
  - interstitial fibrosis.

### Further reading

Ferrans VJ. (1989) Pathologic anatomy of the dilated cardiomyopathies. *Am J Cardiol.* **64**: 9C–11C.

# Screening for familial DCM

In the absence of another recognized pathology, DCM is likely to be secondary to an inherited genetic defect and screening of first-degree relatives is thus encouraged. The hereditary nature of the DCM should be discussed with the proband to allow assessment of other family members who may be at risk. Asymptomatic individuals undergoing screening should be counselled appropriately.

### Criteria for familial disease

The diagnosis of familial DCM requires:
- two or more affected individuals in a single family, *or*
- a first-degree relative with unexplained sudden death at <35 years of age.

### Clinical screening for familial DCM

- Screening consists of history taking, clinical examination, electrocardiography and two-dimensional echocardiography.
- Electrocardiographic changes may precede the development of DCM.
- Echocardiographic or electrocardiographic abnormalities with no obvious alternative diagnosis have a high probability of being the expression of the same gene mutation seen in the proband.
- Affected first degree relatives can be diagnosed using the following criteria (Table 8.9):
  - major criterion i.e. conventional diagnostic criteria for DCM
  - left ventricular dilatation (>117% predicted) and one minor criterion
  - three minor criteria.
- Disease expression is time-dependent requiring long-term follow-up.

### Genetic screening

- If the disease causing mutation has been identified in the proband, then relatives can be genetically screened.
- Carriers require long-term clinical assessment for disease expression.
- Relatives who do not carry the gene mutation can be reassured.
- The genetic heterogeneity of fDCM and the high incidence of private mutations have hindered the development of reliable genetic testing.

### Further reading

Mestroni L., et al. (1999) Guidelines for the study of familial dilated cardiomyopathies. *Eur Heart J* **20**: 93–102.

**Table 8.9** Screening criteria for DCM in first-degree relatives

**Major criterion**

Impaired left ventricular function and dilatation satisfying the diagnostic criteria for DCM (hence no other features are required to make the diagnosis)

**Minor criteria**

Unexplained supraventricular or ventricular arrhythmias, or frequent ventricular ectopy (>1000/24h) before the age of 50

Left ventricular dilatation >112% of the predicted value

Ejection fraction <50% or fractional shortening <28%

II or III atrioventricular conduction block, left bundle branch block, sinus node dysfunction

Unexplained sudden death or stroke before 50 years of age

Unexplained regional wall motion abnormalities

Modified from Mestroni L. et al. (1999) *Eur Heart J* **20**: 93–102.

# Genetics of familial DCM

A diverse group of gene mutations has been implicated in DCM. The exact mechanism by which most of these mutations cause DCM is not known and the genotype-phenotype relationships are poorly understood.

Familial DCM exhibits incomplete penetrance, and thus not all carriers of the affected gene develop disease. In addition, a particular gene mutation shows variable expression both within and between families. Accurate pedigree analysis can provide the mode of inheritance and narrow down candidate genes. *De novo* mutations are probably responsible for some apparently non-inherited DCM.

## Autosomal dominant fDCM

Up to 90% of fDCM cases are inherited in an autosomal dominant mode and the following genes have been implicated.

### Sarcomeric protein genes
- Cardiac actin: uncommon, no well-defined phenotype.
- a-Tropomyosin: uncommon, may be associated with SCD.
- β-Myosin heavy chain: common, and associated with early-onset disease and SCD.
- Troponin T and C: associated with early-onset disease and SCD.
- Myosin-binding protein-C: uncommon, no well-defined phenotype.
- Titin (connectin): conduction system disease and arrhythmias have been reported.
- Telethonin: associated with early-onset disease and SCD.

### Cytoskeletal protein genes
- Desmin: associated with SCD, and some mutations may cause a skeletal myopathy.
- Metavinculin: variable phenotype.
- δ-Sarcoglycan: no well-defined phenotype.
- Cardiac muscle LIM protein: variable phenotype.
- α-Actinin: no well-defined phenotype.
- Cypher/ZASP: left ventricular non-compaction.

### Nuclear membrane genes
- Lamin A/C gene (LMNA).
  - One of the commonest causes of fDCM.
  - Associated with arrhythmias, conduction system disease and SCD.

### Ion channel protein genes or genes regulating Ca2+metabolism
- ABCC9: associated with severe disease and SCD.
- SCN5A: DCM associated with arrhythmias. Mutations of this gene also cause the Brugada and long QT syndrome.
- Phospholamban: associated with early-onset disease.

## Autosomal recessive fDCM
- Not a common pattern of inheritance.
- Cardiac troponin I mutations have been associated with severe, early onset disease.

## X-linked fDCM

- Approximately 5% of fDCM cases exhibit X-linked inheritance.
- Dystrophin mutations:
  - the same gene implicated in Duchenne and Becker muscular dystrophy can cause DCM with no clinical skeletal muscle involvement
  - increased serum creatine kinase often seen in patients and carriers
  - males have a variable course, but typically heart failure develops in the second and third decade of life and progresses rapidly
  - female carriers may also develop DCM later on in life but disease is usually milder.
- Tafazzin mutations:
  - Associated with left ventricular non-compaction
  - Barth syndrome: X-linked recessive disease causing DCM, skeletal myopathy, growth retardation, and neuropenia associated with high mortality during infancy from heart failure and sepsis.

## Matrilineal (mitochondrial) inheritance

- Hypertrophic cardiomyopathy is typically associated with the mitochondrial cytopathies, but DCM has also been reported in:
  - MELAS (mitochondrial encephalomyopathy, lactic acidosis and stroke-like episodes)
  - Kearns–Sayre syndrome
  - MERFF (myoclonus epilepsy with ragged red fibres).

## Further reading

Burkett E.L. and Hershberger R.E. (2005) Clinical and genetic issues in familial dilated cardiomyopathy. *J Am Coll Cardiol* **45**: 969–981.

# Echocardiography in DCM

Cardiac ultrasound (echocardiography) is used routinely to confirm, quantify and characterize ventricular function in dilated cardiomyopathy.

## 2D Echocardiography

LV dimensions should be recorded and ejection fraction (EF) calculated using the biplane Simpson's method (Figure 8.10). Less accurate measures of EF can be obtained using fractional shortening (which represents basal function only) or by giving a visual estimation. It should be recognized that left ventricular ejection fraction does not truly represent contractility and is influenced by preload, afterload, valve function and heart rate. Nonetheless EF is widely used to risk stratify and monitor response to therapy. Typical changes found in dilated cardiomyopathy include:

- LV end diastolic diameter >55–60mm
- EF <45–50%
- global hypokinesis of LV walls
- change in LV geometry (from elliptical to spherical shape)
- alteration in spatial arrangement of mitral valve apparatus.

## Doppler echocardiography

Diastolic function is assessed using mitral inflow patterns and pulmonary vein Doppler. Three abnormal patterns exist and correlate with worsening prognosis:

- impaired relaxation (↓E velocity, ↑A velocity, ↓E/A)
- pseudo normal pattern (E/A ratio and E deceleration time is normal but TDI and pulmonary vein Doppler is abnormal)
- restrictive filling (↑E velocity, ↓E deceleration time, ↑E/A).

Indices derived from Doppler echocardiography can also be used to assess LV systolic function and are less influenced by loading conditions:

**dP/dT:** is measured from the mitral regurgitant Doppler signal (Fig. 8.10) and correlates with dyssynchony and survival in heart failure.

**Myocardial performance (Tei) Index:** is the ratio between the (isovolumic contraction time + isovolumic relaxation time)/ejection time. It reflects global myocardial performance and is useful in DCM where systolic and diastolic function often co-exist.

## Tissue Doppler imaging

TDI permits the quantitative and reproducible assessment of myocardial velocity and deformation. Mitral annular velocities reflect longitudinal systolic function and can be combined with mitral inflow velocity to provide a non-invasive assessment of LV filling pressure (E/E'). LV dyssynchrony can also be assessed using TDI.

## Transoesophageal echocardiography

TOE may be useful to assess complex valve pathology in DCM, look for LV thrombus or exclude endocarditis.

## Stress echocardiography

Dobutamine or dypridamole stress echocardiography has been used in DCM to assess contractile reserve, which correlates with prognosis.

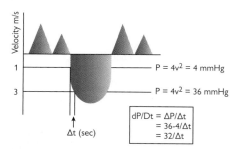

**Fig. 8.10** Measurement of dP/dt from the CW Doppler signal. The time interval between 1m/s and 3m/s is measured in seconds and converted to a pressure using the simplified Bernoulli equation. Reproduced from Kolias TJ *et al.* (2000) Doppler-derived dp/dt and dp/dt predict survival in congestive heart failure. *J Am Coll Cardiol*, 36:1594–1599, with permission from Elsevier.

# Cardiovascular magnetic resonance in DCM

The morphology and functional abnormalities of DCM can be clearly demonstrated and quantified by CMR.

### Diagnosis

- CMR can characterize the myocardium with the LGE technique to highlight focal interstitial expansion.
- With the use of gadolinium based contrast agents areas of focal fibrosis or interstitial expansion from other causes (e.g. amyloid).
- CMR aids in the diagnosis of DCM by exclusion and is ideally suited to identify multiple aetiologies including ischaemia, hypertrophic cardiomyopathy, sarcoid, iron overload and myocarditis.
- The majority of cases of DCM show no LGE but when it does occur it often has a characteristic mid-wall pattern.
- CMR can identify thrombus formation in both the left and right ventricle with high sensitivity and specificity.
- Signs of heart failure may also be seen with dilated IVC, hepatomegaly, ascites and pleural effusions.

### Risk

- Mid-wall fibrosis has important prognostic implications being associated with an increased risk of sudden cardiac death and ventricular tachycardia (VT), independent of other more traditional markers of increased risk.
- CMR has high spatial and temporal resolution and can identify myocardial infarction (MI) missed by other techniques such as single photon emission computerised tomography (SPECT). Importantly, patients with normal coronary angiography and LGE (unrecognized ischaemic heart disease (IHD) labelled as DCM) have the same adverse prognosis as patients with ischemic cardiomyopathy.

### Thalassemia

- Additional benefits of CMR in DCM are to exclude cardiac iron overload, mainly from transfusion-related, iatrogenic iron overload in thalassaemia major.
- This can be rapidly progressive and death may occur within months.
- CMR can identify patients at higher risk using a T2* measurement to quantify cardiac iron. This allows chelation therapy to be increased in a timely manner.
- T2* measurements below 20ms indicate a high cardiac iron burden and incipient cardiac failure.

# DCM and laminopathies

## Isolated DCM secondary to lamin AC gene mutations

Caused by mutations in lamin AC (□ see Chapter 16, Cardiac manifestations in inherited skeletal muscle disease).
- Conduction system disease:
  - early-onset first-degree heart block and other mild conduction abnormalities with progression to complete heart block
  - approximately one-third of patients beyond the third decade of life require antibradycardia pacing.
- Arrhythmias:
  - early-onset atrial fibrillation
  - supraventricular arrhythmias become common with increasing age
  - ventricular arrhythmias can cause SCD which is the commonest mode of death affecting almost half of all carriers at a mean age of 46 years
  - preliminary data suggest that carriers with conduction system disease benefit from an ICD for the primary prevention of SCD.
- Cardiomyopathy:
  - heart failure develops after the conduction system disease develops
  - may have an independent course from conduction system disease
  - heart failure occurs in 64% of patients over the age of 60 years.

## fDCM with skeletal muscle disease secondary to LMNA mutations

Less often LMNA mutations cause fDCM associated with skeletal muscle involvement:
- autosomal dominant Emery–Dreifuss muscular dystrophy
- limb-girdle muscular dystrophy type 1B

The risk of SCD is probably the same as in isolated fDCM

## fDCM associated with other laminopathies

DCM has been reported in:
- partial lipodystrophy
- axonal neuropathy
- lipoatrophy with diabetes, disseminated leukomelanodermic papules and liver steatosis.

### Further reading

Sylvius N. and Tesson F. (2006) Lamin A/C and cardiac diseases. *Curr. Opin. Cardiol* **21**: 159–165.

# DCM and deafness

The combination of familial sensorineural hearing loss (SNHL) and DCM raises the possibility of the following diagnoses:

## Epicardin disease
- Autosomal-dominant with age-related penetrance.
- Caused by mutations in the *EYA4* gene in chromosome 6.
- SNHL overt by the second decade of life.
- Asymptomatic DCM develops by the third decade of life.
- Severe heart failure leading to death in fifth and sixth decade.

## Mitochondrial diseases
- Progressive SNHL occurs frequently in mitochondrial diseases.
  - MERRF syndrome (myoclonic epilepsy and ragged red fibres).
  - MELAS syndrome (mitochondrial encephalopathy with lactic acidosis and stroke-like episodes).
  - Kearns–Sayre syndrome.
- HCM is more common than DCM.

## Alström syndrome
- Rare autosomal recessive disease.
- Caused by mutations in the *ALMS1* gene on chromosome 2.
- SNHL.
- Childhood obesity.
- Blindness due to congenital retinal dystrophy.
- Hyperinsulinemia and early-onset type 2 diabetes.
- DCM affects ~60% and occurs at any age.
- DCM is the most common cause of death in the infantile period.

## Further reading
Schonberger J., Levy H., Grunig E., Sangwatanaroj S., *et al.* (2000) Dilated cardiomyopathy and sensorineural hearing loss: a heritable syndrome that maps to 6q23–24. *Circulation* **101**: 1812–1818.

# DCM/ARVC overlap

Desmosomal gene mutations, classically associated with ARVC have recently been described in patients with predominantly left ventricular disease. Desmosomal gene mutations cause a spectrum of pathology that extends from the classic ARVC phenotype, to biventricular involvement and a primarily left ventricular cardiomyopathy with minimal right ventricular involvement. The following features may suggest desmosomal disease in cases with DCM phenotypes:

- Mode of presentation
  - Palpitation and syncope are commoner than heart failure symptoms.
- ECG
  - T waves inversion in the inferolateral leads.
- Arrhythmia
  - Ventricular arrhythmia of left ventricular origin (right bundle branch block morphology) or arrhythmias out of proportion to the severity of the left ventricular dysfunction/dilatation.
- CMR
  - Left ventricular late gadolinium enhancment in a epicardial/midmyocardial distribution, with variable right ventricular involvement.

## Further reading

Sen-Chowdhry S., Syrris P., Ward D., Asimaki A., *et al.* (2007) Clinical and genetic characterization of families with arrhythmogenic right ventricular dysplasia/cardiomyopathy provides novel insights into patterns of disease expression. *Circulation* **115**: 1710–1720.

# Peripartum cardiomyopathy

Peripartum cardiomyopathy (PPCM) complicates 1 in 3000 deliveries and is an important cause of maternal mortality. Diagnosis rests on finding a decline in cardiac function during the last month of pregnancy or up to five months afterwards. There must be echocardiographic evidence of LV systolic impairment in the absence of pre-existing cardiac disease or another cause of heart failure.

## Clinical features

Fatigue, oedema and exertional dyspnoea occur commonly in the last trimester of pregnancy and may mask symptoms of congestive heart failure due to PPCM. Signs of increased cardiac filling pressures (raised JVP, pleural effusions, hepatomegaly, peripheral oedema) and low cardiac output (hypotension, cool peripheries, and reduced organ perfusion) are usually evident. Heart failure due to pre-existing cardiac disease typically presents earlier, i.e. second trimester. A high index of suspicion is needed to differentiate PPCM from pulmonary emboli, pre-eclapmsia or anaemia. Echocardiography should be performed to confirm the diagnosis and to look specifically for LV thrombus.

Risk factors for PPCM include:
- maternal age >30 years old
- multiparity and/or multigravida
- geography: sub-Saharan Africa (1 in 100 Nigeria), Haiti (1 in 400)
- obesity
- pregnancy induced hypertension
- tocolytics (drugs used to suppress premature labour).

## Pathophysiology

The precise mechanisms that underlie PPCM are not known. Serum markers of inflammation, apoptosis and oxidative stress are elevated in PPCM and are used to support autoimmune, viral, and hormonal theories. The familial occurrence of PPCM and wide variation in geographical incidence support a genetic predisposition although no specific mutations have been identified.

## Management

An antenatal diagnosis of PPCM should prompt escalation of obstetric care to a centre with anaesthetic and cardiac support. Treatment is similar to other forms of systolic heart failure with ACE inhibitors, beta-blockers and diuretics though during pregnancy hydralazine and nitrates are usually preferred (ACE inhibitors are teratogenic). Patients are at high risk of thromboembolism so anticoagulation with heparin must be considered. There is some support for immune modulation given the potential inflammatory nature of PPCM. Prolactin inhibition with bromocriptine has also been reported to improve LV function.

## Prognosis

Is variable ranging from complete recovery in 23% to progressive heart failure and mortality of 15%. Spontaneous recovery usually occurs in the first 6 months, however if LV function remains impaired future pregnancies are discouraged because of the high risk of recurrence. Advice on contraception must be given.

## Further reading

Hilfiker-Kleiner D. *et al.* (2007) A cathepsin d-cleaved 16 kDa form of prolactin mediates postpartum cardiomyopathy. *Cell* **128**: 3, 589–600.

Hilfiker-Kleiner D. *et al.* (2008) Peripartum cardiomyopathy: recent insights in its pathophysiology. *Trends in CV Medicine* **18**: 5, 173–179.

Silwa K. *et al.* (2006) Peripartum cardiomyopathy. *Lancet* **368**: 687–693.

# Pharmacological treatment of DCM

Treatment of familial dilated cardiomyopathy is based on inferences drawn from general heart failure (HF) drug trials where the underlying aetiology is usually classified as ischaemic or non-ischaemic. Standard HF management (Table 8.10) is initiated according to the severity of symptoms or signs. Further understanding of genotype phenotype correlation in DCM may identify more specific HF treatment targets in the future.

## Diuretics

Recommended in patients with symptoms and signs of congestion. Since diuretics activate the renin–angiotensin system they should be used in combination with ACEi/A2RB. A loop diuretic (frusemide, torasemide, bumetanide) is used first line and a thiazide diuretic (bendrofluazide, metolazone, indapamide) added if required. Doses must be adjusted on an individual patient basis to avoid dehydration, hypovolaemia, electrolyte losses and decline in renal function.

**ACE inhibitors (ACEi):** should be used in all patients with LVEF <=40%. There is robust evidence that they improve LV function, reduce hospital admission rates and prolong survival (CONSENSUS, SOLVD-Treatment trials). Contraindications include creatinine >220µmol/L, potassium >5mmol/L, bilateral renal artery stenosis, angioedema and aortic stenosis.

**Beta-blockers (BB):** should be used together with ACEi if LVEF<=40%. They improve both morbidity and mortality outcomes (COPERNICUS, CIBIS II, MERIT-HF trials). Patients should be clinically stable before initiating treatment to prevent worsening HF due to the negative inotropic effect. Asthma and high degree AV block are contraindications.

**Angiotensin 2 receptor blockers (A2RB):** are used in patients intolerant of ACEi (due to cough, hypotension or worsening renal function) or in patients with EF< = 40% who remain symptomatic despite treatment with ACEi and BB (Val HEFT and CHARM trials). A2RB should not be used in those receiving ACEi and aldosterone antagonist.

**Aldosterone antagonists:** should be added to HF treatment in all patients with EF< = 35% in NYHA Class III or IV. They reduce hospital admission and prolong survival (RALES study). Contraindications include creatinine >220µmol/L, potassium >5mmol/L or a combination of ACE and A2RB. Eplerenone is associated with less breast discomfort in men.

**Hydralazine and isosorbide dinitrate:** can be used as an alternative to ACEi/A2RB or in addition to an ACEi alone if A2RB or aldosterone antagonist is not tolerated. The greatest benefit is seen in those of African descent.

**Digoxin:** where EF< = 40% digoxin is useful for AF rate control either used alone or alongside a BB. For a patient in SR there is no evidence digoxin improves survival though hospital admission are less (DIG trial).

## Early disease

Clinical screening of families with DCM has identified an asymptomatic cohort with echocardiographic LV enlargement or mild systolic impairment. It is not known whether pharmacological intervention at this stage may prevent or attenuate progression of heart failure but clinical trials in this group are underway.

**Table 8.10** Common drugs used in heart failure

|  | Starting dose (mg) |  | Target dose (mg) |  |
|---|---|---|---|---|
| **ACEI** |  |  |  |  |
| Captopril | 6.25 | t.i.d. | 50–100 | t.i.d |
| Enalapril | 2.5 | b.i.d. | 10–20 | b.i.d. |
| Lisinopril | 2.5–5.0 | o.d. | 20–35 | o.d. |
| Ramipril | 25 | o.d. | 5 | b.i.d. |
| Trandolapril | 0.5 | o.d. | 4 | o.d. |
| **ARB** |  |  |  |  |
| Candesartan | 4 or 8 | o.d. | 32 | o.d. |
| Valsartan | 40 | b.i.d. | 160 | b.i.d. |
| **Aldosterone antagonist** |  |  |  |  |
| Eplerenone | 25 | o.d. | 50 | o.d. |
| Spironolactone | 25 | o.d. | 25–50 | o.d. |
| **β-Blocker** |  |  |  |  |
| Bisoprolol | 1.25 | o.d. | 10 | o.d. |
| Carvedilol | 3.125 | b.i.d. | 25–50 | b.i.d. |
| Metoprolol succinate | 125/25 | o.d. | 200 | o.d. |
| Nebivolol | 1.25 | o.d. | 10 | o.d. |

ESC guidelines (2008).

# Pacing in DCM

DCM and conduction disease may co-exist in some families. Conduction system disturbances (sinus bradycardia, atrioventricular conduction block, atrial fibrillation) may precede ventricular dysfunction and necessitate pacemaker implantation before the onset of DCM in later life. Electrophysiological studies ± ICDs should be considered in those with syncopal episodes, and/or a strong family history of sudden death.

Causes of familial DCM associated with conduction disease include:

- Lamin A/C (LMNA)
- Desmin (DES)
- Sodium channelopathies (SCN5A)
- myotonic dystrophy
- mitochondrial disease.

LNMA mutations appear to be highly penetrant, associated malignant arrhythmias and adult-onset heart failure. If early conduction disease is present there is a low threshold for recommending defibrillator therapy.

## Cardiac resynchronization therapy (CRT)

Conventional indications for pacing apply to patients with DCM where single or dual chamber pacemakers are used to treat atrial fibrillation, AV block or chronotropic incompetence. In patients with DCM and HF symptoms, CRT should be considered as well. CRT with pacemaker (CRT-P) or defibrillator (CRT-D) function is recommended to reduce morbidity and mortality in patients in NYHA Class III or IV. Selection of patients for CRT is challenging in particular identify the cohort of non-responders.

Current NICE guidelines recommend CRT be considered if:

- NYHA Class III to IV
- LVEF <= 35%
- QRS >120ms
- on optimal medical therapy.

Due to the effectiveness of ICD therapy in reducing sudden cardiac death in DCM, CRT-D is commonly preferred in clinical practice provided life expectancy exceeds 1 year.

Following device implantation, CRT optimization is usually performed using echocardiography to select the best AV delay and the interval between left and right ventricular activation for efficient diastolic filling and to maximize cardiac output. No long-term data is available to suggest echo optimization improves outcome.

# Implantable cardioverter defibrillators in DCM

A number of clinical trials have demonstrated the superiority of ICDs over anti-arrhythmic drugs in prevention of death from ventricular arrhythmias.

## Indications

In non-ischaemic DCM an ICD is recommended for primary and secondary prevention of sudden cardiac death[1]:

| Primary prevention | Secondary prevention |
| --- | --- |
| NYHA Class II or III and LVEF < = 35% (on medical treatment) with expected survival >1 year | Prior cardiac arrest or haemodynamically unstable VT/VF and LVEF < = 40% (on medical treatment) with expected survival >1 year |

## Contraindications

- Reversible cause of ventricular fibrillation/VT (e.g. drugs, metabolic disorder).
- Patient choice.
- Non-compliance with follow-up.
- Co-morbidity and expected survival <1 year.

## Procedure and complications

ICDs were originally implanted via a thoracotomy and defibrillator patches applied to the epicardium. Most devices nowadays are implanted transvenously similar to pacemakers. Both dual and single chamber systems are available and contain intravascular spring or coil electrodes, which are used to defibrillate. Patients should be counselled about device complications including infection, lead displacement and inappropriate shocks, which occur in around 10% patients.

## Mechanism of action

ICDs usually use heart rate criteria to discriminate rate, rhythm and morphology of ventricular arrhythmias. The following features can help distinguish VT and VF from benign sinus and atrial arrhythmias:
- rate detection (usually HR >200/min)
- rate stability (VT is associated with little inter-beat rate variation)
- detection cycle (the number of consecutive beats)
- sudden onset (sinus tachycardia is usually of gradual onset).

ICDs may be programmed to overdrive pace haemodynamically stable VT (ATP = anti-tachy pacing) prior to delivering shock therapy. Numbers of attempts at ATP and detection zones are usually set on an individual patient basis and exercise testing may help identify appropriate parameters. Patients with HF are less likely to tolerate tachyarrhythmia due to their lower stroke volume and blood pressure.

1. Task force for Diagnosis and Treatment of Acute and Chronic Heart Failure 2008 of European Society of cardiology. ESC Guidelines for the diagnosis and treatment of acute and chronic heart failure. *European Heart Journal.* **29**, 2388–2442.

# Cardiac transplant indications

Cardiac transplantation is recommended for advanced, irreversible heart failure with a limited life expectancy. Organ shortage currently dictates availability of the procedure but there are currently 3,500 cardiac transplants performed per year worldwide.

## Indications

- Symptomatic HF despite optimal medical and device therapy.
- Free from significant co-morbidities.
- Able to tolerate immunosuppression.
- Refractory life-threatening arrhythmias.

The patient must be well-informed, motivated, emotionally stable and capable of complying with immunosuppressant treatment and follow-up.

## Contraindications

- Irreversible pulmonary hypertension or parenchymal lung disease.
- Irreversible hepatic failure.
- Irreversible cerebrovascular disease.
- Life expectancy limited by systemic disease.
- Ongoing alcohol or substance misuse.

## Relative contraindications

Renal impairment (eGFR <40ml/min), malignancy, diabetes with end-organ damage, age (>70 years), obesity (BMI>30), smoking, active peptic ulcer disease, hepatitis B, C or HIV.

## Transplant procedure

Donor compatibility is primarily determined by ABO blood group. Human leukocyte antigen (HLA) matching is not usually performed to minimize ischaemic time though graft survival has been shown to significantly improve with HLA compatibility. Height and weight are also important for size matching the donor and recipient. In the majority of cases an orthotopic transplant is performed although heterotopic (where the recipients heart is not removed) procedures are preferred if the donor heart is small or mildly impaired or if the recipient has pulmonary hypertension.

## Prognosis

Allograft rejection accounts for the majority of transplant-related deaths (15% mortality) in the first 12 months. Long-term outcome is determined primarily by the consequences of immunosupression (infection, malignancy, renal failure and coronary artery disease) and 5-year survival rate is around 70% regardless of underlying HF aetiology.

# Arrhythmogenic right ventricular cardiomyopathy

Arrhythmogenic right ventricular cardiomyopathy (ARVC) is an inherited heart muscle disease characterized by:
- myocyte loss with fatty or fibro-fatty replacement predominately of the right ventricle (30% also have left ventricular involvement)
- ventricular arrhythmias
- congestive heart failure and sudden cardiac death.

ARVC has been reported as a common cause of sudden death in the young, including athletes.

The estimated prevalence is 1:2500/1:5000.

Five genes encoding important desmosomal proteins have been associated with the disease:
- plakoglobin (*JUP*)
- desmoplakin (*DSP*)
- plakophilin-2 (*PKP2*)
- desmoglein-2 (*DSG2*)
- desmocollin-2 (*DSC2*).

## Diagnostic criteria

The Task Force of the Working Group Myocardial and Pericardial Disease of the European Society of Cardiology proposed in 1994 the criteria for the clinical diagnosis of ARVC. These criteria have recently been modified (Table 8.11). The criteria are based on the identification of:
- right ventricular functional and structural abnormalities
- fibro-fatty replacement of the right ventricular myocardium
- electrocardiographic repolarization abnormalities
- electrocardiographic depolarization abnormalities
- arrhythmias of right ventricular origin
- familial disease
- genetic mutations.

Diagnostic criteria are classified as **major or minor**, according to their specificity for the disease. The diagnostic terminology for the revised criteria is:
- **Definite diagnosis:** *two major*, or *one major and two minor* or *four minor* criteria from different categories
- **Borderline diagnosis:** *one major and one minor* or *three minor* criteria from different categories
- **Possible diagnosis:** *one major* or *two minor criteria* from different categories.

**Table 8.11** 2010 Task force criteria for the diagnosis of ARVC

**I Global and/or regional dysfunction and structural alterations**

*Major*

**By 2D echo**: regional RV akinesia, dyskinesia, or aneurysm *and* 1 of the following (end diastole):
- PLAX RVOT $\geq$ 32 mm (corrected for body size [PLAX/BSA] $\geq$19mm/m$^2$)
- PSAX RVOT $\geq$ 36 mm (corrected for body size [PSAX/BSA] $\geq$21mm/m$^2$)
- *or* fractional area change $\leq$33%

**By MRI**: regional RV akinesia or dyskinesia or dyssynchronous RV contraction *and* 1 of the following:
- Ratio of RV end-diastolic volume to BSA $\geq$110mL/m$^2$ (male) or $\geq$100mL/m$^2$ (female)
- *or* RV ejection fraction $\leq$40%

**By RV angiography**: regional RV akinesia, dyskinesia, or aneurysm

*Minor*

**By 2D echo**: regional RV akinesia or dyskinesia *and* 1 of the following (end diastole):
- PLAX RVOT $\geq$29 to <32mm (corrected for body size [PLAX/BSA] $\geq$16 to <19mm/m$^2$)
- PSAX RVOT $\geq$32 to <36mm (corrected for body size [PSAX/BSA] $\geq$18 to <21mm/m$^2$)
- *or* fractional area change >33% to $\leq$40%

**By MRI**: regional RV akinesia or dyskinesia or dyssynchronous RV contraction *and* 1 of the following:
- Ratio of RV end-diastolic volume to BSA $\geq$100 to <110mL/m$^2$ (male) or $\geq$90 to <100mL/m$^2$ (female)
- *or* RV ejection fraction >40% to $\leq$45%

**II Tissue characterization of walls**

*Major*

Residual myocytes <60% by morphometric analysis (or <50% if estimated), with fibrous replacement of the RV free wall myocardium in $\geq$1 sample, with or without fatty replacement of tissue on endomyocardial biopsy

*Minor*

Residual myocytes 60–75% by morphometric analysis (or 50–65% if estimated), with fibrous replacement of the RV free wall myocardium in $\geq$1 sample, with or without fatty replacement of tissue on endomyocardial biopsy

**III Repolarization abnormalities**

*Major*

Inverted T waves in right precordial leads ($V_1$, $V_2$, and $V_3$) or beyond in individuals >14 years of age (in the absence of complete right bundle-branch block QRS $\geq$120ms)

*Minor*

Inverted T waves in leads $V_1$ and $V_2$ in individuals >14 years of age (in the absence of complete right bundle-branch block) or in $V_4$, $V_5$, or $V_6$

Inverted T waves in leads $V_1$, $V_2$, $V_3$, and $V_4$ in individuals >14 years of age in the presence of complete right bundle-branch block

*(Continued)*

**Table 8.11** (Contd.)

**IV Depolarization/conduction abnormalities**

*Major*

Epsilon wave (reproducible low-amplitude signals between end of QRS complex to onset of the T wave) in the right precordial leads (V₁ to V₃)

*Minor*

Late potentials by SAECG in ≥1 of 3 parameters in the absence of a QRS duration of ≥110ms on the standard ECG: filtered QRS duration (fQRS) ≥114ms; duration of terminal QRS <40μV (low-amplitude signal duration) ≥38ms; root-mean-square voltage of terminal 40ms ≤20μV

Terminal activation duration of QRS ≥55ms measured from the nadir of the S wave to the end of the QRS, including R', in V₁, V₂, or V₃, in the absence of complete right bundle-branch block

**V Arrhythmias**

*Major*

Non-sustained or sustained ventricular tachycardia of left bundle-branch morphology with superior axis (negative or indeterminate QRS in leads II, III, and aVF and positive in lead aVL)

*Minor*

Non-sustained or sustained ventricular tachycardia of RV outflow configuration, left bundle-branch block morphology with inferior axis (positive QRS in leads II, III, and aVF and negative in lead aVL) or of unknown axis

>500 ventricular extrasystoles per 24 hours (Holter)

**VI Family history**

*Major*

ARVC/D confirmed in a first-degree relative who meets current Task Force criteria

ARVC/D confirmed pathologically at autopsy or surgery in a first-degree relative

Identification of a pathogenic mutation categorized as associated or probably associated with ARVC/D in the patient under evaluation

*Minor*

History of ARVC/D in a first-degree relative in whom it is not possible or practical to determine whether the family member meets current Task Force criteria

Premature sudden death (<35 years of age) due to suspected ARVC/D in a first-degree relative

ARVC/D confirmed pathologically or by current Task Force Criteria in second-degree relative

PLAX, parasternal long-axis view; RV, right ventricular; RVOT, right ventricular outflow tract; BSA, body surface area; PSAX, parasternal short-axis view; aVF, augmented voltage unipolar left foot lead; aVL, augmented voltage unipolar left arm lead.

Modified from Marcus F.I., McKenna W.J. *et al. Eur Heart J* 2010; **31**: 806–814, published with permission of the Editor.

## Electrocardiography

The electrocardiogram (ECG) plays a key role in the diagnosis of ARVC (see Fig. 8.11). Typical ECG abnormalities in ARVC include:

- **T-wave inversion (TWI) in right precordial leads (V1–V3)** in individuals beyond the age of 12 years and in absence of right-bundle bunch block has been described in up to 80% of patients with ARVC. This pattern is highly specific, being present in less than 3% of healthy adult subjects. Extension of TWI to left precordial leads (V4–V6) is often a sign of left ventricular involvement and presence of TWI only in these leads has been described in forms of the disease with prevalent left ventricular involvement. TWI may also be present in inferior leads, but its role for the diagnosis of ARVC is not clear.

- **Localized prolongation of QRS complex in V1–V3 >110msec** is believed to be related to delayed repolarization of the right ventricle due to myocardial areas of fibro-fatty replacement. It has been described in up to 70% of the ARVC patients.

- **A prolongation ≥55msec of the terminal part of the QRS**, from the nadir of the S wave to the isoelectric line, in V1–V3 has been observed in a highly symptomatic population with ARVC and may be a marker in the late stage of the disease.

- **Epsilon waves** are defined as a low-amplitude deflection occurring between the end of the QRS and the beginning of the T wave and are described in up to one-third of patients with ARVC. They probably derive from slow conduction in localized areas of the right ventricle.

### Other ECG features of ARVC

- **QRS dispersion**, defined as a difference ≥40msec between the QRS duration in right precordial leads and V6; it has been reported as a strong predictor of sudden cardiac death.

- **QRS duration ratio**, defined as the ratio between QRS duration in right and left precordial leads (V1+V2+V3)/(V4+V5+V6) >1.2.

- **Poor R-wave progression** in the right precordial leads, often associated with TWI in the same leads.

- **Low voltages of the QRS complex** in the limb leads and, sometimes, also in the precordial leads, often a sign of diffuse and extensive disease.

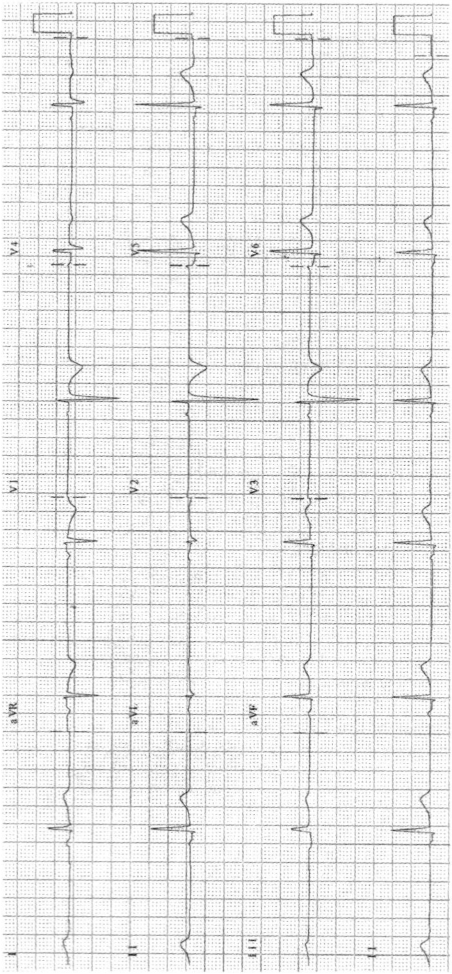

**Fig. 8.11** 12-lead electrocardiogram from a patient with ARVC, showing the typical T-wave inversion in right precordial leads. Poor R-wave progression is also present.

## Echocardiography

Right ventricle (RV) is very difficult to image, due to its complex shape, orientation, geometry, position close to the anterior chest wall, composite mechanical activation, and thin walls. This leads to high inter-observer and intra-observer variability.

Comprehensive echocardiographic assessment of ARVC patients includes:

- RV global size and function
- RV regional wall motion abnormalities
- RV focal dilatation and aneurysms
- LV size, function and regional wall motion abnormalities

Fig. 8.12 shows the standardized planes for the full evaluation of the RV.

- **RV dilatation** in ARVC may be global or focal. The latter usually involves the 'triangle of dysplasia': the inferior wall, RVOT or the apex. In the presence of global dilatation, differential diagnosis should include shunts (i.e. atrial septal defects), tricuspid regurgitation, pulmonary hypertension. Competitive athletes may exhibit a degree of RV dilatation and may represent a challenge for the diagnosis of ARVC and complete clinical evaluation is mandatory.
- **Regional wall motion abnormalities** are classified as hypokinesia, akinesia and dyskinesia. When analysing wall motion, care should be taken for particular areas like moderator band insertion point, which often results in false positive abnormalities. Regional diastolic bulging, caused by structural weakness secondary to fibro-fatty infiltration, may be present.

Other features described in patients with ARVC are **hyperreflective moderator band** and **excessive/abnormal RV trabeculations**, but their role (sensitivity and specificity) for the diagnosis of ARVC is controversial.

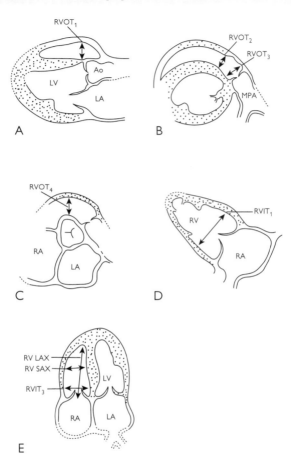

**Fig. 8.12** Standardized planes for RV evaluation. Modified from Foale R *et al*. Echocardiographic measurement of the normal adult right ventricle. *Br Heart J* 1986; **56**: 33–44, with permission from BMJ Publishing Group (See this article for reference values).

## Cardiac magnetic resonance in ARVC

Cardiac magnetic resonance (CMR) has emerged as an important tool for the diagnosis of ARVC (Fig. 8.13). The main advantages of this technique for imaging the RV are: three-dimensional visualization of the heart and its relation with thoracic structures, no need of geometrical assumptions for the quantification of the RV and LV volumes, excellent spatial and temporal resolution, ability to scan every possible plane, tissue characterization and detection of fatty infiltration and fibrosis. However, there are also limitations: the RV wall is very thin and partial volume effect may affect the image; differentiation between pericardial fat and fatty infiltration may be difficult; there is lack of knowledge about the normal spectrum of the RV morphology, which potentially could lead to over-diagnosis; arrhythmias, like ventricular ectopics or atrial fibrillation, motion and breathing artefacts, blood flow may influence the image quality; there are some absolute contraindication (metallic devices; cerebral shunts, clips, claustrophobia, etc.).

A comprehensive CMR evaluation of patients with possible ARVC should include:

- **Functional abnormalities**, assessed by bright blood sequences, like steady-state free procession gradient echo (SSFP GE) cine images in long axis, short axis and axial views:
  - global RV/LV function and dimensions
  - regional wall motion abnormalities: hypokinesia (wall thickening <40%), akinesia (wall thickening <10%); dyskinesia (paradoxal outward movement during systole); aneurysm (dyskinetic or akinetic area with diastolic bulging). Minor regional wall motion abnormalities are commonly seen in proximity of the moderator band insertion point and should be interpreted with caution to avoid over-diagnosis.
- **Morphological abnormalities**, assessed by dark blood sequences, like double-inversion recovery turbo spin echo (TSE):
  - intramyocardial fat, detected by T1-w TSE with fat suppression technique. However, fat infiltration on CMR is not part of the diagnostic criteria
  - focal RV wall thinning (RV wall thickness <2mm), which has particular significance if associated with regional function abnormalities
  - localized dilatation, usually in the RVOT
  - trabecular disarray (increased and prominent RV trabeculations), which is, however, difficult to quantify
  - intramyocardial fibrosis, assessed by late gadolinium enhancement (LGE) technique, which can be difficult to detect in the thin RV wall. Presence of LGE in the LV should also be assessed. As for fatty infiltration, fibrosis detected by LGE is not part of the current diagnostic criteria.

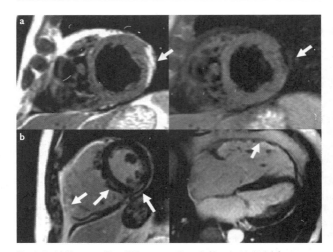

**Fig. 8.13** (a) Short axis T1-w TSE images without (left) and with (right) fat suppression from an ARVC patient with LV involvement. Arrows indicate fat infiltration in the left ventricle. (b) Late gadolinium enhancement images from a different patient with ARVC showing areas of fibrosis in the RV and LV (arrows) (left, short axis, right, 4 chambers).

## Electrophysiological study in ARVC

Electrophysiological study (EPS) has an important role in the management of selected patients with ARVC. EPS has been proposed as a diagnostic, prognostic and therapeutical tool.

### Diagnostic applications of EPS

Areas of low amplitude endocardial voltages, secondary to myocardial atrophy and fibro-fatty replacement, the hallmark of ARVC, can be detected by three-dimensional electro-anatomic voltage technique. A catheter with a magnetic sensor on its tip is introduced under fluoroscopic guidance in the RV and it is positioned in different places of the RV endocardium and it is localized through a very low magnetic field. After contact of the catheter tip to the endocardial surface has been assured, bipolar and unipolar voltages are recorded and displayed in a color scale. Electro-anatomical scar is defined as an area ≥1cm² comprehending at least three adjacent points with bipolar signal amplitude <0.5mV. Electro-anatomical mapping has been shown to improve the accuracy of the diagnosis of ARVC and to differentiate ARVC from myocarditis mimicking ARVC, as well as early stage of ARVC from benign RVOT tachycardia. In addition, electro-anatomical mapping can be used as guidance for improving sensitivity of endomyocardial biopsy. Non-contact mapping techniques can also be used (Fig. 8.14).

## Prognostic value of EPS

The prognostic role of EPS is still controversial. Several studies[1–3] showed that inducibility of VT/VF during EPS is not a statistically significant independent risk factor for arrhythmic events, although another study[4] demonstrated that a positive EPS was associated with increased arrhythmic risk. Different population characteristics, different protocols, multicentre vs unicentre studies, may explain this discrepancy. Overall, it appears that the prognostic role of EPS in ARVC is limited.

## Therapeutical role of EPS

Transcatheter radiofrequency ablation is an invasive therapeutic option for ARVC patients with ventricular tachycardia refractory to medical treatment. Electro-anatomical mapping or non-contact mapping may help the localization of the origin of the VT and may be used to target the VT ablation. VT morphology is commonly multiple. Rarely, in difficult cases, pericardial ablation has to be employed. Although, peri-procedural success rate is usually high, VT typically tends to be recurrent and several procedures are required. Severe patients with VT storms, refractory to medical treatment and multiple radiofrequency ablations, need consideration for heart transplantation. EPS can also be performed to test the efficacy of antiarrhythmic drugs in selected ARVC patients.

## Further reading

Corrado D., Leoni L., Link M.S., et al. (2003) Implantable cardioverter defibrillator therapy for prevention of sudden death in patients with arrhythmogenic right ventricular cardiomyopathy/dysplasia. *Circulation* **108**: 3084–3091.

Lemola K., et al. (2005) Predictors of adverse outcome in patients with arrhythmogenic right ventricular dysplasia/cardiomyopathy: long term experience of a tertiary care centre. *Heart* **91**: 1167–1172.

Roguin A., et al. (2004) Implantable cardioverter-defibrillators in patients with arrhythmogenic right ventricular dysplasia/cardiomyopathy. *J Am Coll Cardiol* **43**: 1843–1852.

Wichter T., et al. (2004) Implantable cardioverter/defibrillator therapy in arrhythmogenic right ventricular cardiomyopathy: single-center experience of long-term follow-up and complications in 60 patients. *Circulation* **109**: 1503–1508.

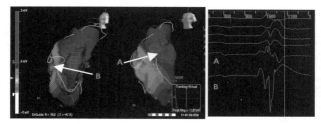

**Fig. 8.14** Non-contact mapping of the right ventricle in a patient with ARVC. This is a voltage map recording the activation of the ventricle from a ventricular ectopic arising in the RVOT. At site A in the anterior RV the electrograms are fractionated and low in amplitude compared to an adjacent site where they are narrower and larger in amplitude indicating the patchy distribution of the disease. See also colour plate section.

### Risk stratification in ARVC

Risk stratification in ARVC, especially for primary prevention of SCD, is a major challenge. Risk markers have been evaluated through small, retrospective studies, usually including cohorts of highly symptomatic patients. Some of these studies derive from ARVC populations with ICD, where the rate of appropriate ICD discharges was up to 22%/year. Prospective data about the natural history and risk stratification from large and unselected ARVC cohorts are lacking.

Annual mortality rate varies according to different centres and it is around 1–3%/year, and includes sudden cardiac death (1–2%/year) and heart failure death.

Bearing in mind the above considerations about the limitations of risk stratifications in ARVC, the following clinical and instrumental parameters are recognized as markers of increased arrhythmic risk:
- previous cardiac arrest (secondary prevention)
- hemodynamically unstable ventricular tachycardia (secondary prevention)
- unexplained syncope
- severe RV dilatation and dysfunction
- left ventricular involvement (defined as LV EF <40%), in the presence of non-sustained or sustained ventricular arrhythmias
- QRS dispersion ≥40msec.

A family history of sudden cardiac death is not recognized as a risk factor.

As for other arrhythmogenic cardiac diseases, the indication for ICD implantation, especially for primary prevention, has to be individualized and weighted against the possible complications (implantation or device related).

# Restrictive cardiomyopathy

Restrictive cardiomyopathy (RCM) is characterized by increased stiffness of the myocardium which causes ventricular pressure to rise steeply with small increases in volume in the presence of normal or reduced diastolic volumes of one or both ventricles, normal or reduced systolic volumes and normal ventricular wall thickness. Restrictive ventricular physiology also occurs in other cardiomyopathies including HCM and DCM. RCM is the least common of all the cardiomyopathies.

## Aetiology

- Restrictive cardiomyopathy is associated with several conditions (Table 8.12).
- In adults, RCM is most commonly caused by amyloidosis in the Western world and endomyocardial fibrosis in the tropics.
- Patients with RCM present with signs and symptoms of biventricular heart failure (shortness of breath, oedema, ascites etc). RCM is often progressive and debilitating and treatment is aimed at retarding progression rather than achieving a cure.

**Table 8.12** Classification and aetiology of restrictive cardiomyopathy

| Familial | Non-familial |
|---|---|
| Familial, unknown gene | Amyloid (AL/prealbumin) |
| Sarcomeric protein mutations: | Scleroderma |
| Troponin I (RCM +/– HCM) | Endomyocardial fibrosis |
| Essential light chain of myosin | Hypereosinophilic syndrome |
| Familial amyloidosis | Idiopathic |
| Transthyretin (RCM + neuropathy) | Chromosomal cause |
| Apolipoprotein (RCM + nephropathy) | Drugs: serotonin, methysergide, ergotamine, mercurial agents, busulfan |
| Desminopathy | |
| Pseuxanthoma elasticum | Carcinoid heart disease |
| Haemochromatosis | Metastatic cancers |
| Anderson–Fabry disease | Radiation |
| Glycogen storage disease | Drugs: anthracyclines |

## Pathology

The macroscopic features of restrictive cardiomyopathy include biatrial dilatation in the presence of normal heart weight, a small ventricular cavity and no left ventricular hypertrophy. However, the morphologic spectrum of primary restrictive cardiomyopathy includes mild ventricular hypertrophy with increased heart weight and mild ventricular dilatation without hypertrophy. Thrombus in the atrial appendages and patchy endocardial fibrosis are common.

The histological features of idiopathic restrictive cardiomyopathy are non-specific with patchy interstitial fibrosis. Myocyte disarray is common in patients with pure restrictive cardiomyopathy. In patients with infiltrative and metabolic cardiomyopathies, there are specific findings appropriate to the condition.

## Investigation

### Electrocardiography

The most frequent abnormalities include:
- p-mitrale and p-pulmonale
- non-specific ST segment and T-wave abnormalities
- ST segment depression
- T-wave inversion, usually in the inferolateral leads
- voltage criteria for left and right ventricular hypertrophy may also be present. Low voltage QRS complexes are seen in amyloid
- conduction abnormalities, including intraventricular conduction delay, and abnormal Q waves may also be seen.

### Chest X-ray

The chest radiograph may show cardiomegaly caused by atrial enlargement, and pulmonary venous congestion. Interstitial oedema may be seen in severe cases.

### Cardiac Catheterization

The characteristic haemodynamic feature on cardiac catheterization is a deep and rapid early decline in ventricular pressure at the onset of diastole, with a rapid rise to a plateau in early diastole ('dip-and-plateau or square root sign'). Left ventricular end-diastolic, left atrial and pulmonary capillary wedge pressures are markedly elevated, and usually 5mmHg or more greater than right atrial and right ventricular end-diastolic pressures. Volume loading and exercise accentuate the difference between left and right-sided pressures.

### Echocardiography
- The hallmarks of RCM can be readily assessed with echo.
- Atrial enlargement occurs as a consequence of chronic elevation of atrial pressure and may be exacerbated by mitral and tricuspid regurgitation.
- Systolic function is usually normal but may be impaired and wall thickness is usually normal but may become thickened in later disease or in specific etiologies.
- Doppler defined restrictive filling is based on transmitral Doppler flow measurement of E/A >2, deceleration time of E<150ms and IVRT<70ms.

### CMR
- Many of the same echocardiographic features are also seen by CMR along with signs of decompensation (such as systemic venous dilatation, hepatomegaly, effusions).
- Clues to aetiology may also be seen with pleural/pericardial effusions (amyloid), specific LGE patterns or hilar lymphadenopathy (sarcoid).

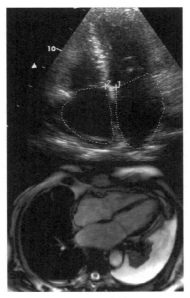

**Fig. 8.15** Two-dimensional echocardiogram (upper panel) and cardiac magnetic resonance scan showing typical biatrial enlargement. See also colour plate section.

# Left ventricular non-compaction

LVNC is a rare cardiomyopathy characterized by excessive trabecula-tions and deep recesses within the myocardium. The typical appearance of a thin compacted layer and thick non-compacted layer arises due to abnormal intrauterine cardiac development and persistence of the fetal myocardial meshwork. Isolated LVNC is classified as a distinct cardiomy-opathy in AHA/ESC guidelines but non-compacted myocardium may also co-exist as a morphological trait in other inherited cardiomyopathies.

## Diagnosis

There is no clear diagnostic standard. Several attempts to quantify the extent of the trabeculations have been made using echocardiography. The most widely used criteria are those described by Jenni et al. (Fig. 8.16), which require a 2:1 ratio of non-compacted to compacted myocardium and colour Doppler evidence of deep perfused intertrabecular recesses. Strictly applying imaging criteria to the general population leads to over-diagnosis of LVNC particularly in those with systolic heart failure of Afro-Caribbean origin. Careful evaluation of symptoms, family history and left ventricular function must accompany imaging investigations.

## Clinical features

Prevalence ranges from 0.014% to 0.25% and is reported to be higher in the paediatric population. The frequency of diagnosis has risen with improve-ments in imaging techniques. Presentation with heart failure, arrhythmias and systemic thromboembolism occurs in all ages and in general complica-tions parallel severity of LV dilatation and systolic dysfuntion.

### Associated conditions

LVNC occurring in isolation is considered a primary cardiomyopathy, however non-compacted myocardium may also be associated with:
- congenital left and right outflow tract abnormalities
- Ebsteins anomaly
- neuromuscular cardiomyopathies.

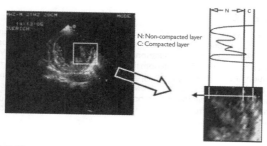

N: Non-compacted layer
C: Compacted layer

**Fig. 8.16** The 2:1 ratio of non-compacted to compacted myocardium is measured at end systole in the parasternal short-axis view. Reproduced from *Heart* Echocardiographic and pathoanatomical characteristics of isolated left ventricular non-compaction: a step towards classification as a distinct cardiomyopathy. Jenni R, Oechslin E, Schneider J, et al. **86**, 666–71 (2001) with permission from BMJ Publishing Group.

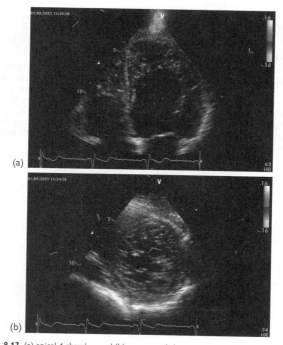

**Fig. 8.17** (a) apical 4 chamber and (b) parasternal short axis 2-dimensional echocardiogram of a patient with LVNC. A mutation in myosin heavy chain was identified.

# Genetics

In around 25% of cases of LVNC there is evidence of familial disease either manifest as a distinct cardiomyopathy or by the presence of hypertrabeculations. Numerous genetic mutations have been associated with LVNC and most are inherited in autosomal dominant pattern necessitating the evaluation and counselling of family members. Sarcomeric protein mutations are found in up to 50% of individuals with LVNC, which represents a departure from their classical association with hypertropic cardiomyopathy and illustrates the diversity between genotype and phenotype across all cardiomyopathies.

### Genetic mutations in proteins associated with LVNC

- α dystrobrevin (DTNA)
- Tafazzin (TAZ/G4.5)
- Cypher/ZASP (LBD3)
- FK506 binding protein (FKBP1A)
- Lamin A/C (LMNA)
- Sodium channel (SCN5A)
- Sarcomeric proteins (MYH7, MYBPC3, TNNI3, TNNT2, ACTC)

### Treatment

There is no specific clinical management for LVNC. Early studies suggested LVNC was associated with high mortality and morbidity due to arrhythmias and heart failure but the incidence of complications is lower than first reported as the condition is now identified at an earlier stage. Heart failure is treated with standard pharmacotherapy. Anticoagulation with warfarin is recommended in the presence of LV dilatation and systolic dysfunction (EF<40%). Arrhythmias should be managed using anti-arrhythmic agents or implantable defibrillators according to guidelines.

# Takotsubo cardiomyopathy

- Also known as stress-induced cardiomyopathy, left ventricular apical ballooning syndrome, ampulla cardiomyopathy or broken heart syndrome.
- First described in Japan in 1991 and named Takotsubo-like LV dysfunction due to the associated LV morphological features (Takotsubo is a Japanese pot with a round bottom and narrow neck used for trapping octopuses).

## Prevalence

- True prevalence remains uncertain.
- Probably accounts for 1–2% all cases of suspected acute MI.

## Diagnosis

- No consensus on diagnostic criteria but Mayo clinic researchers proposed criteria in 2004 for Takotsubo cardiomyopathy where patients must fulfill all of these:
  - transient hypokinesis, akinesis or dyskinesis in the LV mid segments with apical involvement
  - regional wall motion abnormalities extending beyond a single vascular distribution
  - often a stressful trigger
  - the absence of obstructive coronary disease or angiographic evidence of plaque rupture
  - new ECG abnormalities or modest elevation in cardiac troponin
  - absence of phaeochromocytoma and myocarditis.

## Patient demographics

- More often found in post-menopausal women (meta-analysis 88% ♀).
- Episode of emotional or physiological stress precedes onset in 65%.
- History of hypertension 43%/diabetes mellitus 11%/dyslipidaemia 25% and current or past smoking 23%.

## Clinical presentation

- Most common presenting symptoms are chest pain and dyspnoea.
- Presentations such as cardiogenic shock and VF are reported.
- Not reliably associated with any specific medical condition or cardiac history in either the patient or their family.

### Electrocardiogram

- Consistent with acute ischaemia.
- Most commonly (anterolateral) ST elevation and T-wave inversion.

### Cardiac biomarkers

- Troponin I or T elevated in 86% of patients and CKMB in 74%.
- Levels not in keeping with the degree of ventricular dysfunction.
- BNP levels elevated in the acute phase but do not correlate with the severity of LV dysfunction or recovery.
- Plasma catecholamines are elevated 2–3 times higher than in acute MI.

### Echocardiography
- Hallmark for the diagnosis of Takotsubo cardiomyopathy.
- Hyperkinetic LV base with mid-ventricular hypokinesis.
- Apical akinesis or dyskinesis resulting in marked apical ballooning and severely reduced ejection fraction.
- Reversible LVOTO reported in 25% (patients are older with a septal bulge associated with reversible SAM of the mitral valve and MR).
- LV thrombus seen in 38% patients—patients with elevated serum C-reactive protein levels at higher risk of developing thrombi.
- In general, all echocardiographic abnormalities resolve fully within days to weeks in all surviving patients.

### Cardiac catheterization
- 80% have normal coronary arteries, remainder have stenosis of <50%.
- Significant LV dysfunction and typical apical ballooning pattern is seen on left ventriculography—completely resolves in all surviving patients.

## Pathophysiology
- This is not yet completely understood.
- Proposed mechanisms include:
  - spontaneous or provokable multi-vessel epicardial
  - abnormalities in coronary microcirculation contribute significantly but it is unclear whether this is the primary cause or a secondary phenomenon
  - direct toxic effect of catecholamines on cardiac myocyte viability (reflecting that apical myocardium may be more responsive to sympathetic stimulation and more vulnerable to sudden catecholamines surges)

## Management
- No double-blind randomized trials to identify best practice.
- Differentiating Takotsubo cardiomyopathy from acute MI is imperative, therefore urgent coronary angiography in suspected cases in order to avoid unnecessary thrombolytic therapy and bleeding risk.
- Treatment should be individualized according to the patient characteristics.
- Cardiogenic shock/decompensated heart failure may require the use of positive inotropes, vasopressors or intra-aortic balloon counter-pulsation.
- Medical therapies include typical heart failure drugs such as nitrates, diuretics, beta-blockers, ACE inhibitors, angiotensin receptor site blockers and aspirin.
- Antiarrhythmic therapy should be instituted where indicated, but patients with may have a prolonged QT interval.
- In patients with LVOTO, beta blockade is highly effective and inotropic agents should be avoided.

Prognosis
- Generally favourable without any form of treatment, provided the patient survives the severe heart failure period.
- Reported mortality rates 0–8%.
- Most commonly reported complication is of left-sided heart failure.
- Other reported complications include:
  - cardiogenic shock—mitral valve dysfunction
  - ventricular arrhythmias—pulmonary embolism
  - LV mural thrombus—LV free wall rupture.
- Recurrence of Takotsubo cardiomyopathy has been reported in up to 10%.

# Chapter 9

# Inherited arrhythmias and conduction disorders

# Familial atrial fibrillation

Atrial fibrillation (AF) is a common condition with the majority of patients having some form of underlying heart disease. Depending on the population studied, 15–30% will have lone AF. A positive familial history of AF has been established in both lone and secondary AF.[1–3]

Multiple families where lone AF segregates as a monogenic trait have been used to map genetic loci.[4]

- Brugada reported the first chromosomal locus to be identified in a family where AF segregated as an autosomal dominant trait.[5] The disease causing gene has not been identified, but several genes encoding for potassium channel subunits (*KCNQ1*, *KCNE2*, *KCNJ2*, and *KCNA5*) at other chromosomal loci have been associated with familial AF.[6]
- Mutations have predominantly resulted in a gain of function effect resulting in a shortening of action potential duration.
- The majority of genes implicated have been reported in Chinese families although studies of Caucasian families have failed to detect these mutations.[6]
- Ethnic variation and low prevalence of identified mutations suggests that other genes, perhaps in different ion channels, will be implicated in familial AF.
- A genetic predisposition to developing or maintaining AF in the context of heart disease is also likely. There is widespread exposure to risk factors for AF and yet not everyone will go on to develop it.
- A number of single nucleotide polymorphisms (SNPs) are associated with AF in patients with underlying structural heart disease or cardiovascular risk factors for AF. SNPs in KCNE1, angiotensinogen and connexin-40 genes have all been identified in patient cohorts.[6]

The genes implicated in both familial AF and AF with underlying heart disease are all biologically plausible given that the initiation and maintenance of atrial fibrillation will depend upon atrial ectopic foci and the propagation of micro-re-entrant circuits around areas of conduction block within the atria. Genes responsible for structural remodelling of the atria including apoptosis and fibrosis are also important candidates facilitating the maintenance of AF.

1. Fox C.X., *et al.* (2004) Parental AF as a risk factor for AF in offspring. *JAMA* **291**: 2851–2855.
2. Darbar D., *et al.* (2003) Familial AF is a genetically heterogeneous disorder. *JACC* **41**: 2185–2192.
3. Ellinor P.T., *et al.* (2005) Familial aggregation in lone AF. *Hum Genet* **118**: 179–184.
4. Darbar D. (2008) Genetics of AF. *Heart Rhythm* **5**: 483–5486.
5. Brugada R., *et al.* (1997) Identification of a genetic locus for familial AF. *N Engl J Med* **336**: 905–911.
6. Tsai C.T., *et al.* (2008) Molecular genetics of AF. *JACC* **52**: 241–250.

# Brugada syndrome

Brugada syndrome is characterized by coved ST elevation in the right precordial leads associated with an increased incidence of sudden death due to ventricular fibrillation in patients with structurally normal hearts.

## Epidemiology

- 5:10 000—but underdiagnosed as ECG pattern often concealed or variable.
- 20% of sudden death in structurally normal hearts.
- Increased prevalence in South East Asia.
- 8:1 ♂ predominance.

## Genetics

- Autosomal dominant inheritance.
- 20% linked to SCN5A mutations—encoding the α subunit of the cardiac Na+ channel.
- SCN5A promoter polymorphisms which reduce Na+ current found to be more common in Asians.
- Mutation in the gene coding for the glycerol-3-phosphate dehydrogenase 1-like protein (GPD1L) has recently been found in a large family.
- Mutations in the α1 and β subunits of the L-type Ca2+ channel (CACNA1C and CACNB2b) have also been associated with the disease (1%).
- KCNE3 ion channel mutation (<1%) affecting the Ito current
- *SCN1B*, which encodes the function-modifying sodium channel beta-1 subunit (<1%).

## Clinical presentation

Patients may present with palpitations, dizziness, syncope or cardiac arrest but are frequently asymptomatic. Arrhythmias typically occur at rest or during sleep.

### Precipitating factors

- Autonomic nervous system imbalance.
- Hypokalaemia.
- Hypothermia.
- Bradycardia.
- Febrile illness.
- Ischaemia.
- Drugs (see box).

### ECG

- Diagnosis relies on 'coved' ST elevation of at least 2mm in 2 right precordial leads with a negative T wave (Type 1 pattern). This may be spontaneous or induced by a sodium channel blocker.
- Type 2 ECGs have a 'saddleback' appearance with high take-off ST elevation of at least 2mm gradually descending and a positive or biphasic T wave.
- Type 3 ECGs have either a 'saddleback' or 'coved' appearance with ST elevation <1mm.

Type 2 and type 3 ECGs are not diagnostic of Brugada syndrome unless conversion to a type 1 pattern after sodium channel blocker administration occurs.

Late potentials on signal averaged electrocardiogram (SAECG) are common and are independent predictors of VF/VT.

Holter monitoring may also detect ST elevation during sleep.

### Pharmacological challenge

Drugs used are ajmaline 1mg/kg over 5 min or flecainide 2mg/kg over 10 min (max. 150mg).

Should be terminated if:
- Type 1 ECG develops
- ST segment in a type 2 ECG increases by >2mm
- arrhythmias develop
- QRS widens to >130% of baseline

In patients at risk of a high degree AV block (ie: 2nd or 3rd degree block) the test should be carried out in an EP lab with a temporary pacing wire inserted.

The sensitivity, specificity, and positive and negative predictive values of the drug challenge were 80%, 94.4%, 93.3%, and 82.9%, respectively in a group of 147 individuals from 4 families with SCN5A mutations.[1]

### Diagnostic criteria

Diagnosis is confirmed by the presence of a type 1 ECG with one of the following:
- documented VF or polymorphic VT
- family history of sudden cardiac death <45 years old
- coved ECGs in family members
- inducibility of VT with programmed electrical stimulation
- syncope or nocturnal agonal respiration.

### Differential diagnosis
- Myocarditis.
- Pericarditis.
- Right-bundle branch block.
- Acute myocardial infarction.
- Pulmonary embolism.
- Dissecting aortic aneurysm.
- Hypo/hyperkalaemia.
- Arrhythmogenic right ventricular cardiomyopathy.
- Hypothermia.

## Pathophysiology

### Role of SCN5A

All the SCN5A mutations that have been studied have been shown to result in a reduction of $I_{Na}$ due to a variety of mechanisms:
- failure of Na+ channel expression
- shift in the voltage dependence of $I_{Na}$ activation or inactivation
- entry into an intermediate state of activation from which it recovers more slowly
- accelerated inactivation of the Na+ channel
- failure of Na channel trafficking to the sarcolemma.

*Electrophysiological mechanisms*

The precise electrophysiological mechanism of Brugada syndrome is uncertain, but two main hypotheses have been proposed:

*Transmural dispersion of repolarization (TDR)[2]*

The transient outward potassium current ($I_{to}$), which drives early repolarization is expressed more strongly in the epicardium compared to the endocardium—so it is more susceptible to the effects of reduced $I_{Na}$. This leads to accentuation of the notch in the action potential and produces a 'spike and dome' shape which is seen as the saddleback ST elevation on ECG. As $I_{Na}$ is further reduced, the epicardial action potential dome is lost. This loss is heterogeneous giving rise to epicardial dispersion of repolarization and creating a vulnerable window for phase 2 re-entry which provides the premature beat to trigger VT/VF between the transmural layers.

*Conduction delay in the RVOT[3]*

This leads to current flowing from the RV to the RVOT when the membrane potential is more positive in the RV. Current then flows back again through the extracellular space. This gives rise to the ST elevation in the right precordial leads. Premature beats that may trigger arrhythmias are thought to originate in the border zone between early and delayed depolarizations.

**Risk stratification and treatment**

- Only established effective treatment is an ICD (see Fig. 9.1 for the 2005 2nd Consensus Document risk stratification recommendations).
- Cardiac arrest survivors have a class I indication for ICD implantation (69% recurrence at 54 months follow up)[4].
- Risk of VF (varies with series):
  - spontaneous Type 1 ECG and syncope: 1.9–8.8%/pa
  - spontaneous Type 1 ECG and no syncope: 0–6.4%/pa
  - asymptomatic Induced Type 1 ECG: 0–0.73%/pa.
- For primary prevention, those at highest risk are men with a spontaneous type 1 ECG (7.7-fold risk compared to pharmacologically provoked type 1 ECG) and a history of syncope[5].
- Asymptomatic patients with a spontaneous type 1 pattern are at intermediate risk—EPS may help although this is becoming increasingly controversial.
- Positive family history or presence of a SCN5A mutation does not predict outcome.
- Patients should avoid drugs that induce the Brugada pattern of ST elevation (see box).

*Role of EPS in risk stratification*

This is controversial—a study by Brugada et al. suggests that inducibility of VT/VF can predict risk—however the majority of investigators have failed to find an association.[4–6] This is most likely due to a lack of standardization in stimulation protocols and patient characteristics. The FINGER Registry is largest series to data reporting 1029 consecutive individuals (745 men; 72%)

with a median age of 45 (35 to 55) years.[6] During a median follow-up of 31.9 (14 to 54.4) months:
- the cardiac event rate per year was 7.7% in patients with aborted SCD
- 1.9% in patients with syncope
- 0.5% in asymptomatic patients overall (0.4%/p.a with drug induced BS ECG and 0,8%/per annum with type 1 resting BS ECG changes)
- symptoms and spontaneous type 1 ECG were predictors of arrhythmic events, whereas gender, familial history of SCD, inducibility of ventricular tachyarrhythmias during EP study, and the presence of an SCN5A mutation were not predictive of arrhythmic events.

### Pharmacological therapy
- Quinidine, a non-specific blocker of $I_{to}$, restores the action potential dome and prevented arrhythmia inducibility by EPS in 76% of patients tested in a small trial[7].
- Isoprenaline and cilostazol, which increase Ca2+ current, have been used to control 'electrical storms' in Brugada patients.

### Drugs that induce Brugada ECG pattern
- Class Ia and Ic anti-arrhythmics
- β blockers
- Tricyclic antidepressants
- Bupivacaine
- Propofol
- Nicorandil
- Lithium
- Cocaine

### Children
- Disease is rare in children and there is little data on prognosis.
- In a recent study of 30 children those with spontaneous type 1 ECG pattern are at greatest risk with no male predominance[8].
- Febrile episodes can trigger arrhythmia.
- ICD implantation carries significant morbidity and quinidine may have a role.

1. Hong K., et al. (2004) Value of electrocardiographic parameters aand ajmaline test in the diagnosis of Brugada syndrome caused by SCN5A mutations. *Circulation* **110**: 3023–3027.
2. Yan G.X. and Antzelevitch C. (1999) Cellular basis for the Brugada syndrome and other mechanisms of arrhythmogenesis associated with ST segment elevation. *Circulation* **100**: 1660–1666.
3. Tukie R., et al. (2004) Delay in right ventricular activation contributes to Brugada syndrome. *Circulation* **109**: 1272–1277.
4. Brugada J., Brugada R. and Brugada P. (2003) Determinants of sudden cardiac death in individuals with the electrocardiographic pattern of Brugada syndrome and no previous cardiac arrest. *Circulation* **108**: 3092–3096.
5. Paul M., et al. (2007) Role of programmed ventricular stimulation in patients with Brugada syndrome: a meta-analysis of worldwide published data. *European Heart Journal* **28**: 2126–2133.

6. Probst V., *et al.* (2010) FINGER Registry. *Circulation* **121**: 635–643.
7. Belhassen B., *et al.* (2004) Efficacy of quinidine in high risk patients with Brugada syndrome. *Circulation* **110**: 1731–1737.
8. Probst V., *et al.* (2007) Clinical aspects and prognosis of Brugada syndrome in children. *Circulation* **115**: 2042–2048.

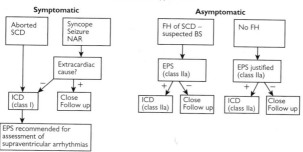

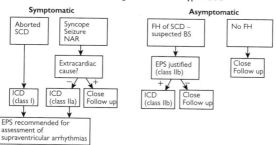

**Fig. 9.1** Indications for ICD implantation in Brugada patients. Class 1, clear evidence treatment is useful or effective; Class II, conflicting evidence on usefulness or efficacy; Class IIa weight of evidence in favour of usefulness or efficacy; Class IIb usefulness or efficacy is less well established. BS, Brugada syndrome; NAR, nocturnal agonal respiration; SCD, sudden cardiac death. Adapted from Antzelevich et al. Brugada Syndrome Report of the Second Consensus Conference, *Circulation* 2005; **111**: 659–670.

# Long QT syndrome

Long QT syndrome (LQTS) is a rare cause of syncope and sudden cardiac death. It is a disease of myocardial ion channels causing delayed repolarization which can lead to torsade de pointes and ventricular fibrillation. Jervell and Lange-Nielsen (1957) described an autosomal recessive familial condition with prolonged QTc, congenital deafness and a high incidence of sudden cardiac death at a young age. Romano (1963) and Ward (1964) then described a similar autosomal dominant condition but without deafness. Both were felt to be similar entities and therefore the unifying diagnosis of LQTS was given.

LQTS can be congenital or acquired. There are several subtypes of congenital LQTS defined by the gene affected. Upper limit of normal (97.5th percentile) for QTc interval in males is 440msec and 460msec in females.

## Epidemiology

- Prevalence is 1 in 5000–6000.
- LQT1 is the commonest form.
- Presentation is in childhood, adolescence or early adulthood.
- Females tend to have a higher diagnostic rate than males which may be due to the relatively longer $QT_C$ interval in females.

## Age

Age at presentation can be gene specific:
- LQT1: youngest to experience cardiac events; 54% of them become symptomatic before age 10; by the age of 20, 86% have had a cardiac event
- LQT2 and LQT3 present later. 50% of LQT2 and LQT3 patients were still asymptomatic at age 16.

## Aetiology

### Congenital

At least twelve genes have been implicated in LQTS. These genes encode cardiac ion channels. 📖 See Genetics.

### Acquired

This is a more common cause of LQTS and is potentially reversible. Acquired causes include electrolyte disturbances or may be drug induced:

*Electrolyte imbalances*
- Hypokalaemia.
- Hypocalcaemia.
- Hypomagnesaemia.

*Drug induced*
- Anti-arrhythmic medications: amiodarone, sotalol, procainamide, quinidine.
- Antibiotics: macrolide antibiotics e.g. erythromycin, quinolones.
- Tricyclic antidepressants.
- Antihistamines: terfenadine, astemizole.
- Antipsychotic medications: haloperidol, quetiapine.

- Gastrointestinal motility drugs: cisapride, domperidone.
- Methadone.
- Major tranquillizers.

*Other*
- Hypothyroidism.
- Anorexia nervosa.
- HIV infection.
- Myocardial infarction.

See ✆ http://www.azcert.org/medical-pros/drug-lists/drug-lists.cfm for fully comprehensive list.

## Pathophysiology

A description of the normal cardiac action potential will help clarify the effect of mutations on ion channels resulting in a prolonged $QT_C$ interval. The ventricular action potential composed of 4 phases (Figs 9.2 and 9.3).

### Phase 0: depolarization
Fast inward sodium channels ($I_{Na}$) open

### Phase 1: fast repolarization
Sodium channels begin to close

### Phase 2: plateau
Slowly activating delayed inward rectifier potassium ($I_{KS}$) channels open giving a net outward current which is matched by the inward flow of calcium ions via the L- type calcium channels, hence a plateau phase.

### Phase 3: repolarization
Rapidly activating delayed inward rectifier potassium ($I_{KR}$) channels open and there is a net outward positive current.

### Phase 4: resting membrane potential
Associated with diastole.

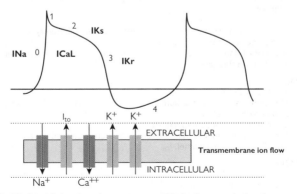

**Fig. 9.2** Principle ion channel currents responsible for the monophasic action potential. See also colour plate section.

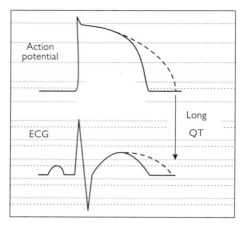

**Fig. 9.3** Relationship of the monophasic action potential to surface ECG.

## Genetics[1]

May affect channel synthesis, function or trafficking to the sarcolemmal membrane. Generally, mutations cause a:

- 'loss of function' of potassium channels *or*
- 'gain of function' of sodium and calcium channels.

### LQT1

- Most common type of LQTS, accounting for 30–35% of cases.
- Due to a mutation in the *KCNQ1* gene.
- Affects the slowly activating delayed inward rectifier potassium channel, $I_{KS}$.
- Gene locates to chromosome 11p15.5.
- Inherited as the autosomal recessive Jervell Lange–Nielsen syndrome associated with congenital deafness.
- Autosomal dominant Romano Ward syndrome is also associated with mutations in this gene.

### LQT2

- 25–30% of cases.
- Due to mutation(s) in the human ether-a-go-go related (*HERG*) gene, also known as *KCNH2*.
- Locates to chromosome 7q35–36.
- Loss of function mutation in the rapidly activating delayed inward rectifier potassium channel, $I_{KR}$.

### LQT3

- Mutation(s) in the SCN5A gene which encodes the sodium channel
- Locates to chromosome 3p21–24.
- Inherited in an autosomal dominant fashion.
- Gain of function mutation in the sodium channel gene.

### LQT4

- Also known as ankyrin B syndrome.
- Autosomal dominant inheritance.
- Mutation in the *ANK 2* or *ANK B* gene.
- Located on chromosome 4 and encodes for ankyrin.
- Ankyrins are adapter proteins which associate with ion channel proteins, for example, the sodium–calcium exchanger.
- A mutation in this leads to the abnormal activity and localization of ion channels, resulting in an increase in intracellular calcium.
- This is an example of where a mutation in a gene encoding for a non-ion channel protein can result in LQTS.

### LQT5

- Autosomal dominant condition.
- Due to mutations in the *KCNE1* gene.
- This is located to chromosome 21q22.1–22.2.
- Encodes for the β subunit of the slowly activating delayed inward rectifier potassium channel.

### LQT6

- The *KCNE2* gene is responsible for LQT6.
- Inherited in an autosomal dominant fashion.
- *KNCE2* has been mapped to chromosome 21q22.
- Encodes the β subunit of the rapidly activating delayed inward rectifier potassium channel.

### LQT7

- This is the Andersen–Tawil syndrome and is considered separately.

### *LQT8 or Timothy's syndrome*

- LQT8 is due to a mutation in the *CACNA12* gene, located to 12p13.
- Gain of function mutation in the voltage dependent L-type calcium channel.
- Timothy's syndrome is characterized by:
  - long QT
  - syndactyly
  - immune deficiency
  - autism.

### LQT9

- Mutations in the caveolin gene.
- Located to 3p25.
- Encodes a scaffolding protein which is involved in the compartmentalization and regulation of the sodium channel.
- Mode of inheritance has not been clarified.
- LQT4 and LQT9 are both due to mutations in proteins associated with ion channels.

### LQT10

- Missense mutation in the *SCN4β* gene, located to 11q24 described in a Mexican family.
- Autosomal dominance inheritance.
- Gain in function in the sodium channel.

Pathophysiology

QT interval represents the time from the onset of depolarization to the end of repolarization (upstroke of the cardiac action potential corresponds to QRS and phase 4 to the downstroke of the T wave) (Fig. 9.2). Prolongation due to:
- 'loss of function' mutations in potassium channels
- 'gain of function' mutations in sodium and calcium channels
- LQTS→ early afterdepolarizations→ torsade de pointes.

### Early after depolarizations (EADs)
- Occur during phase two of the action potential.
- Due to reactivation of L-type calcium channels caused by delayed repolarization.

Therefore, torsade de pointes is initiated by EAD triggered beats and is maintained by re-entrant mechanisms.
- ↑adrenergic drive e.g.: with exercise or stress→ $I_{KS}$ channel mutation prevents rapid repolarization at rapid heart rates→ ↑cardiac events in LQT1 and LQT2.
- ↑vagal drive e.g.: during sleep→ cardiac events in LQT3.

### After depolarization (Fig. 9.3)
- Depolarizing after potential which occurs in tissue which is NOT excitable
- Cause of VT or atrial arrhythmias in LQTS.
- Can be early or delayed.

### Early after depolarization (EAD)
- Occurs during phase 2 or 3 of the action potential.
- Reactivation of L- type calcium channels due to adrenergic stimuli.

### Delayed afterdepolarization (DAD)
- Occurs during phase 4 of the action potential.
- Net depolarizing current occurs due to spontaneous calcium release following repolarization via the Na/Ca exchanger.
- Important for initiation of VT in CPVT.

EADs

DAD

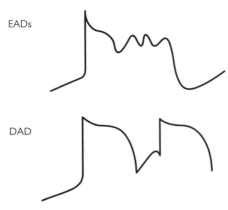

**Fig. 9.4** Early (EAD) and delayed after depolarizations (DAD).

Presentation
- Asymptomatic—incidental finding on the ECG.
- Syncope.
- Epilepsy.
- Sudden death.

Syncope and sudden death is due to torsade de pointes and ventricular fibrillation.

Patients with LQTS can develop symptoms in characteristic situations:
- LQT1 exercise and swimming
- LQT2 sudden, acoustic stimuli or stress
- LQT3 rest or sleep.

A family history of the following should raise suspicion of the diagnosis in a person presenting with palpitations, dizziness or syncope and an abnormal ECG:
- LQTS in relatives
- sudden death
- recurrent syncope
- epilepsy
- deafness.

Diagnosis
- Can be challenging; clinical criteria identify 38% of gene positive cases.
- Misdiagnosis of epilepsy common.
- Proportion of gene-positive patients have a normal $QT_C$ interval.
- The Schwartz score has been used to give a probability of LQTS based upon ECG and clinical characteristics.[2] Score ≥4 high probability of LQTS; 2–3 intermediate probability; and ≤1 low probability.

**Table 9.1** LQTS diagnostic criteria (Schwartz score)

| ECG findings (in absence of medications known to affect QTc) | Points |
|---|---|
| QTc calculated by Bazett's formula | |
| ≥480msec | 3 |
| 460–470msec | 2 |
| 450msec (in males) | 1 |
| Torsade de pointes | 2 |
| T wave alternans | 1 |
| Notched T wave in three leads | 1 |
| Bradycardia (resting rate <2nd percentile for age) | 0.5 |
| **Clinical history** | |
| Syncope with stress (or) without stress | 2 (or) 1 |
| Congenital deafness | 0.5 |
| **Family history** | |
| Family members with definite LQTS (score ≥4) | 1 |
| Unexplained sudden cardiac death <age 30yrs in immediate family | 0.5 |

Adapted from Schwartz et al *Circulation* 2001; **103**: 89–95.

### ECG
#### Calculation of the QTc interval
Accurate diagnosis important due to lifestyle and treatment implications. Longer $QT_C$ interval→ the greater the risk of torsade de pointes and sudden cardiac death.
- Begins at Q wave and ends at the end of the T wave.
- Best calculated in lead II or V5, although the lead with longest measurable QT should be used.
- The corrected QT interval is calculated; this corrects the QT interval for heart rate as it shortens with heart rate in normal individuals.
- Calculated using Bazett's formula:
  - $QT_C$ (sec) = QT (sec)/$\sqrt{RR}$ (sec)
- The tangent 'method' used to prevent overestimation (Fig. 9.5):
  - draw horizontal line across the baseline
  - draw a tangent along the steepest part of the T wave
  - the QT interval ends where the tangent crosses the baseline.
- Broad and bizarre T wave morphologies can be characteristic, although not diagnostic of the type of LQTS (see Fig. 9.6):[3]
  - LQT1broad-based, late onset or normal
  - LQT2low amplitude, notched or bifid.

- LQT3late onset, peaked, biphasic, asymmetrical peaked
- LQT4inverted, bifid, low amplitude
- LQT5insufficient data
- LQT6insufficient data
- LQT7prolonged terminal T down slope, prominent U wave
- LQT8T wave alternans

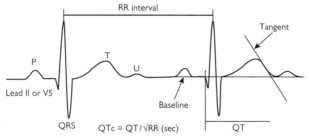

**Fig. 9.5** Tangent method for estimating QTc. Reprinted from Postema *et al.* Heart Rhythm 2008; **5**:1015–1018.

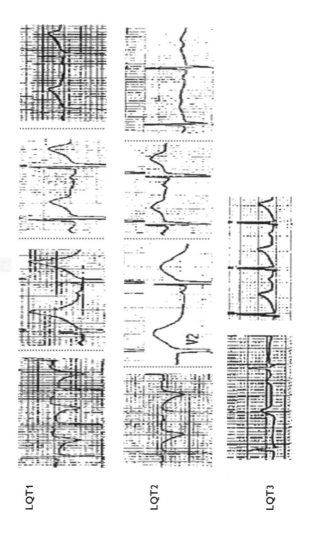

LQT1

LQT2

LQT3

**Fig. 9.6** Examples of typical T wave morphology of long QT 1–3. Adapted from Zhang L, et al. *Circulation* 2000; **102**: 2849–2855.

### Torsade de pointes

- Polymorphic ventricular tachycardia first described by Desertenne in 1966.
- The rotational nature of the tachycardia along an imaginary isoelectric line lends to this tachycardia being termed torsade de pointes.
- Usually terminates after 10–12 cycles due to refractoriness and thus is usually self-limiting.
- Can degenerate into VF in a minority of cases.
- Responds poorly to conventional therapy for VT and class Ia and III can exacerbate it.
- Increase in heart rate→ prevents torsade de pointes by shortening the $QT_C$ interval; consider overdrive atrial pacing, magnesium and isoprenaline.

## Investigations

### Exercise ECG

- In healthy, ↑heart rate→ ↓$QT_C$ to facilitate optimal diastolic filling.
- In LQT1, the $QT_C$ interval on exercise does not shorten as much as in normal individuals and this may be easiest to appreciate in the immediate recovery phase.

### Holter

- Diurnal variation may be present; in LQT3, marked prolongation of the $QT_C$ interval may be seen overnight.
- T wave changes, not apparent at rest, may be identified.
- Ventricular ectopics, torsade de pointes and even non-sustained VF may occur.

### Adrenaline challenge

- Helpful in identifying individuals with LQT1 and unknown mutations.
- Administered by intravenous bolus and brief infusion[4] or an escalating dose protocol (Mayo protocol[5]).
- An increase of ≥30ms in QT had a sensitivity of 92.5%, specificity of 86%, positive predictive value of 76%, and negative predictive value of 96% for LQT1 status with Mayo protocol[6].
- Can reveal T-ave notching in LQT2[7].
- Shimizu protocol:
  - differential assessment of adrenaline at peak dose (bolus) and steady state (infusion)
  - important because in LQT2, for example, the QT interval can lengthen then shorten
  - epinephrine (0.1mcg/kg/min) was employed. The sensitivity by ECG diagnostic criteria was lower in LQT1 (68%) than in LQT2 (83%) or LQT3 before epinephrine and was improved with steady state epinephire in LQT1 (87%) and LQT2 (91%) but not in LQT3 (83%), without the expense of specificity (100%). The sensitivity and specificity to differentiate LQT1 from LQT2 were 97% and 96%; those from LQT3 were 97% and 100% and those from Control were 97% and 100%; respectively, when Δ mean corrected Q-Tend ≥ 35 ms at steady state was used. The sensitivity and specificity to differntiate LQT2 from LQT3 or Control were 100% and 100% respectively, when Δ mean corrected Q-Tend > 80 ms at peak
  - suggest may be useful to differentiate LQT subtypes according to QT response.

- The false positive adrenaline challenge:
  - a paradoxical increase with low-dose adrenaline followed by shortening of the QTc interval can be seen in LQT1 and LQT2. Genetic testing should follow
  - where a U wave cannot be clearly differentiated from T wave, a baseline QTU measurement should be compared with the peak adrenaline QTU measurement.
- Safe and well tolerated. There is a theoretical risk of torsade de pointes and VF. Patients should be appropriately counselled and study performed in an electrophysiology laboratory.

### Genetic screening
- In families with LQTS, important to identify all mutation carriers for risk stratification and preventative measures.
- Also important in families where there has been sudden cardiac death.
- Costly and diagnosis does tend to be clinical.

## Treatment
### ACC/AHA/ESC recommendations for treatment[8]
*Class I*
(1) Lifestyle modification (clinical and/or molecular) (Level of Evidence: B)
(2) Beta blockers (ie in the presence of prolonged $QT_C$ interval) (Level of Evidence: B)
(3) ICD along with use of beta-blockers recommended for LQTS patients with previous cardiac arrest who have reasonable expectation of survival with good functional status for more than 1 year (Level of Evidence: A)

*Class IIa*
(1) Beta blockers to reduce SCD in patients with a molecular LQTS diagnosis and normal $QT_C$ interval (Level of Evidence: B)
(2) ICD with beta blockers to reduce SCD in LQTS patients with syncope and/or VT while receiving beta blockers and who have reasonable expectation of survival with a good functional status for more than 1 year (Level of Evidence: B)

*Class IIb*
(1) Left cardiac sympathetic nerve denervation considered for LQTS patients with syncope, torsade de pointes, or cardiac arrest while receiving beta blockers (Level of Evidence: B)
(2) ICD with beta blockers considered for prophylaxis of SCD for patients with higher risk of cardiac arrest eg certain LQT2 and LQT3 cases and who have reasonable expectation of survival with a good functional status for more than 1 year (Level of Evidence: B)

### Lifestyle
- Avoid competitive sport.
- LQT1—swimming under supervision or avoided; can trigger an event in 33%.
- LQT2—avoidance of acoustic stimuli especially during sleep. Telephones and alarm clocks should be removed from the bedroom
- Avoidance of drugs that prolong the $QT_C$ interval and those that deplete potassium and magnesium.

### Medication
*Beta blockers*
- Mainstay of drug treatment—strong evidence base for LQT1 and 2—contentious in LQT3 (due to limited data in smaller population).
- Shorten QTc.
- Anti-adrenergic and more useful in LQT1 and LQT2, than LQT3.
- If silent mutations, prophylaxis to decrease sudden cardiac death.
- Used throughout pregnancy in symptomatic mothers.
- Care in LQT3 as vagal stimulation predisposes to cardiac events and pause dependent torsade de pointes occurs—useful in combination with pacing and preventing EAD's.
- In LQT3: Schwartz approach is to use β-blockers, beginning with propranolol (2.0 to 3.0 mg/kg/day according to symptoms and heart rate), and then switching to nadolol for better compliance, in the following groups: asymptomatic patients (with few exceptions depending on age and QT duration) and all symptomatic patients.[9]

Channel specific therapy does not, at present, form the mainstay of treatment but is under investigation:

*Mexilitine*[10]
- Class 1b anti-arrhythmic drug.
- Sodium channel blocker and therefore could be useful in LQT3.
- Has been shown to decrease the $QT_C$ interval in humans.

*Nicorandil*[10]
- Potassium channel opener and can facilitate repolarization in LQT1 and LQT2.

### Pacing
- Atrial pacing at increased heart rates of 80/min helps shorten the $QT_C$.
- Useful for pause dependent or bradycardia induced VT (class 1 recommendation[11]).
- Allows up-titration of beta blockers without causing symptomatic bradycardia.

### Implantable cardiac defibrillators (ICD)
Beta-blockers are effective in 70%, leaving 30% of patients at an increased risk of cardiac events. Beta blockers and pacing do not prevent sudden death in those with continued symptoms despite therapy. 1 cardiac arrest→ high risk of another within 5 years. Children under 10 years and patients with syncope are at risk of aborted cardiac arrest and death

ICDs are used as secondary prevention in patients with syncope, VT, aborted cardiac death and cardiac arrest.
- Primary prophylaxis for high risk groups with LQT3 with the following features:
  - QTc >550msec–600msec
  - T wave alternans
  - sinus pauses.
- ICD implantation in neonates and children can be challenging or not feasible.

- The long QT interval or abnormal T wave morphology coupled with small R waves can lead to inappropriate shocks due to T-wave oversensing. This can be overcome by decreasing the sensitivity of the device or programming the R wave detection threshold and gain decay profiles to help overcome this.
- Prolonging the VT detection time to allow brief self-terminating episodes of torsades de pointes to end spontaneously may prevent excessive therapies for VT and may reduce the incidence of recurrent cycles of VT/VF due to high adrenergic drive induced by ICD shocks.

### Surgery: left cardiac sympathetic nerve denervation (LCSD)

- Reduces incidence of syncope and aborted cardiac arrest.
- Left cervical sympathectomy should be considered in patients failing beta blocker therapy. Recent experience with VATS cervical sympathectomy has shown good efficacy for both primary and secondary prevention of ventricular arrhythmia in both LQT and CPVT.[12]
- LCSD is used in conjunction with beta blockers or ICD's
- Should be considered as an appropriate therapeutic option especially in children as opposed to an ICD with its attendant long term complication risks.

### Clinical dilemmas

#### Asthma and LQTS[13]

- Beta agonists are used in the treatment of asthma→ predispose to ventricular arrhythmias.
- Beta blockers can cause bronchospasm.
- Treatment for either condition should not be denied and cardioselective beta blockers should be used.

#### Gene positive with a normal $QT_C$ interval

- Silent mutation carriers are highest among patients with LQT1 (36%)[14].
- Mutations in the LQT3 gene are less likely to cause a normal QTc (10%)[14]
- 'Silent' carriers are treated with beta blockers which act as prophylaxis and prevent life-threatening arrhythmias.

#### Children

- Children are treated in a similar way to adults.
- Implications of permanent pacemaker and ICD insertion should be carefully considered:
  - remain implanted lifelong
  - several box changes and new leads may be required
  - implant not without risk
  - venous access for new lead placement may become an issue.
- Genetic screening should take place if there is a family history.
- Asymptomatic children who are carriers and parents may find it psychologically challenging to deal with 'carrier status'.

#### Athletes[15]

- Significance of isolated $LQT_C$ in athletes is unknown.
- It may represent increased left ventricular hypertrophy characteristic of an athletic heart but may be the only manifestation of an ion channel mutation and predisposition to sudden cardiac death.

- Bazett's formula may not be relevant to elite athletes.
- One study has shown that:
  - asymptomatic athletes with a $QT_C$>500, lengthened their $QT_C$ on exercise or had a first-degree relative with LQTS
  - $QT_C$<500 but >460 had no typical features on exercise testing or Holter, no family history of LQTS and an intermediate score on the Schwartz score
  - study suggests that only elite athletes with a $QT_C$ interval >500 should be restricted from sport and that genotyping may help in making a decision about participation.
- The ACC/AHA/ESC presently suggests that such people should avoid competitive sport.

## Long QT syndrome in pregnancy and labour

Pregnancy→ ↑cardiac output and heart rate→ ↑arrhythmias. Multidisciplinary approach involving obstetricians, cardiologist and anaesthetist, along with a birth plan. Diagnosis should be made at the antenatal clinic. Little known about incidence of arrhythmias in pregnant patients with LQTS. A retrospective study has shown that the risk of arrhythmias in the post partum period is 10%.[16] Possible aetiology: ↑oestrogen and progesterone →↑adrenergic drive → ↑mutant ion channel function.

### General principles

- Pain, hypoxia, hypercapnia, shivering, anxiety, hypothermia, hypoglycaemia and hyperglycaemia should be avoided.
- Pain and stress→ ↑ adrenergic drive→ ↑ risk of arrhythmias.
- Avoid drugs which prolong $QT_C$.
- Electrolytes should be checked and replaced.
- In LQT1 and LQT2, beta blockers should continue as they are not teratogenic but may cause intrauterine growth restriction, bradycardia and hypotension in the fetus. These are excreted into breast milk which confers a negligible risk to a healthy neonate.
- In LQT3, bradycardia should be avoided.
- Valsalva can prolong the $QT_C$ in healthy individuals and therefore the second stage of labour should be shortened by assisted labour.
- If there is an ICD or PPM:
  - bipolar diathermy should be used
  - otherwise, reprogramme device to asynchronous pacing.

### Anaesthesia and analgesia in labour and delivery[13]

- Opioids can be given although these may not give relief.
- Regional anaesthesia decreases adrenergic drive.
- Epidural, spinal, and combined epidural and spinal anaesthesia may be used.

### Caesarean section

- Regional anaesthesia.
  - Advantage over epidural anaesthesia as the level of block can be controlled which decreases the risk of hypotension.
- General anaesthesia.
  - Anaesthetic agents, both intravenous and inhalational, prolong the $QT_C$ (Table 9.2).
  - Catecholamine release prevented by anxiolytics, e.g. midazolam.

**Table 9.2** Effects on the QT interval of anaesthetic agents

| | Prolong QT interval | DO not prolong QT |
|---|---|---|
| Induction agents | Ketamine | Etomidate |
| | Thiopental | Methohexital |
| | | Propofol |
| Inhalation anaesthetics | Desflurane | |
| | Enflurane | |
| | Halothane | |
| | Isoflurane | |
| Neuromuscular blockers | Pancuronium | Atracurium |
| | Succinylcholine | Vecuronium |
| | | Cisatracurium |
| Opioids | Methadone | Alfentanil |
| | Sufentanil | Fentanyl |
| | | Morphine |
| Benzodiazepines | | Midazolam |
| Neuromuscular block reversal agents | Neostigmine | |
| | Atropine | |
| Anti-emetics | Ondansetron | Cyclizine |
| Sympathomimetics | Adrenaline | Phenylephrine |
| | Noradrenaline | |
| | Dopamine | |
| | Dobutamine | |
| | Isoproterenol | |

Adapted from Drake E, et al. Can J Anaesthesia 2007; **54**: 561–572.

Prognosis
- Mortality with the first episode of syncope is 30%.
- Boys under 10 years have a higher mortality rate which is then similar in males and females.
- LQT3 tends to be more lethal.

Risk stratification
- QTc duration most powerful predictor of risk.

In an analysis of 647 LQT1, LQT2, and LQT3 mutation carriers,[17] the incidence of syncope or sudden death by 40 years of age in those with a QTc interval in the lowest quartile (<446msec) was less than 20%, whereas it was more than 70% among those in the highest quartile (>498msec). In the same study, features identifying patients at particularly high risk (>50% risk of an event before 40 years of age) included:

• QTc interval of more than 500msec in carriers with LQT1 and LQT2.
• Male sex in carriers with LQT3.

Predictors of lower risk (<30% risk of an event before 40 years of age) included:

• QTc interval of less than 500 msec in carriers with LQT1
• male sex in carriers with LQT2.

Although some of the subgroups were small and the effects of therapy were not controlled, these findings underscore the concept that risk is a continuum in this disease. Mutations that appear to be especially severe have been reported, although the numbers of affected patients and families are small.

1. Saenen B., Vrints C.J. (2008) Molecular aspects of the congenital and acquired long QT syndrome: clinical implications. *Journal of Molecular and Cellular Cardiology* **44**P: 633–646.
2. Schwartz P.J., et al. (2001) Genotype-phenotype correlation in the long-QT syndrome, gene-specific triggers for life-threatening arrhythmias. *Circulation* **103**: 89–95.
3. Modell S.M., Lehmann M.H. (2006) The long QT syndrome family of cardiac ion channelopathies: A HuGE review. *Genet Med* **8**: 143–155.
4. Shimizu W., et al. (2004) Diagnostic value of epinephrine test for genotyping LQT1, LQT2, and LQT3 forms of congenital long QT syndrome. *Heart Rhythm* **1**: 276–283.
5. Ackerman M.J., et al. (2002) Epinephrine-induced QT interval prolongation: a gene-specific paradoxical response in congenital long QT syndrome. *Mayo Clin Proc* **77**: 413–421.
6. Vyas H., et al. (2006) Epinephrine QT stress testing in the evaluation of congenital long QT syndrome: diagnostic accuracy of the paradoxical QT response epinephrine QT stress testing in the evaluation of congenital long-QT. *Circulation* **113**; 1385–1392.
7. Khositseth A., et al. (2005) Epinephrine induced T-wave notching in congenital long QT syndrome. *Heart Rhythm* h **2**: 141–146.
8. ACC/AHA/ESC 2006 Guidelines for prevention SCD *JACC* 2006; **48**: 1064–1108.
9. Schwartz P.J., Spazzolini C. and Crotti L. (2009) All LQT3 patients need an ICD-true or false? *Heart Rhythm* **6**: 113–120.
10. Ruan Y., et al. (2008) Therapeutic strategies for long QT syndrome: does the molecular substrate matter? *Cir Arrhythmia Electrophysiol* **1**: 290–297.
11. ACC/AHA/HRS (2008) Guidelines for Device-Based Therapy of Cardiac Rhythm Abnormalities. *J Am Coll Cardiol* **51**: e1–e62
12. Collura C.A., et al. (2009) Left cardiac sympathetic denervation for the treatment of long QT syndrome and catecholaminergic polymorphic ventricular tachycardia using video-assisted thoracic surgery. *Heart Rhythm* **6**: 752–759.
13. Thottathil P., et al. (2008) Risk of cardiac events in patients with asthma and long-QT syndrome treated with beta(2) agonists. *Am J Cardiol* **102**: 871–874.
14. Priori S.G., et al. (2003) Risk stratification in the long-QT syndrome. *NEJM* **348**: 1866–1874.
15. Basavarajaiah S., et al. (2007) Prevalence and significance of an isolated long QT interval in elite athletes. *European Heart Journal* **28**: 2944–2949.
16. Rashba E.J., et al. (1998) Influence of pregnancy on the risk for cardiac events in patients with hereditary long QT syndrome. *Circulation* **97**: 451–456.
17. Drake E., Preston R., Douglas J. (2007) Brief review: anesthetic implications of long QT syndrome in pregnancy. *Canadian Journal Of Anaesthesia* **54**: 561–572.

# Short QT syndrome

Since 2000, short QT syndrome (SQTS) has been identified as a disease entity in its own right.[1] Gaita et al. made the definitive link between short QT syndrome and sudden death in 2003.[2]

It is characterized by:
- syncope
- paroxysmal atrial fibrillation
- ventricular arrhythmias and sudden cardiac death.

## Genetics

SQTS is due to *gain in function* mutations in potassium ion channels, which shorten the action potential duration. Three genes have been implicated.[3–5] Inheritance is autosomal dominant.

### SQT1: HERG (also known as KCNH2)
- Encodes for the rapidly activating delayed rectifier potassium channel, $I_{KR}$.

### SQT2: KCNQ1
- Encodes for the slowly activating delayed rectifier potassium channel, $I_{KS}$.

### SQT3: KCNJ2
- Encodes for the inward potassium rectifier channel, $I_{KJ}$.

A clinical entity with overlapping phenotypes of Brugada syndrome and short QT syndrome has been described with loss of function missense mutations in CANCNB2b and CACNA1C encoding α1- or β2b-subunits of the cardiac L-type calcium channel.[6]

## Clinical symptoms and signs
- Commonly presents in the very young.
- Cause of sudden cardiac death in neonates.
- Shortened action potential duration can predispose to ventricular fibrillation.
- Palpitations due to atrial fibrillation.
- Family history of sudden death or atrial fibrillation.
- Severity of symptoms and signs represent a spectrum from no symptoms to sudden cardiac death.

## Diagnosis

There are no firm diagnostic criteria.

## ECG
- QTc interval <330ms which does not change with heart rate.
- Upright, tall, peaked T waves.
- Well separated U waves have been reported.
- Atrial fibrillation.

The diagnosis is not made on QTc alone (0.4% of the normal population have QTc<340msec) but must include T-wave morphology and QT adaptation. All confirmed cases of SQTS to date have had QTc<320msec.[7]

### Electrophysiology studies

- Reveals short atrial and ventricular refractory periods.
- Easily inducible ventricular fibrillation on programmed electrical stimulation.

### Management

- No clear genotype–phenotype correlation.

### Drug therapy

- Quinidine may be helpful in KCNH2 mutation carriers to prolong repolarization and prevent VF. Disopyramide may also have beneficial effects. There is currently no clinical drug efficacy data available for the other mutations.
- There are no randomized clinical trials given the small patient numbers.
- There is no specific drug available to block the $I_{KS}$ or $I_{KI}$ channels.

### ICD

- This is first line therapy particularly in those with failed sudden death.
- ICD implantation in neonates and children can be challenging or not feasible.
- The short QT interval can lead to inappropriate shocks due to T-wave oversensing. This is due to short coupled T waves but decreasing the sensitivity or programming the R wave detection threshold and gain decay profiles may help overcome this.

1. Gussak I., et al. (2000) Idiopathic short QT interval: a new clinical syndrome? *Cardiology* **94**: 99–102.
2. Gaita F., et al. (2003) Short QT Syndrome: a familial cause of sudden death. *Circulation* **108**: 965–108:970.
3. Brugada R., et al. (2004) Sudden death associated with short-QT syndrome linked to mutations in HERG. *Circulation* **109**: 30–35.
4. Bellocq C., et al. (2004) Mutation in the KCNQ1 gene leading to the short QT-interval syndrome. *Circulation* **109**: 2394–2397.
5. Priori S.G., et al. (2005) A novel form of short QT syndrome (SQT3) is caused by a mutation in the KCNJ2 gene. *Circ Res* **96**: 800–807.
6. Antzelevitch C., et al. (2007) Loss-of-function mutations in the cardiac calcium channel underlie a new clinical entity characterised by ST-segment elevation, short QT intervals, and sudden cardiac death. *Circulation* **115**: 442–449.
7. Crotti L., et al. (2010) Congenital short QT syndrome (Review). *Indian Pacing Electrophysiol J* **10**: 86–95.

# Catecholaminergic polymorphic VT

Catecholaminergic polymorphic ventricular tachycardia (CPVT) is an inherited arrhythmia disorder in structurally normal hearts that predisposes to a characteristic VT morphology provoked by exercise or catecholamine stress.

### Genetics

Pathological mutations in two genes located on chromosome 1:
- RyR2 gene encoding cardiac ryanodine receptor, responsible for approximately 50% of CPVT. Autosomal dominant inheritance (CPVT1)
- CASQ2 gene encoding cardiac calsequestrin, responsible for rarer form. Autosomal recessive inheritance (CPVT2).

Molecular autopsy of 49 cases of sudden unexplained death detected pathological mutations of RyR2 in 17% of cases.[1] Family history of unexplained sudden cardiac death is present in a third of CPVT cases.[2]

### Pathophysiology

Ryanodine receptor 2 is a sarcoplasmic reticulum (SR) channel protein expressed in cardiac tissue. Calsequestrin is a calcium storage protein in the SR. Both play critical roles in regulating intracellular calcium-mutations that can result in excessive calcium release during adrenergic stimuli, triggering delayed after depolarizations providing the substrate for arrhythmogenesis.

### Presentation

The characteristic presentation is syncope precipitated by exercise or catecholaminergic stress. The age of onset ranges from 2–38 years with a mean of 7–14 years in published case series.[2–4] Established RyR2 mutations are more common in males and associated with an earlier age of symptom onset. A significant delay in diagnosis can occur given the presentation of childhood syncope and normal findings on initial investigation.

### ECG

Patients with CPVT have a normal resting ECG. The characteristic arrhythmia is a polymorphic VT with an 180° rotating axis on a beat to beat basis (bidirectional VT—typically RBBB morphology with alternation R and L axis deviation). This occurs consistently on exercise with ventricular ectopy first observed once heart rate exceeds 110bpm (beats per minute), progressing to more frequent and complex ventricular arrhythmia with increasing exercise.[5] Ventricular ectopy on stress testing or Holter recordings during times of increased sympathetic activity should raise suspicion of the condition. Reproducibility of this exercise response makes exercise testing an effective tool for monitoring the efficacy of therapy to suppress ectopic activity and VT.

### Investigation

- Exercise test and 24hr Holter.
- Provocation testing with adrenaline can be more effective than exercise testing in eliciting arrhythmia.[6]

- Echocardiography to exclude other causes of syncope and VT.
- Genetic testing (diagnostic yield of 50%, but recommended given significance of a positive result).[7]
- Programmed electrical stimulation unhelpful as only non-sustained arrhythmia is inducible in a minority of cases.

## Treatment

- Lifestyle advice to avoid exercise and stress-related triggers.
- Beta blockers for both those with clinically diagnosed CPVT and asymptomatic gene positive CPVT.[8] A long-acting, non-selective agent such as Nadolol is preferred. Exercise testing to monitor efficacy and titrate dose.
- Verapamil alone and in combination with beta blockers has been used without consistent success and not currently recommended.
- Amiodarone not effective in suppressing arrhythmia in CPVT.
- Sodium channel blockers historically have not been effective in CPVT; however recent success has been reported with Flecainide in a mouse model of CPVT and in two patients.[9]
- ICD indicated for survivors of cardiac arrest and those with syncope or documented VT whilst on beta blockers.[8] Beta blockers are continued following ICD implant.
- Cervical sympathectomy has been shown to suppress VT/VF in patients unresponsive to beta blockers or with recurrent VF storm.[10]

## Prognosis

Family studies of CPVT have estimated the mortality of untreated cases at 30–50% by the age of 30yrs.[11] Established medical therapy is not completely effective. Up to half of patients on beta blockers have had demonstrable arrhythmia and 50% of those who went on to have an ICD implanted with continuation of their beta blocker still received an appropriate shock for ventricular tachyarrhythmia.[2]

## Dilemmas

Asthmatics with CPVT pose a significant challenge given their intolerance to beta blockers. Patients are evaluated on a case by case basis and an in-patient trial of beta blocker should be considered. If this fails then consider less established therapies such as verapamil. There is now an increasing trend to recommend ICDs in these patients due to concerns regarding adequate protection if beta blocker doses are missed. There is a significant risk of inappropriate shocks in these patients due to bigeminny on exercise—this can be reduced with programming prolonged detection for VT and a VF only zone.

1. Tester D.J., et al. (2004) A molecular autopsy of 49 coroner's cases. *Mayo Clin Proc* **79**: 1380–1384.
2. Priori S.G., et al. (2002) Clinical and molecular characterisation of CPVT. *Circulation* **106**: 69–74.
3. Leenhardt A., et al. (1995) CPVT in children. *Circulation* **91**: 1512–1519.
4. Sumitomo N., et al. (2003) CPVT: electrocardiographic characteristics and optimal therapeutic strategies to prevent sudden death. *Heart* **89**: 66–70.
5. Napolitano C., et al. (2007) Diagnosis and treatment of CPVT. *Heart Rhythm* **4**: 675–678.

6. Krahn AD, *et al.* Diagnosis of unexplained cardiac arrest. Circulation 2005; **112**:2228–2234.
7. Heart Rhythm UK Familial Sudden Death Syndromes Statement Development Group (2008) Clinical indications for genetic testing in familial SCD syndromes: an HRUK position statement. *Heart* **94**: 502–507.
8. Zipes D.P., *et al.* (2006) ACC/AHA/ESC 2006 guidelines for management of patients with ventricular arrhythmias and the prevention of sudden cardiac death. *Europace* **8**: 746–837.
9. Watanabe H., *et al.* (2009) Flecainide prevents CPVT in mice and humans. *Nature Medicine* **15**: 380–383.
10. Wilde A.A.M., *et al.* (2008) Left cardiac sympathetic denervation for CPVT. *New Engl J Med* **358**: 2024–2029.
11. Francis J., *et al.* (2005) Catecholaminergic polymorphic ventricular tachycardia. *Heart Rhythm*, **2**: 550–4

# Inherited conduction system disorders

Inherited conduction system disorders are often associated with other diseases such as congenital heart disease or cardiomyopathy but can rarely be an isolated finding.

### Lev–Lenègre disease (progressive cardiac conduction defect)

- ECG shows prolonged PR and QRS intervals progressing to complete AV block, causing syncope and sudden death.
- Prolonged HV but normal AH intervals are seen at electrophysiological study.
- Associated with SCN5A mutations (encodes α subunit of Na+ channel).
- Acquired form in elderly due to fibrosis of conducting system tissue.

### Sinus node dysfunction

- Manifests as intermittent sinus pauses, prolonged sinus arrest.
- Associated with mutations in the hyperpolarization-activated cyclic nucleotide gated channel 4 (HCN4) gene—1 of 4 genes that encodes If ('funny' current) and is responsible for the spontaneous depolarization of pacemaker cells.
- Also associated with CASQ2 mutations (calsequestrin gene) in autosomal recessive catecholaminergic polymorphic ventricular tachycardia.
- SCN5A mutations have also been identified in this disease.

### Myotonic dystrophy

- 📖 See Myotonic dystrophy, pp. 332–335.
- Patients at highest risk of cardiac events are >40yo and PR>240msec. Should have frequent follow up.
- Recommend HV measurement at EP study if: 1st degree AV block/ QRS>100msec, palpitations, presyncope, pre-op general anaesthetic.
- Permanent pacing recommended if HV>70msec at EP study.
- Small proportion of myotonic dystrophy patients with HV prolongation and PPM develop VT due to bundle branch re-entry of intra-mural re-entry resulting in further syncope/sudden death.
- VT stimulation studies may have a role to identify patients needing permanent pacemaker at risk of VT and hence an ICD as primary prophylaxis in suitable cases.
- Recommend monitoring of VT at PPM checks in permanently paced patients to identify high-risk patients.

### AMP kinase (PRKAG2 gene)

- AMP kinase-activated by increases in adenosine monophosphate/ATP ratio to reduce ATP utilization.
- Induces hypertrophy, abnormal MV/TV annulus formation—WPW (68%)
- Rarely develop AV re-entrant tachycardias.
- 38% require pacing for progressive conduction disease and sick sinus syndrome by mean age of 38yrs[1].
- Low incidence VT.

## Lamin A/C
📖 See DCM and laminopathies, p.195

### Neuromuscular disorders

The following conditions are associated with an increased risk of conduction disease:

- Kearns–Sayre syndrome (oculocraniosomatic disease—triad of chronic progressive external opthalmoplegia, bilateral pigmentary retinopathy and cardiac conduction abnormalities)
- Erb's dystrophy (limb girdle)
- peroneal muscular dystrophy.

These patients should be monitored closely for evidence of 1st, 2nd and 3rd degree AV block and fascicular block. Progression to complete AV block is unpredictable.

1. Murphy R., et al. (2004) Adenosine monophosphate-activated protein kinase disease mimicks hypertrophic cardiomyopathy and Wolff–Parkinson–White syndrome. Natural history. *Journal of American College of Cardiology* **45**: 922–930.

# Inherited disorders of connective tissue

# Introduction

The phenotype of inherited disorders of connective tissue is extensive and may involve multiple body systems. In most cases, the clinical picture is that of a progressive disease with mild to severe dermatological, osteo-articular, ocular, and cardiovascular manifestations. The spectrum of cardiovascular manifestations ranges from a mild strucural abnormality (for example, mitral incompetence) to life-threatening complications (for example, aortic dissection) (Table 10.1). This section provides a general guide to diagnosis and management of cardiovascular manifestations in the common inherited disorders of connective tissue.

**Table 10.1** Cardiovascular phenotype of inherited disorders of connective tissue

| Disorder (OMIM#) | Cardiovascular phenotype |
|---|---|
| Marfan syndrome (154700) | Mitral valve prolapse, mitral regurgitation, dilatation of the aortic root, aortic regurgitation; major life-threatening cardiovascular complications—aneurysm of the aorta and aortic dissection |
| Loeys–Dietz syndrome (609192LDS1; 608967LDS2) | Aortic aneurysm; aortic dilatation; arterial tortuosity |
| **Beals–contractual** | |
| Arachnodactyly (121050) | Mitral valve prolapse; mitral incompetence, aotic dilatation |
| **Ehlers–Danlos syndromes** | |
| EDS II (130010) | Aortic dilatation, mitral incometence |
| EDS III (130020) | Mitral valve prolapse; mitral incompetence |
| EDS IV (130050) | Aortic and arterial rupture; vascular fragility |
| **Osteogenesis imperfecta** | |
| OI I (166200) | Mitral valve proplase and mitral regurgitation; aortic dilatation with aortic regurgitation |
| OI III (259420) | Uncommon; chronic heart failure secondary to severe deforming kyphoscoiosis |
| Cutis laxa (123700) | Multiple vascular anomalies; pulmonary srtery stenosis; aortic dilatation; coarctation of aorta |

# Clinical approach to inherited connective disease

## Family history

It is essential to obtain a detailed three generation family history.

Several minor and non-specific symptoms and illnesses in the family raise suspicion of a familial connective disease:

- joint laxity—mild, moderate, severe (recurrent dislocations); enquire about hobbies like gymnastics and ballet dancing indicating social and personal advantage of having lax joints
- arthritic symptoms—mild to moderate recurrent and chronic joint pains without associated significant signs of inflammation (swelling, effusion and restricted movements)
- skin laxity—usually around neck, axilla, abdomen, elbows, forearms, and knees
- scars and marks of fresh and old bruises—ask specifically for cigarette paper-thin scars on lower legs
- delayed healing of cuts and wounds (including surgical procedures)
- acute medical events such as severe chest pain, stroke, rapid loss of vision, acute abdomen and emergency surgical intervention for a major life-threatening event.

## Clinical examination

The following plan for clinical examination provides sufficient information for making a clinical diagnosis and, if necessary, proceeding to specific investigations:

### General inspection

- Appearance older than chronological age.
- Expressionless face due to lax facial skin.
- Thin and long face.
- Unusual joint shape and deformity.
- Unusual position of arms and legs.
- Tall thin build.
- Long fingers and toes.

### Measurements (whenever possible, record as gender/age equivalent percentile)

- Vertical height.
- Arm span—calculate vertical height/span ratio.
- Total hand length.
- Middle-finger length.
- Total foot length.

### Skin

- Texture—velvety, smooth.
- Laxity—usually behind elbows, forearms, front of knees.
- Scars—thin cigarette-paper like.
- Marks of old and fresh bruises.
- Striae—shoulders, side of abdomen, back, ilaic region.

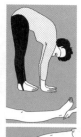

1. Score one point if you can bend and place you hands flat on the floor without bending you knees.

2. Score one point for each knee that will bend backwards.

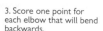

3. Score one point for each elbow that will bend backwards.

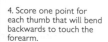

4. Score one point for each thumb that will bend backwards to touch the forearm.

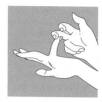

5. Score one point for each hand when you can bend the little finger back beyound 90°.

Fig. 10.1 Beighton Hypermobility Score.

### Joints
- Shape.
- Deformity.
- Laxity—expressed as Beighton score (maximum 9): see Fig. 10.1).
- Scars for surgical procedures.

### Spine
- Shape—kyphosis/scoliosis/lordosis.
- Bony deformity.
- Mobility.

### Dental
- Crowded/unusual-shaped teeth.
- Unusual palate shape/size.
- Abnormal appearnace—thin mottled enamel.
- Unusual, early loss of teeth.

### Eyes
- Myopia—often moderate to high.
- Unusual iris movements on examination—iridodenesis.
- Unusual lens appearnace/position including signs of lenticular opacity.
- History of opthalmological procedures including surgery (for example retinal detachment).

### Systemic examination
- Respiratory:
  - shape of thorax
  - scars for drains, surgical procedures

- movements (restricted on the side of pneumothorax)
- Respiratory sounds.
- Cardiovascular:
  - signs of congestive heart failure
  - blood pressure measurements, if appropriate separately for upper and lower limbs
  - heart sounds
  - murmurs, mitral imcompetence (EDS 1, EDSIII), aortic incompetence (Marfan).
- Abdomen:
  - shape
  - palpation, pulsatile mass (abdominal aortic aneurysm)
  - hernia—inguinal, femoral, para-umbilial.
- Nervous system:
  - look for sensory and/or motor deficit (cord compression; dural ectasia).

Investigations

History and examination are usually sufficient for diagnosis but in some cases further laboratory and radiological investigations are necessary.

### Radiological

- Post-anterior chest X-ray.
- Anterior and lateral X-ray spine.
- Cervical spine X-ray to exclude atlanto-axial instability.
- Skeletal survey might be necessary to exclude underlying skeletal dysplasia. This normally includes skull (anterior and lateral views), Chest to include shoulders, one uppper arm at elbow, pelvis to include femoral heads and one lower leg to include the knee.
- MRI or a computed tomography (CT) scan of spine should be considered to exclude dural ectasia in Marfan syndrome.

### Laboratory

- Chromosomes, particularly when learning difficulties and developmental delay.
- Molecular genetic mutation analysis for some inherited connective tissue disorders: Fibrillin-1 (Marfan); TGFBR1/2 (Marfan, Loeys–Dietz syndrome; thoracic aortic dissection); COL3A1 (EDSIV).
- Histopathology—skin biopsy for both light and electron microscopy to demonstrate collagen fibre abnormality.
- Clinical biochemistry.
- Collagen studies on skin fibroblasts to include collagen protein gel electrophoresis.
- Urinary excretion of collagen metabolites.

# Cardiovascular phenotypes in connective tissue disorders

It is important to carry out a thorough cardiovascular examination in all cases of proven or suspected inherited connective tissue disease. However, in most cases, the cardiovascular involvement is mild and does not require any close surveillance except for 3–5 yearly review by the family doctor with the option of specialist cardiology consultation.

Major cardiovascular manifestations are encountered in Marfan syndrome and the vascular type Ehlers–Danlos syndrome (type IV) (Table 10.1). Only these two conditions are discussed in this chapter. This section also includes non-syndromic thoracic aortic dilatation and aneurysms that may be familial and clinically overlap with Marfan syndrome and vascular EDS.

# Marfan syndrome: general features

Marfan syndrome (MIM 154700) is a clinically variable, progressive auto-somal dominant disorder of connective tissue whose cardinal features affect the cardiovascular system, eyes, and skeleton:

- the minimal birth incidence is around 1 in 9800 and the prevalence may be around 1/5000
- personal or family history of tall/thin body habitus, unsual chest shape, long/thin fingers or toes, long arms, lens subluxation, aortic dissection or rupture in a young person
- tall thin-built person with a positive thumb sign and wrist sign (Figs 10.2 and 10.3)
- progressive aortic dilatation, typically maximal at the sinus of Valsalva
- aortic valve incompetence
- aortic dissection or rupture and is the principal cause of mortality in many cases
- mitral valve prolapse with incompetence may be present
- ocular features include lens dislocation and progressive myopia
- arthralgia associated with chronic joint laxity.
  Other minor features include:
- high arched palate with dental crowding
- skin striae
- recurrent hernia
- recurrent pneumothorax may increase suspicion. Family history may be helpful, but around 27% of cases arise from new mutation.

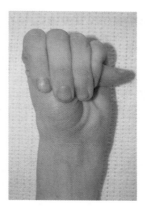

**Fig. 10.2** Long thumb protruding out of closed hand—the 'thumb sign' in Marfan syndrome. Reprinted from *Principles and Practice of Clinical Cardiovascular Genetics*, Oxford University Press, New York, 2010, Fig. 11.2, page 159.

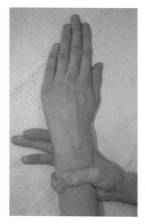

**Fig. 10.3** Positive 'wrist sign' in Marfan syndrome—thumb overlapping the whole nail of the little finger. Reprinted from *Principles and Practice of Clinical Cardiovascular Genetics*, Oxford University Press, New York, 2010, Fig. 11.2, page 159.

# Marfan syndrome: molecular genetics

Between 66 and 91% of Marfan syndrome patients have an identifiable fibrillin-1 (FBN1) mutation. Fibrillin-1 mutations also cause some other Marfan-like disorders or fibrillinopathies, usually with a better prognosis:
- MASS phenotype (MIM 604308; myopia, mitral valve prolapse, mild non-progressive aortic dilatation, skin and skeletal features)
- Isolated ectopia lentis (MIM 129600).

In addition to fibrillin-1, mutations in the TGFbeta receptor 2 (*TGFβR2*) gene on chromosome 3 and in the *TGFβR1* gene on chromosome 9 were recently found in some families with apparent Marfan syndrome (type 2). Marfan syndrome type 2 (MIM 154705) families are less likely to have ectopia lentis.

*TGFβR2* mutations at the R460 codon have also been described in families with the chromosome 3-linked form of familial thoracic ascending aortic aneurysm (FTAA3, MIM 608967), and *TGFβR1* and 2 mutations are found in Loeys–Dietz syndromes type 1 and 2.

# Diagnosis of Marfan syndrome

The diagnosis of Marfan syndrome (MFS) is largely clinical based on the international Ghent criteria. In the Ghent nosology, clinical features are assessed within seven body systems, to determine whether that system provides a major criterion, or only system involvement (Table 10.2). The revised Ghent MFS diagnostic criteria (see Further reading) are applicable in the absence of family history and systemic involvement with a proven disease-causing FBNI mutation. These may also be helpful in clarifying MFS in children. A new scoring system has also been recommended that is not yet sufficiently validated.

**Table 10.2** Ghent diagnostic criteria. Having one of the features listed constitutes a major criterion or system involvement for all systems except the skeletal system, where more than one feature is needed

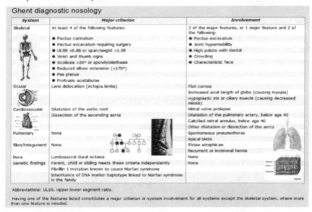

**Ghent diagnostic nosology**

| System | Major criterion | Involvement |
|---|---|---|
| Skeletal | At least 4 of the following features:<br>● Pectus carinatum<br>● Pectus excavatum requiring surgery<br>● ULSR <0.86 or span:height >1.05<br>● Wrist and thumb signs<br>● Scoliosis >20° or spondylolisthesis<br>● Reduced elbow extension (<170°)<br>● Pes planus<br>● Protrusio acetabulae | 2 of the major features, or 1 major feature and 2 of the following:<br>● Pectus excavatum<br>● Joint hypermobility<br>● High palate with dental<br>● Crowding<br>● Characteristic face |
| Ocular | Lens dislocation (ectopia lentis) | Flat cornea<br>Increased axial length of globe (causing myopia)<br>Hypoplastic iris or ciliary muscle (causing decreased miosis) |
| Cardiovascular | Dilatation of the aortic root<br>Dissection of the ascending aorta | Mitral valve prolapse<br>Dilatation of the pulmonary artery, below age 40<br>Calcified mitral annulus, below age 40<br>Other dilatation or dissection of the aorta |
| Pulmonary | None | Spontaneous pneumothorax<br>Apical blebs |
| Skin/Integument | None | Striae atrophicae<br>Recurrent or incisional hernia |
| Dura | Lumbosacral dural ectasia | None |
| Genetic findings | Parent, child or sibling meets these criteria independently<br>Fibrillin 1 mutation known to cause Marfan syndrome<br>Inheritance of DNA marker haplotype linked to Marfan syndrome in the family | None |

Abbreviations: ULSR, Upper:lower segment ratio.

Having one of the features listed constitutes a major criterion or system involvement for all systems except the skeletal system, where more than one feature is needed.

Courtesy of Dr. Andrew Fry, Academic Trainee in Clinical Genetics, University Hospital of Wales, Cardiff, UK.

- In a proband, the diagnosis of Marfan syndrome requires a major criterion in two systems and involvement of a third.
- The cardiovascular, ocular and skeletal systems provide major criteria, or system involvement, the pulmonary system and skin/integument can provide only system involvement, the dura and family/genetic history provide only major criteria.
- The cardiovascular assessment requires measurement of the aortic diameter at the sinuses of Valsalva, usually by transthoracic echocardiography and comparison with normal values based on age and body surface area, calculated from height and weight (Figs 10.3 and 10.4).

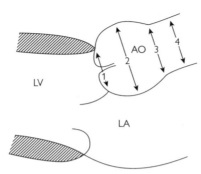

**Fig. 10.4** Measurement of the aortic root at the sinus of Valsalva. Reprinted from *Principles and Practice of Clinical Cardiovascular Genetics*, Oxford University Press, New York, 2010, Fig. 11.3, page 160.

- Other imaging techniques such as transoesophageal echocardiography, or MRI scanning (Fig. 10.6) may be helpful in some cases, including those with severe pectus deformity. Assessment of the skeletal system should include pelvic X-ray to detect protrusio acetabulae. In some cases a lumbar MRI scan may reveal dural ectasia.
- Ocular evaluation for myopia (due to increased globe length, measured by ultrasound), corneal flattening (measured by keratometry), hypoplastic iris or iris muscle and lens subluxation requires ophthalmology assessment.

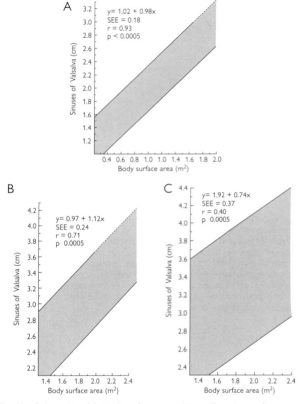

**Fig. 10.5** Relationship of the body surface area and 'normal' aortic root diameter measured at sinuses of Valsalva (from under 1.2 cms to 3.6 cms). Reprinted from *Principles and Practice of Clinical Cardiovascular Genetics*, Oxford University Press, New York, 2010, Fig. 11.4, page 161.

## Differential diagnosis

In some cases, the diagnosis of Marfan syndrome may be doubtful due to lack of family history and/or clinical findings sufficient to meet the Ghent criteria. In such cases other clinical disorders with Marfan-like features should be considered. The term 'Marfanoid' is often used which should be avoided as this is misleading and may result in erroneous interpretation and inaccurate genetic advice. The differential diagnosis of a tall young person with Marfan-like skeletal features includes:

- homocystinuria (MIM 236300)
- Beals syndrome or congenital contractural arachnodactyly (MIM 121050)
- Marshall–Stickler syndrome (MIM 108300, 604841, 184840)
- Ehlers–Danlos syndrome (MIM 130050), specifically type EDS IV or Vascular EDS (see EDS section in this chapter)
- MASS phenotype—myopia mitral valve prolapse, mild non-progressive aortic dilatation, skin and skeletal features (MIM 604308), occasionally mitral valve prolapse may be the only manifestation in a tall thin build person (mitral valve prolapse syndrome (MVPS))
- familial thoracic aortic aneurysm (FTAA) (MIM 607086)—other features of Marfan syndrome (mainly skeletal)—may or may not be present. Additional clinical findings may include bicuspid aortic valve
- Shprintzen–Goldberg syndrome (MIM 182212)—Marfan-like with craniosynostosis, intellectual impairment
- Loeys–Dietz syndrome type 1 (MIM 609192)—arterial tortuosity or widespread aneurysms, hypertelorism, bifid uvula/cleft palate, craniosynostosis
- Loeys–Dietz syndrome type 2—arterial tortuosity or widespread aneurysms, visceral rupture, joint hypermobility, thin skin with atrophic scarring
- Lujan–Fryns syndrome (MIM 309520)—intellectual impairment, velopharyngeal insufficiency.

# Management of Marfan syndrome

The initial evaluation of patients with possible Marfan syndrome requires a multidisciplinary approach including clinical genetics, cardiology, ophthalmology and radiology.

A positive Marfan diagnosis in the family by genetic testing (linkage or mutation testing) can provide a major criterion.

Because many Marfan features (for example, echocardiographic findings, ectopia lentis, scoliosis, upper:lower segment ratio, protrusio acetabulae) are age-dependent in their occurrence, younger patients with a family history of Marfan syndrome who do not fulfil the diagnostic criteria, and younger Marfan-like patients with no family history who fail to meet the diagnostic criteria by one system, should be offered repeat evaluations periodically at 5 yearly intervals (for example, ages 5, 10, and 15 years) until age 18.

## Cardiovascular management

All patients with a confirmed diagnosis of Marfan syndrome should be regularly followed up by a cardiologist with a special interest in inherited cardiovascular conditions. The key issues in the cardiovascular management of Marfan syndrome are:

- beta blocker therapy should be considered at any age if the aorta is dilated, but prophylactic treatment may be more effective in those with an aortic diameter of less than 4cm. There is evidence for the prophylactic use of angiotensin-receptor blocking agents (for example, Losartan) in preventing progression of aortic dilatation and possibly reducing the risk for aortic dissection. Large randomized studies are under way
- risk factors for aortic dissection include aortic diameter greater than 5cm, aortic dilatation extending beyond the sinus of Valsalva, rapid rate of dilatation (>5% per year, or 1.5mm/year in adults), and family history of aortic dissection
- at least annual evaluation should be offered, comprising clinical history, examination and echocardiography. In children, serial echocardiography at 6–12 month intervals is recommended, the frequency depending on the aortic diameter (in relation to body surface area) and the rate of increase
- prophylactic aortic root surgery should be considered when the aortic diameter at the Sinus of Valsalva exceeds 5cm
- in pregnancy, there is an increased risk of aortic dissection if the aortic diameter exceeds 4cm. Frequent cardiovascular monitoring throughout pregnancy and into the puerperium is advised.

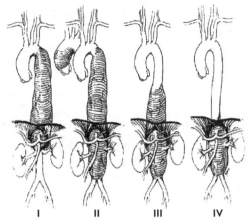

**Fig. 10.6** The Crawford classification of thoraco-abdominal aortic aneurysms type I to IV. Reprinted from *Principles and Practice of Clinical Cardiovascular Genetics*, Oxford University Press, New York, 2010, Fig. 12.1, page 172.

# Vascular Ehlers–Danlos syndrome (EDS IV)

The Ehlers–Danlos syndromes represent a group of inherited connective tissue conditions caused by mutations in genes encoding different collagen proteins. There at least 10 clinically recognizable types of EDS with over-lapping clinical features.

The common clinical features in most EDS types are variable degree of skin laxity, a tendency for easy bruising and delayed healing and variable degree of joint hypermobility. Most EDS forms manifest with a range of cardiovascular manifestations that are also seen in other connective tissue disorders. Cardiovascular complications in EDS include:

- bundle branch block—left and partial right bundle branch block
- aortic stenosis and incompetence
- tricuspid regurgitation
- abnormal looking mitral valve—nodular thickening, floppy with mitral incompetence
- associated CHD—ASD, VSD and TOF.

Various studies record wide distribution of cardiovascular complications from around 5–30%. Beighton (1970) recorded benign systolic murmurs (10%), mitral incompetence (1%), ASD (1%), right-sided aortic arch (1%), aortic stenosis and incompetence (1%), mitral incompetence (1%). In most cases, patients are asymptomatic and the cardiovascular signs are incidentally detected. However, the presence of a cardiac sign may warrant long-term surveillance.

This section describes only the vascular type of EDS (EDS IV) that is recognized by moderate to severe cardiovascular manifestations including risk of sudden death and stroke due to aortic/arterial rupture. Details of other EDS types can be found elsewhere.

## Clinical

The clinical picture in EDS IV may be entirely normal. Important clinical features include:

- vascular fragility dominates EDS IV or vascular EDS, often causing lethal arterial rupture or dissection
- severe phenotype may include pre-tibial ecchymoses and haemosiderosis, thereby sometimes causing confusion with EDS types I/II and EDS VIII
- the skin may be prematurely thinned and less extensible compared to EDS type I/II. Skin thinning may be focal, and limited to the face, shoulders and forearms or more generalized and even complete
- widespread skin thinning is accompanied by specific facial features, including large eyes, variably thin lips, lobeless ears—the Madonna face. The combination of prematurely thin skin over the dorsum of hands and feet together with the facial appearance is termed acrogeria (Fig. 10.7)
- the extensive premature acral dermal atrophy and bruising may be Accompanied by metacarpal subluxations and can be misdiagnosed as rheumatoid degeneration with steroid atrophy (Fig. 10.7)

- premature thinning of scalp hair (metageria) may be confused with progeria
- other more variable clinical signs include acro-osteolysis, elastosis perforans serpiginosa, keloid scars, premature hip or other joint dislocations, bilateral premature talipes in children, or spontaneous colonic perforations in adults.

## Pathology of EDS IV

Pathological features in EDS IV include vascular changes, evidence of connective tissue changes, abnormal type 3 collagen profile and mutations in *COL3A1* gene.

### Vascular pathology

- Aneurysms of small- and medium-sized arteries, such as the renal, splenic, coeliac axis, brachial, subclavian, femoral, popliteal, internal carotid, and carotid cavernous sinus vessels (Fig. 10.7).
- Occasionally, coronary aneurysms have also been described.
- Aortic aneurysms involving the aortic arch, descending and abdominal aorta are much more frequent than coronary pathology and fatal aortic dissections may occur.

### Histopathology

- Light microscopy characteristically shows marked dermal thinning, collagen depletion and elastic proliferation (Fig. 10.7) and are sufficiently specific as to be diagnostic.
- Electron microscopy of dermal collagen fibres shows altered collagen fibril diameters, in contrast to the normal evenly distributed size distribution.

### Biochemistry

- More severe dominant–negative type only 1/8th of collagen trimers are normal and abnormal trimers remain intracellular.
- The haploinsufficient type, collagen type III secretion is close to 50% and abnormal protein is not produced or retained. Protein patterns may match the general clinical appearance and overall severity (Fig. 10.7).

### Molecular genetics

Several different collagen type III gene (*COL3A1*) mutations are descibed with minimal clinical correlation:

- triple helical glycine substitutions
- exon skips
- small and large deletions
- occasional non-helical C propeptide mutations have also been described.

## Management of vascular EDS

Cardiovascular complications are a major feature in vascular EDS, compared with other EDS subtypes. In EDS IV, catastrophic and frequently fatal, arterial rupture or dissection is common. Very few examples are published in other EDS subtypes, despite the relatively common occurrence of aortic root dilatation in EDS types I, II, and III.

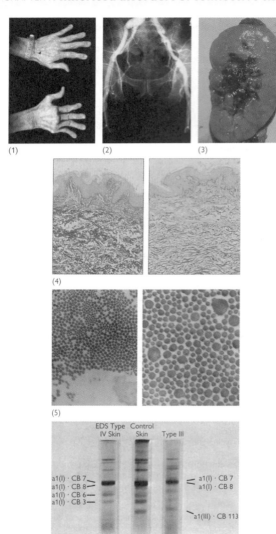

(1)
(2)
(3)
(4)
(5)

| EDS Type IV Skin | Control Skin | Type III |
| --- | --- | --- |
| a1(I) · CB 7 | | a1(I) · CB 7 |
| a1(I) · CB 8 | | a1(I) · CB 8 |
| a1(I) · CB 6 | | |
| a1(I) · CB 3 | | a1(III) · CB 113 |

(6)

**Fig. 10.7** Vascular Ehlers-Danlos syndrome (EDS IV): 1. Prematurely aged hands clearly demonstrate the remarkable dermal thinning, reminiscent of steroid atrophy; 2. Arterial pathology includes diffuse aortic-iliac tortuosity and dilation;

**Fig. 10.7** (*Cont.*)3. A medium-sized ruptured renal artery necessitating total nephrectomy to control bleeding; 4. Light microscopy of acrogeric skin with collagen depletion and elastic proliferation; 5. Electron microscopy shows variably sized collagen fibrils in both arterial (L) and skin samples (R); 6. Direct collagen protein analysis from cultured skin fibroblasts, show collagen type III deficiency in EDS IV. Reproduced from Kumar and Elliott (eds). *Principles and Practice of Clinical Cardiovascular Genetics*, with permission from Oxford University Press.

Unlike the Marfan syndrome in which the value of aortic root diameter monitoring and prophylaxis with either beta blockade or transforming growth factor (TGF) beta inhibitors, in retarding aortic dilatation is well proven, vascular EDS produces sudden arterial failure without evidence of gradual deterioration.

The management of the arterial complications of vascular EDS are immediate and not prospective. Vascular surgery is potentially hazardous, as haemostasis can be very difficult to establish, given the friability of the aneurysmal or dissected vessels. Varicose vein surgery should be avoided whenever possible.

The following approaches may be applicable:
- conservative control of bleeding—generally successful in managing smaller aneurysms and small arteries
- coil embolization—for example, carotid cavernous sinus aneurysms, causing acute exophthalmos and III cranial nerve paresis with Horner's syndrome can be successfully managed by coil embolization
- resection of aneurysms within the help of non-angiographic arteriography, to localize the source
- surgical repair—grafting and endovascular repair
- factor VIIA infusions—this approach has been tried with limited success in controling the bleeding.

# Thoracic aortic aneurysms

- Most cases of thoracic aortic dilatation with or without aneurysm occur in otherwise healthy persons without any physical features of a connective tissue disorder (non-syndromic/isolated thoracic aortic dialtation/aneurysm). Tragically, the first presentation may be sudden unexplained death and diagnosed at post-mortem examination.
- Approximately 20% of patients with thoracic aortic aneurysms and dissections may have a genetic predisposition.
- Most follow autosomal dominant mode of inheritance with incomplete penetrance and variable clinical presentation.
- Associated structural abnormalities may include bicuspid aortic valve and abnormal aortic annulus.
- Dilatation and aneurysms involving the medium/small sized peripheral arteries may be accompanied with thoracic aortic aneurysm (TAA) manifesting with myocardial infarction, stroke, rupture, and paralysis.

## Classification

TAA are classified according to the anatomical segment involved (Fig. 10.8).

- *Aneurysmal dilatation of the proximal part of the thoracic aorta* (may be associated with congenital abnormality of the aortic valve, for example bicuspid aortic valve).
- *Ascending aortic aneurysms* (occur anywhere from the aortic valve to the innominate artery).
- *Aortic arch aneurysms* (include thoracic aneurysms that involve the brachiocephalic vessels).
- *Descending thoracic aneurysms* (anywhere distal to the left subclavian artery but confined to the thoracic aorta).
- *Thoraco-abdominal aneurysms* (arise anywhere distal to the left subclavian artery extending to the abdominal aorta.

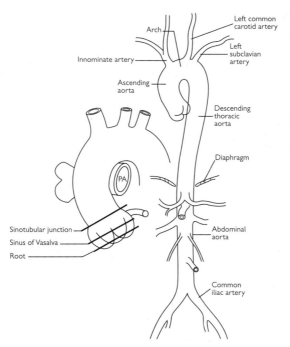

**Fig. 10.8** The anatomy of thoracic and abdominal aorta. Reprinted from *Principles and Practice of Clinical Cardiovascular Genetics*, Oxford University Press, New York, 2010, Fig. 12.1, page 171.

### Crawford classification

In addition to anatomic position, the Crawford classification (Fig. 10.9) provides guidance to the likely aetiology, indications:

I. Involves all or most of the descending thoracic aorta and the upper abdominal aorta above the renal arteries.

II. Involves all or most of the descending thoracic aorta and the upper abdominal aorta above the renal arteries.

III. Involves all or most of the descending thoracic aorta and all or most of the abdominal aorta below the renal arteries.

IV. Involves the distal half or less of the descending thoracic aorta (usually below T6) with varying segments of the abdominal aorta.

**Aortic dissection**
- An aortic dissection occurs when blood separates the inner and outer layers of the vessel, producing a false lumen or double-barrelled aorta, which can occlude major aortic branches.
- Dissections can result in rupture or formation of an aneurysm.
- Aortic dissection affects around 10 per 100 000 of the population per year and has a high mortality. If left untreated, 62–91% of patients die in one week.

Aortic dissections are classified according to either DeBakey (types I, II, IIIa, IIIb) or Stanford (types A and B) classification (Fig. 10.9) according to the part of the aorta that has been affected by the dissection.
- A proximal dissection (DeBakey Types I and II, Stanford A) involves the ascending aorta; a distal dissection (DeBakey Type III, Stanford B) only affects the aorta distal to the left subclavian artery.
- Dissections are acute if they present within 14 days and chronic if the presentation is longer.
- Early death is more common with proximal dissections affecting the ascending aorta and arch compared with distal dissections involving the descending thoracic aorta.

**Clinical and molecular genetics**
- Several gene loci are mapped on different chromosomal locations (Table 10.3).
- Mutations in TGFBR1, TGFBR2, MYH11 and ACTA2 account for a large proportion of genetic TAA, including those manifesting with aortic dissections thoracic aortic aneurysm with dissection (TAAD); TGFBR1 is less likely to be causative for non-syndromal TAA/TAAD.
- Some mutations may predispose to aortic dissections but there are no proven genotype–phenotype correlations.
- Genetic counselling is necessary and should include discussion on inheritance pattern, genetic risks, need for long-term surveillance of 'at-risk' close relatives, option for predictive genetic testing, and reproductive choices.
- Clinical management and surveillance should be co-ordinated and supervised by a dedicated multidisciplinary team consisting of cardiologist, specialist cardiac nurse, clinical geneticist, cardiac genetic counsellor, cardio-thoracic surgeon, imaging experts, and counselling support to deal with psychosocial implications.

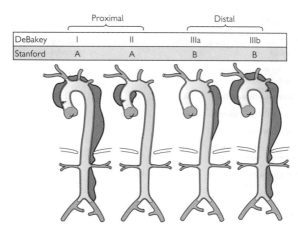

**Fig. 10.9** Classification of aortic dissections—proximal and distal. DeBakey and Stanford classification systems. (Reproduced with permission from *Textbook of Cardiovascular Medicine*, Third Edn, Eric J. Topol, Ed.)

## Genetic counselling

Genetic counselling for familial thoracic aortic aneurysm/dissection is recommended in all cases. This should follow the standard format as for any other incompletely penetrant and clinically variable autosomal dominant inherited disorder. The following guidelines may assist the genetic counsellor or clinician dealing with the affected person or a close relative.

- The majority of individuals diagnosed with familial TAA/TAAD may have an affected parent. It is appropriate to evaluate both parents for manifestations of thoracic aortic aneurysms by performing a comprehensive clinical examination and an echocardiogram to image the ascending aorta and the sinuses of Valsalva and cardiac valves.
- The risk to the sibs of the proband depends upon the status of the parents. If a parent is affected, the risk to the sib of inheriting the disease-causing mutation is 50% (1 in 2); however, because of reduced penetrance, the likelihood that the sib will develop TAA/TAAD is slightly reduced, with increasing risk as the individual increases in age.
- If there are other affected individuals in the extended family, reduced penetrance and variable expression of the disease raise the possibility that sibs could be at risk even if the parents are unaffected.
- The children of an affected parent are at 50% risk of inheriting the mutant allele and the disorder.
- Since the penetrance of TAA/TAAD is reduced, the offspring who inherit a mutant allele from a parent may or may not develop thoracic aortic aneurysms.
- The risk to other family members depends upon the status of the proband's parents, siblings, and offspring. If a parent is found to be affected, other family members are at risk.

**Table 10.3** Inherited thoracic aortic aneurysms

| Designation synonyms/ symbol | OMIM# | Ininheritance | Locus gene allelic variants |
|---|---|---|---|
| Familial thoracic aortic aneurysm type 1; | | | |
| Annulo-aortic ectasia | 607086 | AD | 11q23.3–q24? |
| Familial thoracic aortic | 607087 | AD | 5q13–q14? |
| aneurysm type 2; TAAD1 | | | |
| Familial thoracic aortic aneurysm type 4 | 132900 | AD | 16p13.13–p13.12 MYH11 IVS32+1G |
| Aortic aneurysm/ dissection with patent ductus arteriosus | 160745 | AD | ARG1758GLN; del72exon28 |
| Familial thoracic aortic aneurysm type 6 | 611788 | AD | 10q22–q24 ACTA2 ARG149CYS |
| • aneurysm type 6 aortic aneurysm with livido reticularis and iris flocculi<br>• thoracic aortic aneurysm with aortic dissections (TAAD3) | | | ARG258HIS; ARG258CYS |
| Familial arterial tortuosity LDS1A/ascending aortic dissections | 609192 | AD | 9q33–q34 TGFBR1 MET318ARG; ASP400GLY |
| Loeys–Dietz syndrome: | | | |
| LDS1B | 610168 AD | 3p22 | TGFBR2;YR336ASN; ALA355PRO; GLY357TRP; ARG528HIS; ARG528CYS; IVS1, A–G, THR200ILE; ARG487PRO; SER241LEU |
| LDS2A | 608967 | AD | 9q33–q34 TGFBR1 ARG487GLN; |
| LDS2B | 610380 | AD | 3p22 TGFBR2; GL; N508GLN; LEU308PRO; SER449PHE; ARG537CYS; ARG460CYS; ARG460HIS |

## Genetic testing

Molecular genetic testing in familial TAA/TAAD is not routine. In syndromal forms, mutations in *FBN1*, *TGFBR1* and *TGFBR2* should be considered to facilitate accurate genetic testing. Mutation analysis in *TGFBR2*, *MYH11* and *ACTA2* may be helpful but this is not yet routinely available in clinical setting. Since it is likely that testing methodology and our understanding of genes, mutations, and diseases will improve in the future, consideration should be given to banking DNA of affected individuals (in accordance with local and national guidelines).

## Predictive genetic testing

- First-degree relatives of an affected person and members of the extended family may wish to undergo predictive genetic testing.
- It is only possible if a disease-causing mutation in either *TGFBR2* or *MYH11* is confirmed.
- Mutations in other genes, such as ACTA2, should be verified for pathogenicity prior to being accepted for predictive genetic testing.
- Genetic counselling of such 'at-risk' family members should focus on prior recurrence risk (50% in a first-degree relative), reliability of the known mutation, sensitivity of the mutation, clinical predictability based on evidence for genotype–phenotype correlation, availability of long-term multidisciplinary cardiology surveillance including option for prophylactic aortic reconstructive surgery (☐ see below section on Surveillance), appreciating and understanding the psychosocial implications, and implications for employment, mortgage, life insurance and any other ethical or legal issues.

## Prenatal and pre-implantation genetic testing

Prenatal diagnosis for pregnancies at increased risk for TAA/TAAD may be the preferred option should one of the parents' be affected. This option is only possible if a disease-causing mutation in either *TGFBR2* or *MYH11* is confirmed (☐ see Chapter 4 Genetic counselling) Ultrasound examination in the first two trimesters is insensitive for detecting manifestations of TAA.

Pre-implantation genetic diagnosis (PGD) may be available for families in which the disease-causing mutation has been identified in an affected family member in a research or clinical laboratory. Where this option was considered then enquiries may be made to relevant IVF/fertility clinics. In the UK, an application would be required for permission from the statutory embryology and fertility authority, such as HEFA in the UK.

## Surveillance

Members considered to be at risk for inheriting the genetic predisposition for TAA/TAAD should be examined serially by transthoracic echocardiogram to evaluate the size of the ascending aorta and sinuses of Valsalva. Other imaging modalities, such as MRA and/or CT, to view the entire aorta should be used every four to five years. The frequency of imaging may vary from 2–3 years, but preferably should be carried out annually. The following general recommendations may be useful and should be incorporated in most cases:

- the variable age of onset of the aortic disease in familial TAA/TAAD makes it necessary to begin imaging the aorta of individuals at risk at a relatively young age
- the ultrasound imaging should begin 10 years before the earliest age of onset in the family. In a child this should commence when the child can undergo an echocardiogram without sedation, usually around age 6–7 years
- because penetrance may be reduced in TAA/TAAD, it is appropriate to image any first-degree relative of an affected individual with a familial form, whether they are the parents, siblings, or offspring of the proband
- imaging of sons of women who are at risk but who have a normal echocardiogram should be considered because of the decreased penetrance in women
- isometric exercise and competitive sports that lead to significant blows to the chest should be avoided because they may accelerate aortic root dilatation
- women with TAA/TAAD are advised to obtain pre-pregnancy counselling from a medical geneticist, a genetic counsellor, a cardiologist familiar with this condition, and a high-risk obstetrician
- it is recommended that women who have TAA/TAAD be followed during pregnancy by a cardiologist and a high-risk obstetrician. Serial monitoring of the aorta may be warranted, depending on the pre-pregnancy assessment of the aorta.

# Abdominal aortic aneurysms

Abdominal aortic aneurysm (AAA) is a multi-factorial disorder resulting from complex interaction of hereditary and environmental factors.

Important features of abdominal aortic aneurysms include:
- 6 times more common in men
- in women tends to present a decade later
- incidence has increased over the last 30 years
- 8:1 preponderance of aneurysms in cigarette smokers compared with non-smokers
- 40% of patients with abdominal aortic aneurysms are hypertensive
- hereditary component in 15–25% cases; however, multiple cases in a family are uncommon probably due to pathogenic effects of mutations in low or incompletely penetrant genes
- in most cases, the inheritance pattern is consistent with multi-factorial/polygenic causation with a broad range of environmental factors including age, hyperlipidaemia, diabetes mellitus, and smoking
- recurrence risks in first degree relatives are usually small
- family history and presence of one or more risk factors may identify an at-risk individual
- surveillance by ultrasound examination is recommended in all at-risk persons aged 50 years or above; individual clinical factors may help in determining the frequency and duration of abdominal ultrasound examinations.

## Clinical genetics and genetic counselling

AAAs usually occur sporadically. Two distinct heritable forms are recognised: AAA1 mapped to 19q13 (OMIM609781) and AAA2 mapped to 4q31 (OMIM609782). Important candidate genes involved in AAA include plasminogen activator inhibitor (*PAI1*), tissue inhibitor of metalloproteinase (*TIMP1; TIMP3*), elastin (*ELN*) and type 3 procollagen (*COL3A1*) 4G allele polymorphism in PAI1 gene is considered to offer a protective advantage while 5G allele may increase genetic susceptibility.

The following information should be used in genetic counselling:
- AAA is much more common in men and presents later in women
- familial cases of AAAs are also encountered (OMIM #10070); associated peripheral arterial aneurysms are likely in some familial cases
- some families may follow autosomal dominant inheritance pattern
- bi-allelic or multi-allelic autosomal recessive inheritance pattern is likely
- most familial clustering indicates multifactorial/polygenic etiology
- histological changes indicate chronic inflammation, destructive remodelling of extra cellular matrix, and depletion of vascular smooth muscle cells
- genetic risks may be guided by the family history alone as no reliable molecular tests exist
- clinical assessment and long-term surveillance may be applicable and should be carried out by the specialist vascular team.

## Further reading

Kumar and Elliott (eds) (2010) *Principles and Practice of Clinical Cardiovascular Genetics.* Oxford University Press, New York, 2010, Chapter 11, pp. 157–170; Chapter 12, pp. 171–188; Chapter 28, pp. 401–420.

Loeys BL, *et al.* (2010) The revised Ghent nosology for the Marfan syndrome. *J Med Genet*, **47**, 476–435.

# Familial hypercholesterolaemia

# Familial hypercholesterolaemia

FH is an inborn error of metabolism that leads to accumulation of LDL-C particles in the blood and premature coronary artery atherosclerosis. In most cases it is caused by defects in the LDL receptor (LDL-R) and a reduced number of functional receptors on the surface of the liver that results in a reduce clearance of LDL-C and thus its accumulation in the plasma. The prevalence of heterozygous FH is 1 in 500 of the population for people of European descent. In heterozygous FH serum LDL-C (and total cholesterol) values are approximately double the usual values. The slower clearance of LDL-C particles also leads to a reduction in LDL particle triglyceride content such that serum total triglyceride values for individuals with FH are usually within the normal range.

High-risk populations for FH include the French Canadian population in Quebec (1 in 120), Norway (1 in 300) and the white Afrikaner population in South Africa (1 in 70), all attributable to a founder gene effect. The prevalence of FH in individuals of black and Asian origin appears to be lower though but his may in part be due to under-diagnosis.

## Genetics

- FH is an autosomal dominant condition caused by mutations in the LDLR gene located at 19p13.2, which encodes the low density lipoprotein-receptor.
- More than 1000 different mutations have been reported worldwide
- 65% of the variants are DNA substitutions, 24% (n = 260) small DNA rearrangements (<100bp) and 11% large DNA rearrangements (>100bp).
- Variants occur in all exons, with the highest number in exon 4, which codes for the critical ligand binding region.
- 3% to 5% of British FH patients, have a single mutation in the APOB gene on chromosome 2p (familial defective ApoB (FDB)), which encodes apolipoprotein B, the major protein of the LDL-C particle and ligand for the LDL-R. It is phenotypically indistinguishable from FH. Although usually milder.
- A third form of monogenic hypercholesterolaemia is caused by gain of function mutations in the gene coding protein convertase subtilisin/ kexin type 9 (PCSK9), an enzyme involved in degrading the LDL-R protein in the lysosome of the cell and preventing it recycling.[1] Gain of function mutations in the PCSK9 gene will therefore cause increased degradation of LDL-Rs, reduced numbers of receptors on the surface of the cell and monogenic hypercholesterolaemia.

## Premature coronary heart disease (CHD)

- The coronary arteries are particularly affected in FH.
- The incidence of clinical CHD by age 50 years in untreated heterozygous males and females is 50% and 30%, respectively.
- Homozygotes often present with CHD in childhood.

- The risk of CHD is influenced by other cardiovascular risk factors (male gender, smoking, low levels of HDL, elevated Lp(a)).
- Carotid intimal thickening can occur in FH, but there is no increased incidence of stroke or peripheral vascular disease.

Valve disease

- Aortic stenosis occurs In homozygous FH aortic stenosis due to lipid deposition; this can sometimes occur to a milder extent in heterozygotes.

1. Kwon Lagace TA *et al* (2008) Molecular basis for LDL receptor secognition by PCSK9, *Proc Natl Acad Sci USA*, **105**, 1820–5.

# Treatment of familial hypercholesteroaemia

## Lifestyle
- Smoking cessation (or prevention in children).
- Dietary measures have a relatively small (less than 10%) effect on serum cholesterol values and excessively restrictive diets should be avoided (particularly in children).
- Nutriceutical products, stanols and sterols, which inhibit cholesterol absorption, can reduce serum LDL-C by approximately 10%.

## HMG-CoA reductase inhibitors (statins)
- HMG-CoA reductase is is the rate limiting step for endogenous cholesterol synthesis.
- Inhibition of HMGCoA reductase In hyperlipidaemic patients including heterozygous FH, leads to an upregulation of LDL-R expression on the cell surface and increased internalization of LDL-C from the blood.
- Statins lower LDL-C concentrations by 30–55%.
- NICE Guideline for FH recommends titration to achieve a greater than 50% reduction of LDL-C from baseline levels.
- Statins are less effective in homozygous FH patients due to the lack (or very low level) of functioning LDL receptors.

## Cholesterol absorption inhibitors (Ezetimibe)
- Ezetimibe is a specific inhibitor of cholesterol absorption in the brush border of the small intestine. This reduces the absorption of dietary cholesterol, blocks the re-uptake of cholesterol secreted in the bile and causes net flux of cholesterol from the liver and a compensatory upregulation of cell surface LDL receptors.
- Ezetimibe has a modest LDL-C lowering action when used as monotherapy, but increases the LDL-C lowering effect of statins by 15–20%.
- NICE guidelines recommend Ezetemibe for FH patients as an adjunct to statins or where statins are not tolerated or are contraindicated.

## Other lipid-lowering medications
- Bile acid sequestrants, nicotinic acid derivatives and fibrates.
- Mostly used as third line agents.

## LDL apheresis
- This is the treatment of choice for individuals with homozygous FH
- It removes LDL from the blood by absorption onto a column via an extra corporeal circulation every two weeks.
- It usually requires an arteriovenous fistula.
- LDL apheresis is occasionally used in heterozygous FH patients for whom medication is ineffective or not tolerated if there is severe and progressive coronary artery disease despite treatment.
- The indications for LDL apheresis have recently been considered by a UK working group[1] and also by the NICE clinical guideline development group on FH.[2]

- Antisense oligonucleotides.
- Experimental treatment for homozygous FH.
- Oligonucleotides directed against messenger RNA for apolipoprotein B inhibit hepatic apoB synthesis and LDL production.
- Oligonucleotides are given as subcutaneous injections. Phase 1 and Phase II studies have demonstrated a significant reduction in plasma LDL-C concentrations (30–50%) with weekly subcutaneous injections and appear to be well tolerated.

## Drug treatment of children

- The timing of therapy in children is debated and depends on clinical judgement, patient preference and family history.
- Nice guidance recommends treatment of children with FH from the age of 10 onwards, especially in families with a history of early onset coronary disease.

## Drug treatment of girls and women of childbearing potential

- Statins in the three months preceding conception or in the early stages of pregnancy may increase in the incidence of congenital fetal abnormalities.
- Current advice recommends treatment of girls from the age of 10 providing that there are clear plans for family planning.

1. Thompson GR, Heart UK LDL Apheresis working group  (2008) Recommendations for the use of LDL apheresis. *Atherosclerosis*, **198**, 247–55.
2. NICE (2008) Familial hypercholesterolaemia. Identification and management of familial hypercholesterolaemia. http://www.nice.org.uk/cg071.

# Coronary artery disease and myocardial infarction

# Introduction

The main causal and treatable risk factors for coronary artery disease (CAD) and myocardial infarction (MI) are hypertension, hypercholesterolaemia or dyslipidemia, diabetes mellitus, and smoking.

Twin and family studies have established that CAD aggregates in families, with a family history of early-onset CAD a risk factor for the disease independent of known risk factors. The highest relative hazard of CAD-related death is seen in monozygotic twins. A history of early-onset CAD in a first-degree relative approximately doubles an individuals risk of CAD (relative risk range 1.3 to 11.3).

High-risk families account for a substantial proportion of early-onset (men aged <55 years, women aged <65 years) CAD cases in the general population (14% of the general population but 72% of early-onset CAD cases).

The common forms of CAD and MI are thought to be multifactorial and determined by many genes, each with a relatively small effect, working alone or in combination with other modifier genes and/or environmental factors.

The 'common disease, common variants hypothesis' proposes that genetic variants present in many normal individuals contribute to overall CAD risk. Susceptibility to some common diseases may be conferred by rarer variants.

# Mendelian disorders associated with coronary artery disease

**Familial hypercholesterolemia**

&#x1F4D6; See Chapter 11, Familial hypercholesterolaemia.

**Tangier disease**

Rare allelic variants of genes influencing high-density lipoprotein (HDL)—cholesterol metabolism, including the ATP-binding cassette, subfamily A, member 1 (ABCA1), apolipoprotein A-I (APOA1), and lecithin-cholesterol acyltransferase (LCAT), are associated with low plasma HDL-cholesterol. Tangier disease is a rare autosomal recessive disorder caused by loss-of-function mutations in ABCA1.

It is characterized by:
- diffuse deposition of cholesterol esters throughout the reticuloendothelial system
- enlarged yellow tonsils
- low plasma HDL-cholesterol
- early onset of CAD.

# Candidate gene studies

Association studies based on the candidate gene approach have revealed a large number of polymorphisms to be associated with the prevalence of MI or CAD (📖 See Further reading).

These include:

**5,10-methylenetetrahydrofolate reductase (MTHFR)**

- Individuals with the 677C→T (Ala222Val) substitution of MTHFR have reduced MTHFR activity and higher plasma homocysteine levels.
- A meta-analysis of the association of the 677C→T (Ala222Val) polymorphism with CAD risk in 11,162 cases and 12,758 controls from 40 studies revealed an odds ratio of 1.16 for CAD in individuals with the TT genotype compared with the CC genotype.
- A second meta-analysis in 26,000 cases and 31,183 controls from 80 studies showed an overall odds ratio of 1.14 for the TT genotype versus the CC genotype but with geographic variation in the risk (odds ratio of 1.0 for Europe, Australia, and North America compared to 2.61 and 1.23 for the Middle East and Asia, respectively).
- Geographic variability may be explained by higher folate intake in Western countries.

**Lipoprotein lipase**

- Lipoprotein lipase (LPL) is the rate-limiting enzyme in lipolysis of triglyceride-rich lipoproteins in the circulation. LPL also plays an important role in the receptor-mediated removal of lipoproteins from the circulation.
- LPL is polymorphic, with amino acid substitutions of the encoded protein affecting triglyceride and HDL-cholesterol levels, which are implicated in atherosclerosis risk.

**Apolipoprotein E**

- Apolipoprotein E (ApoE) has an important role in lipid transport and metabolism.
- Three common alleles (ε2, ε3, and ε4) encode the three major isoforms (E2, E3, and E4) of ApoE, which differ at amino acid positions 112 and 158.
- Allelic variation of APOE accounts for variability in total cholesterol and LDL-cholesterol concentrations (ε4 and ε2 alleles increased and decreased LDL-cholesterol levels, respectively).
- A meta-analysis of 15,492 subjects with CAD and 32,965 controls from 48 studies showed that carriers of the ε4 allele had a higher risk for CAD (odds ratio 1.42), than those with the ε3/ε3 genotype; the ε2 allele was not associated with CAD risk.

## Genome-wide association studies

GWAS have identified a number of susceptibility genes for CAD and MI. In 2007, independent GWAS based on the use of SNP chips identified four SNPs on chromosome 9p21.3 that were associated with CAD or MI in several white cohorts. Several SNPs at 9p21.3 that were significantly associated with type 2 diabetes mellitus in white populations in England, Finland and Sweden were also identified.

The underlying mechanism of this association is still unknown. The region is defined by two flanking recombination hot spots and contains the coding sequences of genes for two cyclin-dependent kinase inhibitors, CDKN2A and CDKN2B. These have an important role in regulation of the cell cycle and belong to a family of genes that have been implicated in the pathogenesis of atherosclerosis through inhibition of cell growth by transforming growth factor—$\beta$1. However, the SNPs associated most strongly with MI or CAD are a long way upstream of these genes.

The high-risk CAD haplotype at 9p21.3 overlaps with exons 13 to 19 of ANRIL, a gene that encodes a large antisense non-coding RNA. ANRIL is expressed in atheromatous human vessels and vascular endothelial cells, monocyte-derived macrophages, and coronary smooth muscle cells. The function of ANRIL is unknown.

### Further reading

Kumar D. Elliott P. (eds) (2010) *Principles and Practice of Clinical Cardiovascular Genetics*, Oxford University Press, New York, pp. 315–328.

# Stroke

# Stroke

## Epidemiology

- Stroke is the third most common cause of death and the most common cause of disability in developed countries.
- Prevalence of stroke in UK is 0.9 million.
- Annual incidence of stroke (first or recurrent) is 133,000.
- 70–80% of strokes are ischaemic caused by atherosclerosis (large-artery disease), cardioembolism, and small-vessel disease (lacunar stroke).
- Approx 13% intracerebral hemorrhage, and 6% subarachnoid hemorrhage.
- Non-modifiable risk factors (age, African and Asian background, male sex) and acquired risk factors (hypertension, cigarette smoking, diabetes, atrial fibrillation, and obesity) account for much of the risk of ischaemic stroke.

## Genetics

- Twin, sibling, and family studies suggest evidence for heritability of common forms of stroke.
- The association is stronger for younger individuals, and those with the large artery disease and small vessel disease subtypes of stroke.
- A family history of myocardial infarction is more common in large-vessel stroke than in other stroke subtypes.
- The incidence of ischaemic and haemorrhagic stroke varies among ethnic groups.

## Single gene causes of stroke

Several conditions in which stroke occur are inherited in a classical Mendelian pattern as autosomal dominant, autosomal recessive, or X-linked disorders. In most, stroke is just one component of the disease phenotype (Table 13.1).

**Table 13.1** Monogenic or single gene disorders causing stroke, classified according stroke subtype

| Stroke subtype | Specific monogenic disease |
| --- | --- |
| Small vessel disease | CADASIL |
| | CARASIL |
| | Cerebrovascular retinopathy and HERNS |
| | COL4A1 small vessel arteriopathy with haemorrhage |
| Large artery atherosclerosis and other arteriopathies | Familial hyperlipidaemias |
| | Moya–Moya disease |
| | Pseudoxanthoma elasticum |
| | Neurofibromatosis type I |
| Large artery disease—dissection | Ehlers–Danlos syndrome type IV |
| | Marfan syndrome |
| | Fibromuscular dysplasia |
| Disorders affecting both small and large arteries | Fabry disease |
| | Homocysteinuria |
| | Sickle cell disease |
| Cardioembolism | Familial cardiomyopathies |
| | Familial arrhythmias |
| | Hereditary haemorrhagic telangiectasia |
| Prothrombotic disorders | |
| Mitochondrial disorders | MELAS |

From Marcus H. (2010) Unravelling the genetics of ischaemic stroke. *PLoS Med* 7(3): e1000225.)

Rare disorders in which it is the prominent or sole clinical manifestation include:

### Cerebral arteriopathy, autosomal dominant, with subcortical infarcts and leukoencephalopathy (CADASIL)

- Caused by mutation of the notch, drosophila, homolog of 3 gene (NOTCH3) (human chromosome 19q12).
- A heritable small-vessel disease.
- Recurrent strokes and transient ischaemic attacks.
- Progressive cognitive impairment and psychiatric disturbance.
- Onset usually in the third to sixth decade.
- About a third of patients develop migraine with aura.

- Neuroimaging similar to sporadic small-vessel disease.
- Bilateral involvement of the anterior temporal white matter characteristic.

### CARASIL (cerebral autosomal recessive arteriopathy with subcortical infarcts and leukoencephalopathy)
- Lacunar stroke, leukoaraiosis, and early-onset vascular dementia.
- Caused by mutations in the HtrA serine protease 1 (*HTRA1*) gene, involved in transforming growth factor-beta (TGF-β) signalling.

### Autosomal dominant retinal vasculopathy with cerebral leukodystrophy
- Microvascular endotheliopathy presenting with visual loss, stroke, and dementia.
- Onset in middle age.
- C-terminal frameshift mutations in *TREX1*, which encodes a DNA-specific 3′ to 5′ exonuclease.

### Autosomal-dominant porencephaly and infantile hemiparesis
- Mutations in *COL4A1*, a gene encoding type IV collagen alpha1 chain.
- Adult-onset white matter ischaemic changes consistent with small vessel disease with microbleeds in the absence of infantile hemiparesis or intracerebral haemorrhage.

### Cerebral hemorrhage with amyloidosis, hereditary
- **Dutch type** (HCHWA-D) caused by mutation in the amyloid beta A4 precursor protein gene (APP).
- **Icelandic type** (HCHWA-I) due to mutations in the gene coding for cystatin 3 (CST3).

These disorders are characterized by the development of cerebral hemorrhage at an age of 40–50 years for HCHWA-D and 20–30 years for HCHWA-I. Both are associated with amyloid deposition in cortical and leptomeningeal arterioles.[1]

### Mutations of the integral membrane protein 2B gene (ITM2B)
Autosomal dominant amyloid angiopathies. Clinically characterized by cerebral hemorrhage and/or vascular dementia.

### The krev interaction trapped 1 gene (KRIT1)
One of the genes responsible for cavernous angiomas.

## Polygenic inheritance
- The genetic contribution to common multifactorial stroke seems to be polygenic.
- There appear to be many alleles with small effect sizes (relative risk <1.5) that may be limited to one or few stroke subtypes vary with depending gender and ethnic origin.
- Candidate gene studies in ischaemic stroke suggest associattions with polymorphisms in: 5.10-methylenetetrahydrofolate reductase MTHFR, ACE, factor V Leiden, prothrombin, PAI1, phosphodiesterase 4D (PDE4D), ALOX5AP.

1. Hademenos GJ, *et al.* (2001) Advances in the genetics of cerebrovascular disease and stroke, *Neurology*, **56**, 997–1008.

# Pulmonary arterial hypertension

# Pulmonary arterial hypertension

## Definitions

- Mean pulmonary artery pressure greater than 25mmHg at rest or greater than 30mmHg during exercise *and* a normal pulmonary artery wedge pressure (less than or equal to 12mmHg at rest).
- Idiopathic pulmonary arterial hypertension (PAH) occurs in the absence of known causes and without a family history of the disease (Box 14.1).
- Familial disease is defined by the presence of two or more relatives with idiopathic disease.

## Epidemiology

- Estimated incidence of one to two per million population per year.
- Prevalence from autopsy studies ranges from 83–1302 per million in unselected cases.
- Higher incidence in of idiopathic PAH in women. Range of estimates1.7:1 to 4.2:1 (females to males).

## Clinical features

Symptoms and signs depend on severity of PAH

- Breathlessness (60%), fatigue (19%), and fainting (8%)
- With progression of disease, patients may experience chest pain, palpitations and other symptoms of right heart failure
- Raynaud's phenomenon (10%)
- Haemoptysis and hoarseness (from left recurrent laryngeal nerve compression by an enlarged pulmonary artery—Ortner syndrome)
- Sudden death
- Central cyanosis (20%)
- Peripheral oedema (32%)
- Raised JVP with prominent *a* and *v* waves
- Right ventricular heave
- Increased pulmonary component of the second heart sound (P2)
- Right-sided third and fourth heart sounds
- Tricuspid and pulmonary regurgitation

**Box 14.1 International symposium classification of pulmonary hypertension, 2003 (Venice) (from Launay, 2003)**

*1. Pulmonary arterial hypertension:*
- Idiopathic
- Familial (at least two affected individuals in one family)
- Related to collagen vascular disease, congenital heart disease, portal hypertension, human immunodeficiency virus, drugs, and toxins
- With significant venous and/or capillary involvement
- Persistent pulmonary hypertension of the newborn

*2. Pulmonary hypertension with left heart disease:*
- Atrial or ventricular disease
- Valvular heart disease

*3. Pulmonary hypertension with lung disease and/or hypoxaemia:*
- Chronic obstructive pulmonary disease
- Interstitial lung disease
- Sleep disorders; alveolar hypoventilation; chronic exposure to high altitude
- Developmental abnormalities

*4. Pulmonary hypertension due to chronic thrombotic and/or embolic disease:*
- Thromboembolic obstruction of proximal pulmonary arteries
- Thromboembolic obstruction of distal pulmonary arteries
- Pulmonary embolism (tumour, parasites, foreign material)

*5. Others:*
Sarcoidosis, histiocytosis X, lymphangiomatosis, pulmonary vessel compression (adenopathies, tumours, fibrosing mediastinitis).

# Familial pulmonary arterial hypertension

- Approximately 6% of patients have at least one first-degree relative with PAH
- More common in females
- Disease expression is age-related (10% by 10 years of age and 92% by 70 years of age)
- Incomplete penetrance and variable clinical expression are common.

## Genetics

- 70% of familial (or heritable) and approximately 20% of idiopathic PAH caused by mutations in bone morphogenic protein receptor type 2 (BMPR2) (member of the TGF-β superfamily that control many cellular functions, including proliferation, migration, differentiation, apoptosis, and extracellular matrix secretion and deposition).
- Population carrier frequency for BMPR2 mutations estimated to be 0.001% to 0.01%.
- Approximately 41% BMPR2 mutations are small deletions or insertions at sites of low-complexity sequence or as a consequence of C>T transitions.
- Two further receptor members of the transforming growth factor (TGF)-β cell signalling superfamily—activin-like kinase-type 1 (ALK1) and endoglin (ENG)—cause hereditary hemorrhagic telangiectasia (HHT) and may rarely cause PAH (see Chapter 15).

## Clinical features of familial PAH

- The clinical, histopathology and prognosis same as sporadic idiopathic PAH.

## Clinical screening of relatives

- Screening is recommended in order to prevent irreversible pulmonary vascular disease
- Screening should include:
  - a thorough history and examination
  - transthoracic echocardiogram
  - exercise stress echo (in specialized laboratories)
  - chest X-ray
  - ECG
- Screen at the time of diagnosis of the index case, if symptomatic or every three years in asymptomatic individuals.
- If estimated pulmonary artery pressure is greater than 40mmHg, cardiac catheterization is recommended.

# Hereditary haemorrhagic telangiectasia

# Introduction

Hereditary haemorrhagic telangiectasia (HHT) was previously known as Osler–Rendu–Weber syndrome.

- Autosomal dominant condition characterized by telangiectasia, arteriovenous malformations of systemic and pulmonary vessels.
- Prevalence estimated to be 1 in 5–8000 people.
- Described in all racial groups but more frequently in the Dutch Antilles, parts of France and the Danish island of Funen and Fyn.
- Frequency same in males and females.

## Genetics

Caused by mutations in genes encoding proteins that modulate transforming growth factor (TGF)-ß superfamily signalling in vascular endothelial cells. Three HHT disease-causing genes have been identified (Table 15.1). There are at least two unidentified genes that can cause classical HHT. ENG mutations are most common (61%) followed by ACVR L1 mutations (37%) and SMAD4 (2%).

**Table 15.1** Identified HHT disease-causing genes

| HHT | OMIM | Chromosome | Gene symbol | Protein |
|---|---|---|---|---|
| HHT type 1 | #187300 | 9 | ENG | Endoglin |
| HHT type 2 | #600376 | 12 | ACVRL1 | Activin receptor-like kinase ALK-1 |
| HT associated with juvenile polyposis | #175050 | 18 | SMAD4 | Smad 4 |
| HHT3 | #601101 | 5 | – | – |
| HHT4 | #610655 | 7 | – | – |

There is the variability between different affected members of the same HHT family.

Prenatal diagnosis is technically feasible is rarely undertaken because of longevity and asymptomatic state of most HHT patients.

A positive molecular diagnosis does not modify management, except in families with a history of gastrointestinal polyps/malignancy and a Smad4 mutation when regular gastrointestinal screening should be performed.

## Clinical features of HHT

- Epistaxis is present in up to 96% of patients and is usually the earliest clinical symptom of HHT.
- Facial and buccal telangiectasia from 3rd decade onwards.
- Arteriovenous malformations (particularly brain, liver and lungs).
- Gastrointestinal haemorrhage.

- Juvenile polyposis.
- Prothrombotic state.
- Immune dysfunction.

### The Curacao criteria

Definite diagnosis of HHT in the presence of at least three separate manifestations:
- spontaneous recurrent nosebleeds
- mucocutaneous telangiectasia (multiple at characteristic
- sites: fingertip pulps, lips, oral mucosa or tongue)
- visceral involvement (gastrointestinal, pulmonary, hepatic, cerebral or spinal arteriovenous malformation [AVM])
- family history: a first-degree relative affected according to these criteria.

An estimated 10% of patients experience major HHT-related complications including:
- Severe anaemia from chronic nasal and gastrointestinal haemorrhage.
- Stroke:
  - (ischaemic and brain abscess from pulmonary AVMs)
  - haemorrhagic from cerebral AVMs).
- Deep venous thromboses.

More rarely:
- Symptomatic liver disease requiring liver transplantation.
- Severe pulmonary hypertension (from multiple secondary causes in HHT or an arterial hypertension phenotype indistinguishable from PAH).
- Pregnancy-related death.
- Spinovascular accidents.

### Treatment

Screening protocols for AVM in asymptomatic patients vary between countries. Most screen for pulmonary AVM using contrast echo and/or CT angiography.
- Iron +/− transfusions for anaemia.
- Nasal humidification; packing in emergencies.
- ENT: laser; surgery.
- Embolization of AVM (particularly lung).
- Systemic: oestrogen–progesterone.
- Antifibrinolytics.
- Liver transplant.

# Cardiac manifestations in inherited skeletal muscle disease

# Introduction

A number of inherited neuromuscular disorders may manifest with cardiac symptoms or signs (Table 16.1). In some cases this may be the first presentation of the neuromuscular disease. A close search for clues in the family history may reveal other individuals affected with a Mendelian neuromuscular condition, for example Duchenne–Becker muscular dystrophy, myotonic dystrophy, Emery–Dreifuss muscular dystrophy etc. This important subject is reviewed by Bushby et al.[1]

Cardiovascular manifestations in inherited neuromuscular disorders are not uncommon. Some disorders are relatively well known to be associated with cardiac involvement. It is possible that the lack of evidence for cardiac involvement in some conditions may reflect gaps in our understanding of the pathogenesis. In some conditions this may be due to insufficient information on the key components such as electrophysiological and histopathological changes. This brief overview provides some basic information on the cardiac involvement in the key inherited neuromuscular conditions (Table 16.2). Cardiac manifestations may be in the form of incidental ECG changes, vague symptoms like palpitation, fatigue, dizzy spells, and generally feeling unwell. Occasionally the individual may be confirmed to have a significant and fairly advanced cardiac pathology like cardiomyopathy or dysrhythmia.

1. Bushby K, Munron F and Bourke SP (2003) 107th ENMC international workshop: the management of cardiac involvement in muscular dystrophy and myotonic dystrophy. 7th–9th June 2002, Naarden, the Netherlands, *Neuromuscul Disord*, **13**, 166–172.

**Table 16.1** Summary of main cardiac findings in neuromuscular disease

| Disorder | OMIM # | Cardiac symptoms/signs | Cardiologic abnormalities |
|---|---|---|---|
| Myotonic dystrophy type 1 (DM1) | 160900 | Dysrhythmia—very common due to selective involvement of the specialized conducting tissue, may present with sudden cardiac death, bradycardia, first-degree heart block and other conduction abnormalities | Bradycardia |
| | | | Prolongation of the PR interval—progression to complete heart block |
| | | Cardiomyopathy—very rare in myotonic dystrophy, except for subclinical evidence on echo or MRI | Left axis deviation (LAD) due to left anterior hemiblock (LAH) |
| | | | Bundle branch block (LBBB or RBBB) |
| | | | Bifasicular block (RBBB and LAH) |
| | | | Atrial fibrillation/flutter |
| Myotonic dystrophy type 2 (proximal myotonic myopathy; PROMM or DM2) | 602668 | Cardiac arrhythmias | ECG/EPS |
| Duchenne muscular dystrophy (DMD) | 310200 | Cardiac death 10–20% usually teens | DMD |
| | | | ECG abnormal >90%, detectable from 6yrs age |
| Becker muscular dystrophy (BMD) | 300376 | Dilated cardiomyopathy | ECHO abnormal >90% HCM and DCM |
| | | X-linked DCM—probably within the BMD spectrum without skeletal muscle involvement | Dysrhythmia |
| | | | Cardiac death 10–20% usually teens |
| | | | BMD |
| | | | ECG abnormal 45%[1]; 90%[2] |

(Continued)

**Table 16.1** (Contd.)

| Disorder | OMIM # | Cardiac symptoms/signs | Cardiologic abnormalities |
|---|---|---|---|
| | | | ECHO abnorm. 17% DCM[1] 65% HCM and DCM[2] |
| | | | Unrelated to phenotype/severity of MD |
| | | | Dysrhythmia |
| | | | Cardiac death up to 50%[2] |
| | | | Manifesting carriers |
| | | | ECG abnormal 21–90%, variable |
| | | | ECHO abnormal 7–11% HCM and DCM |
| | | | Dysrhythmia |
| | | | Very disproprtionate to skeletal involvement |
| | | | Cardiac death:?%. Successful transplants reported[2] |
| | | | Unaffected carriers 10% develop CCF[3] |
| X-linked cardiomyopathy (CMD3B) | 302045 | Dilated cardiomyopathy with minimal skeletal muscle involvement | Echo/MRI changes of HCM/DCM |
| Congenital muscular dystrophy (MDC) | | Rarely cardiac arrhythmias | ECG/ECHO |
| • Merosin (laminin α2 chain) positive | 609456 | | |

| Condition | OMIM | Features | Cardiac |
|---|---|---|---|
| • Merosin negative<br>• Fukuyama type<br>• (Walker–Warburg (with muscle, eye and brain abnormalities) | 607855<br>253800<br>236670 | | |
| Emery–Dreifuss muscular dystrophy: X-linked (EDMD1) | 310300 | No pseudohypertrophy; contractures around elbow, hands, knees—usually before 10yrs, cardiac involvement the rule, symmetrical limb weakness (adult onset)—proximal UL, distal LL; Cardiac conduction defect may manifest with sudden cardiac death | Cardiac—>95% ECG abnormal by 30yrs<br>Dysrhythmia—characteristic atrial standstill (AV block), bradycardia, prolonged PR, AF/flutter<br>Atrial involvement- risk of TIA/CVA (anticoagulate)<br>Cardiomyopathy—exceptionally rare<br>SCD common in unpaced individuals, preventive pacemaker RECOMMENDED (mean age 24yrs)<br>Death rare after pacemaker insertion (X-linked)<br>Carriers—periodic ECG surveillance recommended |
| Emery–Dreifuss: autosomal dominant type (EDMD2) | 181350 | >95% conduction anomalies by 30yrs<br>35% DCM 19–55yrs<br>Mean age at pacing 32yrs (19–57)<br>SCD in 50% (despite pacing)<br>Implantable defibrillators may be more approp. | Duboch—69 deaths,[4]<br>32 sudden (12 paced)<br>Ventric dysrhythmia suspected<br>Van Berla et al in Banne et al reviewed 20 publications<br>Heart failure—26% (64% >50yrs) |

(Continued)

**Table 16.1** (Contd.)

| Disorder | OMIM # | Cardiac symptoms/signs | Cardiologic abnormalities |
|---|---|---|---|
| | | | Conduction anomaly—61% (91% >30yrs) |
| | | | Pacemaker (PM) —44% >30yrs |
| | | | 38% paced died vs 21% without |
| | | | Pacemaker DID NOT prevent sudden cardiac death in LMNA |
| | | | PM not recommended but ICD |
| Emery–Dreifuss autosomal recessive type (EDMD3) | 604929 | Probably less common cardiac involvement | Normal cardiologic investigations in the affected and normal consanguineous parents |
| Limb-girdle muscular dystrophy | | | |
| LGMD2A | 253600 | 'LGMD' is a phenotypic description | |
| LGMD2B | 253601 | LL before and more severe than UL | |
| | | Symmetrical | |
| LGMD2C | 253700 | AR, most childhood, often severe (SCARMD) | |
| LGMD2D | 608099 | Wide range of proteins—mainly structural | |
| LGMD2E | 604286 | Sarcoglycans (LGMD2C-2F) | |
| LGMD2F | 601287 | Cardiac involvement in 20% (ECG, HCM, DCM)[1] | |
| LGMD2G | 601954 | | |
| LGMD2H | 254110 | | |

| | | | |
|---|---|---|---|
| Limb-girdle muscular dystrophy<br>LGMD2J | 608807 | Titin-related dilated cardiomyopathy<br>Progessive heart failure<br>Skeletal muscle weakness of the limb-girdle type | Echo/MRI changes of DCM |
| Desminopathies<br>MFM/RCM11<br>RCM2 | 601419<br>609578 | Restrictive cardiomyopathy<br>Cardiac conduction blocks<br>Arrythmias | ECG/EPS studies—dysrrhythmias<br>Echo/MRI changes of DCM |
| Limb-girdle muscular dystrophy<br>LGMD2I Fukutin-related protein (FKRP) | 606596 | AR—widely availble variable phenotype<br>a. More severe phenotype<br>   Onset <2yrs, hypotonia<br>b. DMD-type onset, waddling gait, mild facial weakness<br>   Cardiomyopathy<br>c. Mild phenotype<br>   Onset 2nd or 3rd decade, CPK 750–10,000<br>   Mild facial weakness, can affect UL>LL<br>   Calf brachioradialis hypertrophy (tongue hypertrophy recorded)<br>d. Can present with cardiomyopathy alone or primarily<br>   Exercise related muscle cramps<br>   European common mutation—C826A exon 4 | More than 50% with cardiac disease[5]<br>symptomatic LVF<br>Responsive to ACE inhibitors and diuretics<br>ECHO—LV impairment<br>ECG SR, frequent atrial ectopics, Q-waves<br>subclinical impairment<br>ECHO—ejection fraction reduced to 50%<br>ECG—notched p waves (PR, QRS, QT norm) |

(Continued)

**Table 16.1** (Contd.)

| Disorder | OMIM # | Cardiac symptoms/signs | Cardiologic abnormalities |
|---|---|---|---|
| Limb-girdle muscular dystrophy | | AD forms of LGMD1A-1E—later onset, wide range of severity | |
| LGMD1A | 159000 | LGMD1B and AD EDMD—same Lamin A/C deficiency | |
| LGMD1B | 159001 | >95% conduction anomalies by 30yrs | |
| LGMD1C | 607801 | 35% DCM 19–55yrs | |
| | | Mean age at pacing 32yrs (19–57) | |
| | | SCD in 50% (despite pacing) | |
| | | Implantable defibrillators may be more appropriate | |
| | | Uncommonly DCM | |
| Facio–scapulo–humeral muscular dystrophy (FSHMD1) | 158900 | Minor/subclinical cardiac conduction abnormalities; minor cardiac muscle involvement; heart failure in late stage probably secondary to generalized weakness | Once thought not to occur |
| | | | More sensitive to electrophysiological stimulation |
| | | | Direct intracardiac programmed electrical stimulation |
| | | | AF or flutter could be induced in 80% FSHD pts vs 17% controls[6] |
| | | | Subclinical impairments |
| | | | SPECT—abnormal fibrosis in 5/7 FSHD (Yamamoto et al. 1988) |
| | | | Tl-201-SPECT—3/4 abnormal, 2/4 abnormal stress test |
| | | | Rogers (2009)[7], of > 100 patients seen, 5 with definite cardiac disease—2 cardiomyopathy, 2 conduction anomalies, 1 undiagnosed CCF; suggests low but definite cardiac risk |

| | | | low but definite cardiac risk | |
|---|---|---|---|---|
| Barth syndrome | 302060 | Skeletal muscle weakness, developmental delay, neutropenia, dilated cardiomyopathy | | ECG/ECHO recommended in affected and carrier females |
| | | Carrier females are generally asymptomatic | | |
| Bethlem myopathy | 158810 | Probably less common; benign disorder with contractures | | ECG; ECHO recommended |

1. de Visser M, de Voogt WG, la Riviere GA (1992) The heart in Becker muscular dystrophy, facioscapulohumeral dystrophy and Bethlem myopathy. *Muscle & Nerve* **15**: 591–596.

2. Bushby K, et al. (2003) 107th ENMC international workshop: the management of cardiac involvement in muscular dystrophy and myotonic dystrophy. 7th-9th June 2002, Naarden, the Netherlands. *Neuromuscul. Disord.* **13**: 166–172.

3. Hoogerwaard EM, et al. (1999) Cardiac involvement in carriers of Duchenne and Becker muscular dystrophy. *Neuromuscul. Disord.* **9**: 347–351.

4. Duboc D, Eymard B, Damian MS (2004). Cardiac management of myotonic dystrophy.*Myotonic dystrophy: present management, future therapy*, Oxford University Press, Oxford (eds. Harper PS, van Engelen BGM, Eymard B and Wilcox DE).

5. Poppe M, et al. (2004) Cardiac and respiratory failure in Limb-Girdle Muscular Dystrophy 2I. *Ann Neurol.* **56**: 738–741.

6. Stevenson WG, et al. (1990) Facioscapulohumeral muscular dystrophy: evidence for selective genetic electrophysiologic cardiac involvement. *JACC* **15**: 292–299.

7. Rogers MT (2009) Facioscapulohumeral muscular dystrophy – a clinical, audiometric and pathological study. Thesis , London University.

**Table 16.2** A short list of the most common muscular dystrophies with prominent cardiac involvement

| Disease | Involvement | Inheritance | Protein | Prevalence/10,000 |
|---|---|---|---|---|
| Duchenne MD | Cardiomyopathy | XL-R | Dystrophin | 8.76 |
| Becker MD | Cardiomyopathy | XL-R | Dystrophin | 7.29 |
| Myotonic dystrophy | Dysrhythmia | AD | DMPK | 10.4 |
| EDMD (XL-R) | Dysrhythmia | XL-R | Emerin | 0.13 |
| EDMD (AD) | Dysrhythmia | AD | Lamin A/C | 0.20 |
| LGMD2I | Cardiomyopathy | AR | Fukutin-related protein | 0.43 |

Since these diseases are primarily diseases of skeletal muscle it is most usual for them to present with primary muscle disease first, and later for the individual to develop signs or symptoms of cardiac disease (e.g. DMD). Occasionally however individuals may present with cardiomyopathy (or respiratory muscle disease) prior to the recognition of skeletal muscle disease (e.g. LGMD2I, or acid maltase deficiency). Similarly diseases that are usually thought to only affect the skeletal muscle may occasionally affect the heart (e.g. facioscapulohumeral muscular dystrophy [FSHD]) and vice versa individuals with cardiomyopathies may develop skeletal muscle weakness.

Family history

Inherited neuromuscular disease may be inherited in a number of different ways. The inheritance pattern will affect the differential diagnosis, investigations and management both for the affected individual and their relatives (particularly first-degree relatives, but sometimes quite distant relatives). At least a three-generation family tree is therefore essential. Particular clues to be looked for in conditions with cardiac involvement:
- a family history of sudden cardiac/unexplained death
- only males affected or males and females equally affected (XL-R or not)
- isolated case or single sibship autosomal recessive (AR) but may be new dominant
- male to male transmission autosomal dominant (AD), and excludes X-linked recessive (XL-R) and mitochondrial inheritance)
- transmission through the female line only (mitochondrial)
- muscle disease more prominent than heart disease
- a family history of pacemakers/ICDs
- older generations with cataracts alone, youngest generation with congenital disease or neonatal death/stillbirth (DM1).

## Summary of key features

- Will usually affect skeletal muscle first.
- Cardiac involvement will tend to narrow the differential diagnosis to a limited number of commoner conditions.
  - Cardiomyopathy—most likely DMD, BMD or limb girdle muscular dystrophy type-2 (LGMD2I).
  - Dysrhythmia—most likely DM1or Emery-Dreiffus muscular dystrophy (EDMD) (AD or XL-R).
  - once these are excluded it is more likely the patient has a rare complication of one of the other dystrophies/myopathies; or a has a rare diagnosis.
- Key clinical features:
  - cardiomyopathy, childhood loss of ambulation, male, calf pseudohypertrophy—DMD
  - heart block, distal weakness, cataracts, balding, facial weakness, ptosis, grip stiffness/myotonia—DM1
  - dysrhythmia, contractures out of proportion to weakness (elbows especially), proximal weakness of upper limb, distal lower limb, pacemaker/ICD, family history (FHx) of sudden death—EDMD
  - cardiomyopathy, proximal weakness of lower limb, pseudohypertrophy of calf, and/or forearm (brachioradialis), macroglossia—LGMD2I.

## Simple immediate investigations

- Creatine kinase (CK)—usually very high in DMD/BMD, LGMD2I and EDMD. Only mildly elevated in DM1.
- Electromyography (EMG)—myopathic in all 4 conditions, but confirms generalized muscle disease, myotonia usually very evident in DM1, but can be absent in DM2.
- Muscle biopsy.

Muscle biopsy should not usually be necessary for the diagnosis of typical cases of DMD, BMD, DM1, LGMD2I or EDMD. However, if initial molecular investigations are normal or the patient has atypical features a muscle biopsy is the most likely way a correct diagnosis will be reached. The correct selection of which muscle to biopsy is very important (a relatively mildly affected muscle is usually best, ideally with prior confirmation that the particular muscle is not severely affected by muscle ultrasound scan (USS) or MRI; the muscle biopsy should only be undertaken in a specialized centre where the sample can be handled appropriately (flash frozen in liquid $N_2$ and orientated properly), therefore only usually undertaken by neuromuscular specialist or neurosurgeon.

- Molecular tests:
  - DMD/BMD—dystrophin
  - DM1—DMPK triplet repeat
  - LGMD2I—testing most usually for the 2 common European mutations
  - EDMD-XL—emerin
  - EDMD-AD—LMNA/C.

Table 16.3 gives a more detailed list of most of the currently known neuromuscular conditions which may present with cardiac involvement.

**Table 16.3** Inherited muscle diseases with cardiac involvement

| Disorder | Gene/locus | Protein |
|---|---|---|
| **Autosomal dominant** | | |
| *Myotonic dystrophy:* | | |
| DM1 | 19q13.2–q13.3 | Myotonin protein kinase (DMPK) |
| DM2/PROMM | 3q13.3–q24 | Zinc finger protein-9 (ZNF9) |
| *Limb girdle muscular dystrophy:* | | |
| LGMD1A | 5q31 | Myotilin |
| LGMD1B | 1q21.2 | Lamin A/C |
| LGMD1C | 3p25 | Caveolin-3 |
| Emery–Dreifuss muscular dystrophy | 1q11–q21 | Lamin A/C |
| Facioscapulohumeral dystrophy | 4q35 | Unknown |
| Bethlem myopathy | 21q22 | CollagenVI (α1;α2) |
| | 2q37 | CollagenVIα3 |
| Nemaline myopathy | | |
| *Desminopathies:* | | |
| Primary desminopathy | 1p36–p35 | Desmin |
| Myofibrillar myopathy (MFM) | 2q35 | Desmin-related |
| **Autosomal recessive** | | |
| *Limb girdle muscular dystrophy:* | | |
| LGMD2A | 15q15.1–q21.1 | Calpain 3 |
| LGMD2B | 2p13.3–p13.1 | Dysferlin |
| LGMD2C | 13q12 | γ-sarcoglycan |
| LGMD2D | 17q12–q21 | α-sarcoglycan |
| LGMD2E | 4q12 | β-sarcoglycan |
| LGMD2F | 5q33 | δ-sarcoglycan |
| LGMD2G | 17q11–q12 | Telethonin |
| LGMD2H | 9q31–q34 | TRIM32 |
| LGMD2I-FKRP | 19q13.3 | Fukutin-related protein |
| LGMD2J | 2q31 | Titin |

**Table 16.3** (Contd.)

| Disorder | Gene/locus | Protein |
|---|---|---|
| *Congenital muscular dystrophy:* | | |
| Fukuyama type (MDC1C) | 19q13.3 | Fukutin |
| Merosin deficient type (MDC1A) | 6q22–q23 | Laminin alpha-2 (LAMA2) |
| Merosin positive type | 4p16.3 | Merosin |
| *Desminopathies:* | | |
| RSMD1 | 1p35–p36 | Desmin |
| *Glycogenoses:* | | |
| GSD II | 17q25.2 | Acid alpha-1,4 glucosidase (GAA) |
| GSD III | 1p21 | Glycogen debrancher enzyme (AGL) |
| GSD IV | 3p12 | Glycogen branching enzyme (GBE1) |
| GSD VII | 12q13.3 | Muscle phosphofructokinase (PFKM) |
| *X-linked:* | | |
| Xp21 dystrophy myopathie: | Xp21 | Dystrophin |
| DMD—surviving longer | | |
| BMD—more active | | |
| Intermediate DMD/BMD | | |
| Manifesting carriers | | |
| X-linked cardiomyopathy | | |
| Emery–Dreifuss muscular dystrophy | Xq28 | Emerin |
| Barth syndrome | Xq28 | Taffazin |
| Danon disease | Xq24 | LAMP2 |

NCBI/OMIM 30 May 2008.

# Myotonic dystrophy type 1 (DM1)

## Genetics

- Caused by the expanding trinucleotide CTG repeat sequence in the untranslated region of the dystrophia myotonica protein kinase (DMPK) gene on chromosome 19q13.3.
- Autosomal dominant inheritance.
- Previous generations commonly more mildly affected and subsequent generations more severely affected—(genetic *Anticipation*).

## Clinical features of DM1

NB: all or only a few of the features may be present in any one individual.

- Congenitally affected individuals are usually more severely affected in all parameters.
- Distal weakness becoming more proximal—e.g. hand grip, wrist flexion and extension, ankle dorsiflexion.
- Myotonia—difficulty relaxing grip, or 'stiffness' of muscles; due to abnormally slow relaxation post contraction.
- Presenile cataracts—characteristically polychromatic 'Christmas tree', but stellate also common.
- Respiratory impairment—a combination of diaphragmatic and extrinsic chest muscle weakness.
- Dysphagia—pharyngeal weakness and/or myotonia—prone to aspiration.
- Endocrine features—male pattern baldness, diabetes mellitus/insulin resistance, hypothyroidism.
- Learning problems—more notable the younger the age of onset.
- Hypersomnolence—is a particular feature and may be due to inherent involvement of the brainstem sleep centre, or be secondary to nocturnal hypoventilation and hypercapnia.
- GI tract involvement is a common but under-recognized feature—young age gallstones, irritable bowel syndrome, delayed gastric emptying.

## Cardiac features

- Cardiac involvement is very common occurring in up to 90% of affected individuals.
- In the majority of cases cardiac involvement is confined to distal AV conduction anomalies most likely due to fatty infiltration of the bundle of His. Dysrhythmia is the predominant feature and very common in DM1.
- Cardiomyopathy is very rare in myotonic dystrophy (but is well recognized and reported in the literature). Detailed studies suggest subclinical evidence of myocardial involvement is quite common.
- Majority of patients asymptomatic but at risk of atrial and ventricular dysrhythmia.
- Sudden death occurs in 10–33% of patients, usually in adulthood but also reported in adolescents as young as 12 years old;[1] but cardiac disease probably not the only cause.[2]

- There is a poor correlation between CTG repeat size or clinical severity and cardiac involvement; this probably reflects the extremely wide tissue variability in CTG repeat size; therefore monitoring is recommended in any patient known to harbour an expanded CTG repeat, even if asymptomatic.

## ECG anomalies in DM1
- Bradycardia.
- Prolonged PR interval, initially within 'normal ranges' progresses to first degree heart block.
- Left axis deviation (LAD) due to left anterior hemiblock (LAH).
- Bundle branch block (LBBB or RBBB).
- Bifascicular block (RBBB & LAH).
- Atrial fibrillation/flutter.

## Recommendations for cardiac monitoring in DM1[3]
### Tests
- Routine 12-lead ECG—even though sensitivity is poor.
- 24hr Holter ECG.
- EPS—invasive elctrophysiological studies (prolongation of HV interval >70msec in 41%, inducible ventricular arrhythmia in 18%)

EPS is controversial and its place in the management of DM1 is not fully established or universally agreed. Those who have a particular interest and expertise in managing cardiac complications in DM1 have published criteria for EPS. Since 90% of DM1 patients will develop first-degree heart block at some point this recommendation would have a significant impact on elctrophysiological departments, and many therefore do not agree that these criteria can be delivered in practice. The evidence suggests however that cardiac involvement is a significant cause of premature death in DM1.

### Criteria for EPS (in DM1)[3]
- 1st degree HB (PR >200ms)—with or without widening of QRS >100ms.
- Palpitations with evidence of dysrhythmia.
- Syncope/near syncope.
- In preparation for major surgery.

## Management guidelines
### Symptomatic
- Pace if HV interval >70ms (but <100ms).
- If severe ventricular dysrrhythmias or HV >100ms consider ICD (implantable cardioverter/defibrillator).

### Asymptomatic—all patients carry an expanded CTG repeats
- Annual ECG.
- Holter 2yrly.
- ECHO every 5 years.

- EPS if 1) PR >0.20s; 2) QRS >0.12; 3) sinus dysfunction or AV block of any kind.
- Aim to establish the absence of infra-Hissian pathology.

1. Harper PS (2001). *Myotonic Dystrophy*, 3rd edition, London, WB Saunders
2. Lazarus A, *et al* (2002). Long-term follow-up of arrhythmias in patients with myotonic dystrophy treated by pacing: a multicenter diagnostic pacemaker study. *J Am Coll Cardiol.* **40**, 1645–52.
3. Lazarus A, *et al* (1999). Relationships among electrophysiological findings and clinical status, heart function, and extent of DNA mutation in myotonic dystrophy. *Circulation.* **99**, 1041–6

# Myotonic dystrophy type 2 (DM2)

Genetics
- A CCTG tetra-repeat expansion in the ZNF9 gene on chromosome 3q21.
- Autosomal dominant.
- Anticipation less frequent than in type 1.

Clinical characteristics
- Similar to type 1 but less severe.
- Cardiac involvement in ~20% but less well defined than type 1.
- Cardiac conduction abnormalities are seen in 20% of patients and include atrioventricular or intraventricular block.
- SCD affects patients with associated DCM.

# Cardiac involvement in Xp21 dystrophies

### Definitions
- Xp21 dystrophy—any of the muscular dystrophies caused by mutations in the dystrophin gene, located at chromosome position Xp21.
- Duchenne MD (DMD)—boys affected with muscular dystrophy, onset 3–5 years of age, loss of ambulation typically by 11–13 years of age, but by definition before 16.[1]
- Becker MD (BMD)—a milder muscular dystrophy, allelic to DMD, onset is later, typically not losing ambulation until after 30, but defined by retention of walking beyond 16, survive into the 60s.
- Intermediate MD—an Xp21 MD intermediate in severity between DMD and BMD.
- Manifesting carrier—a female carrying a dystrophin mutation, usually an adult woman (exceptionally a girl) showing signs of muscle involvement (cardiac or skeletal).
- Exceptionally mutations at the first exon–intron boundary of the dystrophin gene have caused XL-R cardiomyopathy without skeletal muscle manifestations.

### Duchenne muscular dystrophy
- Onset in early childhood—delayed early motor milestones, walking delayed >18 months age.
- High CK—×200–300 normal (in the thousands).
- Unable to run, hop, skip.
- Proximal weakness starting in the lower limbs, progressing more rapidly distally and into the upper limb.
- Scoliosis common.
- Respiratory impairment—due to respiratory muscle weakness +/– scoliosis.
- Calf pseudohypertrophy common.
- Mild learning problems in 1/3.
- Cardiomyopathy—often asymptomatic (because of inactivity).
- Death typically late teens to early 20s untreated; but life expectancy and quality of life extended by supportive care, scoliosis surgery and non-invasive ventilation.

#### Cardiac features in DMD
- ECG abnormal in >90%, detectable from as early as 6yrs of age.
- Echo abnormal in >90% either HCM or DCM, >50% by 13 years of age.
- Dysrhythmia (as a function of or without overt cardiomyopathy).
- Lateral and basal-posterior wall motion abnormalities are common.
- Sudden cardiac death occurs in 10–20%—usually teens.
- Angiotensin inhibitors (ACEi) have been shown to delay progression of LV dysfunction even in those with late diagnosis of cardiomyopathy.
- ACEi alone or in combination with β-blockers (+/– sprironolactone for its antifibrotic effect) are effective when started at the first sign of LV dysfunction (leading to normalisation in >half treated in some studies).
- Evidence is emerging that prophylactic use of ACEi even before presymptomatic signs of LV dysfunction, can delay the onset of cardiac disease in DMD.

Becker muscular dystrophy

- Onset usually in second decade/adolescence, but milder variants may not be symptomatic until 6th decade or later, childhood motor milestones usually normal.
- High CK—but much more variable than DMD.
- Proximal weakness starting in the lower limbs, progressing more slowly distally and into the upper limb.
- Respiratory impairment—a late feature.
- Calf pseudohypertrophy often striking.
- Cardiomyopathy—a major cause of morbidity because much more physically active than DMD.

### Cardiac features in BMD
- ECG abnormal in 45%;[2] 90%;[3] ECHO abnormal in 17% DCM;[2] 65% HCM and DCM.[3]
- Unrelated to severity of MD.
- Dysrhythmia.
- Cardiac death occurs in up to 50%.[3]

Manifesting carriers[3]
- ECG abnormal in 21–90%, but very variable.
- ECHO abnormal in 7–11% HCM and DCM.
- Dysrhythmia.
- Very disproprtionate to skeletal involvement (because of random Lyonization).
- Successful transplants reported.

Unaffected carriers
- 10% develop CCF.[4]

1. Bushby KMD (1995). Diagnostic criteria for the limb-girdle muscular dystrophies: report of the ENMC consortium on limb-girdle dystrophies. *Neuromusc Disord.* **5**, 71–74.
2. de Visser M, de Voogt WG, la Riviere GA (1992). The heart in Becker muscular dystrophy, facioscapulohumeral dystrophy and Bethlem myopathy. *Muscle & Nerve* **15**, 591–596
3. Bushby K, Muntoni F, Bourke JP (2003). 107th ENMC international workshop: the management of cardiac involvement in muscular dystrophy and myotonic dystrophy. 7th-9th June 2002, Naarden, the Netherlands. *Neuromuscul Disord* **13**, 166–172.
4. Hoogerwaard EM, et al (1999) Cardiac involvement in carriers of Duchenne and Becker muscular dystrophy. *Neuromuscul Disord.* **9**, 347–351.

# X-linked Emery–Dreifuss muscular dystrophy

Caused by mutations of the Emerin (EMD) gene on chromosome Xq28.

Key features
- Symmetrical limb weakness (adult onset).
- Proximal UL, distal LL.
- No pseudohypertrophy.
- Contractures of elbow and spine (knee, finger).
- Onset usually before 10yrs.
- Cardiac involvement is the rule.

Cardiac involvement
- Cardiac involvement in >95%.
- ECG abnorm by 30yrs.
- Dysrhythmia - characteristic atrial standstill (AV block), bradycardia, prolonged PR, AF/flutter.
- Cardiomyopathy - exceptionally rare.
- SCD common in unpaced individuals.
- Preventive pacemaker RECOMMENDED (mean age 24yrs).
- Death rare after pacemaker insertion.
- Carriers also at risk—periodic ECG surveillance recommended.

# LGMD1B and AD EDMD (laminopathies)

Genetics
- Lamin A and C are alternative splice products of the Lamin A/C gene (*LMNA*) on chromosome 1p1.
- *LMNA* mutations are associated with a diverse number of diseases collectively known as the laminopathies:
  - LGMD 1B
  - familial partial lipodystrophy
  - mandibuloacral dysplasia
  - hutchinson–Gilford progeria
  - atypical Werner's syndrome
  - lipoatrophy with diabetes, hepatic steatosis, HCM and leakomelanodermic papules
  - isolated dilated cardiomyopathy (📖 see Chapter 8, Cardiomyopathies).

Cardiac involvement in AD EDMD
- >95% conduction anomalies by 30yrs.
- 35% DCM 19–55yrs.
- Mean age at pacing 32yrs (19–57).
- SCD in 50% (despite pacing).
- Implantable defibrillators may be more appropriate.

# Limb girdle muscular dystrophy (LGMD) 2A-2J

'LGMD' is a phenotypic description of muscular dystrophy involving the muscles of the pelvic and shoulder girdles. Symptoms and signs affect the proximal LL muscles before and more severely than the proximal UL.

## Key features

- Nearly always symmetrical (compare with FSHD).
- Majority are autosomal recessive.
- Onset is usually in childhood.
- Often severe (hence previous name SCARMD—severe childhood AR muscular dystrophy).
- Wide range of proteins—mainly structural sarcoglycans.
- Cardiac involvement occurs in 20%, but is more common in some (ECG, HCM, DCM).[1]

## LGMD2I–FKRP

- Wide range in age of onset (from congenital to adulthood.
- 2 founder European mutations, particularly 'common' in the United Kingdom, and account for the majority in UK cases.
- Sometimes presents with cardiomyopathy before limb-girdle weakness is recognised (although it is usually apparent on examination).
- Typically associated with pseudohypertrophy of calf, brachioradialis, and tongue (macroglossia).
- >50% of patients develop cardiac impairments.[2]

1. Bushby K, Muntoni F, Bourke JP (2003). 107th ENMC international workshop: the management of cardiac involvement in muscular dystrophy and myotonic dystrophy. 7th-9th June 2002, Naarden, the Netherlands. *Neuromuscul Disord* **13**, 166–172.
2. Poppe M et al, (2004). Cardiac and respiratory failure in Limb-Girdle Musculr Dystrophy 21 *Ann Neurol* 56, 738–741.

# Facioscapulohumeral muscular dystrophy (FSHD)

- AD - 4q35.
- Characteristic myopathic facies.
- Limbgirdle and facial involvement.
- Upper Limb before prox Lower limb.
- Typically asymmetrical.
- Not typically associated with cardiac disease.

## Cardiac involvement in FSHD

- A rare feature, NOT definitely established as attributable to FSHD, once thought not to occur.
- 5% of patients in some series show overt cardiac features.
- No single characteristic cardiac problem.
- May be more prone to cardiac dysrhythmia.
- Following direct intracardiac programmed electrical stimulation AF or flutter could be induced in 80% FSHD pts vs 17% controls.[1]
- subclinical impairments.
  - SPECT - abnormal fibrosis in 5/7 FSHD.[2]
  - Tl-201-SPECT - 3/4 abnormal, 2/4 abnormal stress test.
  - ECG anomalies.[3]
  - 38% minor abnormalities.
  - 4% - age related changes.
- 5% 'significant' conduction defects.
- Sudden death, cor pulmonale, abnorm ECHO, cardiomyopathy described.[4]

## Management

- Screening with electrocardiography and echocardiography is suggested, and long term follow-up is guided by the clinical condition.

1. Stevenson WG et al. (1990) Facioscapulohumeral muscular dystrophy: evidence for selective genetic electrophysiologic cardiac involvement. JACC **15**: 292–299.
2. Yamamoto S et al. (1988) A comparative study of thallium-201 single photon emission computed tomography and electrocardiography in Duchenne and other types of muscular dystrophy. Am J Cardiol **61**: 836–843.
3. Laforêt et al. (1998) Cardiac involvement in genetically confirmed facioscapulohumeral muscular dystrophy. Neurology **51**: 1454–1456.
4. Rogers MT. (2009) Facioscapulohumeral muscular dystrophy - a clinical, audiometric and pathological study. Thesis, London University.

# DCM and limb-girdle muscular dystrophies (LGMD)

- Genetics:
  - genetically heterogeneous
  - autosomal dominant or recessive.
- Clinical characteristics:
  - weakness and wasting of the shoulder and pelvic girdle muscles, calf hypertrophy and reduced tendon reflexes.
  - cardiac involvement is limited primarily to LGMD2 types C to F (sarcoglycan gene mutations) and LGMD2I (*FKRP* gene mutations).
  - cardiac involvement is not well defined
  - common electrocardiographic abnormalities include incomplete right bundle branch block, dominant R-wave in $V_1$, left anterior hemiblock, and repolarization abnormalities
  - DCM can develop
  - LGMD2C-F and LGMD2I patients should be followed up in a manner similar to patients with Duchene muscular dystrophy.
  - the value of ongoing cardiac screening in other types of LGMD is probably limited.
- Management recommendation for all muscular dystrophies:
  - regular ECG (usually annually)
  - Holter if indicated
  - regular Echo (1–5 yearly)
  - further cardiological assessment as indicated
  - preventive management
    - pacing
    - defibrillator
    - ACE-Inhibitor
  - transplantation.

## Further reading

Bushby K., Muntoni F. and Bourke JP. (2003) 107th ENMC international workshop: the management of cardiac involvement in muscular dystrophy and myotonic dystrophy. 7th-9th June 2002, Naarden, the Netherlands. *Neuromuscul.Disord.* **13**: 166–172.

Finsterer J. and Stollberger C. (2008) Primary myopathies and the heart. *Scand. Cardiovasc. J* **42**: 9–24.

Muntoni F. (2003) Cardiomyopathy in muscular dystrophies. *Curr. Opin. Neurol.* **16**: 577–583.

# Mitochondrial disease

# Introduction

Cardiovascular conditions resulting from pathological changes in the mitochondrial genome are increasingly diagnosed with the advances in molecular diagnostic techniques. Cardiovascular manifestations are a major component of clinical syndromes that follow mitochondrial inheritance (📖 see Chapter 2, General principles) and present with the most challenging situations in cardiovascular medicine and clinical genetics. Genetic counselling is often difficult as a precise diagnosis may not always be possible.

# Clinical approach

### History

- Three-generation pedigree with specific enquiry about muscle weakness, hearing, vision, breathlessness, fainting, chest disomfort, and neurological problems.
- Extend the family tree as far as possible through the maternal line.
- Obtain detailed information on individual affected family members. Mitochondrial disorders often display unusual and marked intrafamilial variability.

### Examination

- Growth parameters—height, weigh occipito-frontal circumference (OFC), record as percentile for age and gender based on current percentile charts.
- Examine eyes, looking for ptosis and nystagmus and testing for external ophthalmoplegia. Ophthalmological examination for pigmentary retinopathy and cataract.
- Cardiovascular system examination including blood pressure measurement and peripheral signs for heart failure.
- Neurolological examination for hypotonia, myoclonus and ataxia.

### Investigations

- Electrocardiogram (12-lead) for conduction defects.
- Echocardiography for any structural changes, specifically cardiomyopathy.
- CMR if echocardiography unhelpful or for clarifying the cardiac involvement.
- Biochemical investigations—CK (usually normal or mildly elevated), blood lactate (high) and blood glucose (high in diabetes mellitus).
- Cardiac enzymes and cardiac troponins may be useful in a patient presenting with acute or sub-acute cardiac symptoms.
- Cerebrospinal fluid (CSF) lactate, specifically when dealing with possible Leigh disease.
- Consider cranial MRI if there are symptoms of encephalopathy— seizures, regression, ataxia, myoclonus, and stroke-like episodes.
- Audiometry.
- Muscle biopsy with Gomori trichrome staining for 'ragged red fibres' and staining for cytochrome c oxidase (COX) (complex IV) and succinate-ubiquinone oxireductase (SDH) (complex II). The muscle biopsy should be undertaken in a specialist unit with expertise for light microscopy, electron microscopy, immunostaining, assay for individual muscle component and DNA extraction and mtDNA mutation analysis. Apart from occasional cases of Leber's hereditary optic neuropathy (LHON) and mitochondrial myopathy, muscle biopsy is the single most important investigation in a mitochondrial genetic disorder

where despite having an underlying pathogenic mtDNA mutation the muscle biopsy may be normal.
- DNA for mutation analysis of mitochondrial genome or nuclear-encoded mitochondrial genes. This is preferably carried out on the muscle tissue as both point mutations and mitochondrial rearrangements are seen in the muscle DNA, whilst only point mutations are detectable on the DNA from peripheral blood leucocytes.

# Heart disease in mitochondrial disorders

Incidence and prevalence of cardiac involvement is unknown and probably under-reported. In early onset of mitochondrial-related disease, neurological sequelae appear to overshadow other organ symptoms including cardiac. This may relate to the rapid fatality of the primary condition that cardiac manifestations do not have time to develop. Age at onset of symptoms and severity of mitochondrial mutation may determine incidence and degree of cardiac abnormalities. Best clinical practice would appear to have a high index of suspicion in all cases of mitochondrial disease for the presence of cardiac pathology and to instigate a surveillance policy.

The cardiac involvement can be assesed using electrocardiography, a chest x-ray, His-bundle electrograms and echocardiography. The spectrum of cardiovascular manifestions may include:

- conduction defects (Kearns–Sayre syndrome)
- left ventricular hypertrophy (MELAS)
- cardiomegaly with septal wall hypertrophy (MERRF)
- ECG abnormalities in ocular myopathy with large mtDNA deletions.

## Cardiovascular phenotypes in mitochondrial disease

### Arrhythmias

- Arrhythmias are common in patients with mitochondrial disease, either as an isolated cardiac feature, or associated with cardiomyopathy.
- Arrhythmias, most commonly ventricular tachycardia, may occur in about 10% patients.
- Cardiac conduction defects are more common, for example in the Kearns–Sayre syndrome (Table 17.1). In some patients second degree heart block remains stable over decades, but sudden death is recognized and cardiac pacing is usually indicated in patients with second degree or third degree atrioventricular block. Conduction defects may also occur as part of a cardiomyopathy in patients with m.3243A>G.
- Accessory pathways and the Wolff–Parkinson–White syndrome (WPW) has been documented in patients with LHON, but it is not clear whether this is a direct aetiological link or simply a chance finding. More recently, a high frequency of WPW has been described in about 13% patients with m.3243A>G mtDNA mutation.
- Asymptomatic individuals do not require active intervention but those with symptomatic tachycardia will require pharmacological management or radiofrequency catheter ablation.

### Hypertrophic cardiomyopathy

The incidence of cardiomyopathy in mitochondrial disease is not known, however it is now recognised that characteristic abnormalities are linked to specific mutations. Hypertrophic cardiomyopathy (HCM) is a common feature of mitochondrial disease and is actually the most frequency cardiac complication. Some of the important observations in HCM and mitochondrial genetics are:

- point mutations of mtDNA can cause sporadic and maternally inherited HCM, which may be the presenting or only feature in patients with the common m.3243A>G MTTL1 mutation first described in MELAS
- left ventricular dysfunction may be the presenting feature in m.3243A>G mutation carriers with neurological features but without evidence of arrythmias on electrocardiography or Holter monitoring.
- MELAS patients may also develop left ventricular hypertrophy with either LV systolic or diastolic dysfunction
- asymptomatic m.3243A>G mutation carriers are not known to manifest with cardiac abnormalities. The natural history of m.3243A>G cardiomyopathy is currently being evaluated. 31P-magnetic resonance spectroscopy (MRS) studies have shown that the myocardial bioenergetic defect precedes the hypertrophic phase and eventually leads to a dilated cardiomyopathy and heart failure which can be fatal. Anecdotal reports support the use of angiotensin converting enzyme inhibitors at an early stage
- other point mutations and mtDNA deletions can also cause HCM, usually as part of a multi-system disorder. For example, HCM is common in patients carrying the m.8344A>G MTTK 'MERRF' mutation, and the MTTI gene encoding tRNAille appears to be a mutation hot spot for HCM
- HCM can be the sole feature of homoplasmic mtDNA tRNA gene mutations, which characteristically cause tissue-specific phenotypes
- HCM has also been described in patients with nuclear gene defects causing a secondary defect of mtDNA, especially mutations in POLG presenting in childhood as part of Alpers–Huttenlocher syndrome or as a late features of autosomal progressive external ophthalmoplegia (PEO)
- HCM has also been described in patients with a mutation in SLC25A4 (which codes for the adenine nucleotide translocase, ANT1) without ophthalmoplegia. This latter finding is mirrored by the cardiomyopathy seen in the transgenic ANT1 knockout mice
- HCM has also been described in Leigh syndrome (LS) (Table 17.1) which can be due to nuclear or mtDNA defects. Infantile HCM dominates the clinical picture in patients with mutations in SCO2 and COX15, which also share features of LS; and mutations in ATP12 also cause LS and cardiomyopathy. More recently, a mutation in the *SLC25A3* gene resulting in mitochondrial phosphate carrier deficiency was reported in two siblings presenting with lactic acidosis, hypertrophic cardiomyopathy, and muscular hypotonia who died within the first year of life. An ATP synthase deficiency in muscle mitochondria was identified correlating with the tissue-specific expression of exon3A.

### Histiocytoid cardiomyopathy

Histiocytoid cardiomyopathy is a rare complication. It is a known manifestation in patients with mutations in the MTCYB gene encoding cytochrome b and presenting in early childhood with respiratory chain complex III deficiency and a propensity for dysrhythmias.

### Left ventricular non-compaction and Barth syndrome

Left ventricular non-compaction (LVNC) is a heterogeneous disease which usually presents with cardiomegaly and congestive cardiac failure in childhood. Some X-linked recessive cases have mutations in TAZ which also causes Barth syndrome, suggesting the two disorders are allelic. Barth syndrome affects young males and presents with congestive cardiac failure, neutropenia and skeletal myopathy, usually associated with abnormal levels of 3-methylglutaconate, 3-methylglutarate, and 2-ethylhydracrylate in the urine.

### Senger's syndrome

Senger's syndrome is a rare autosomal recessive mitochondrial disease charactersized by congenital cataracts, HCM and skeletal myopathy with a defect of cytochrome c oxidase in muscle. The aetiology of Sengers syndrome is not known, but presumed secondary abnormalities of ANT have been described at the gene expression and protein levels. A patient with HCM due to Sengers syndrome has received a successfully cardiac transplant.

### Congenital heart defects (CHD)

Congenital structural heart defects have been documented in patients with mitochondrial disease. Conversely, biochemical abnormalities of mitochondrial function have been described in patients with complex congenital heart defects. These are likely to be secondary to the primary pathology, and their significance has yet to be established.

**Table 17.1** Clinical syndromes associated with mitochondrial disease

| Syndrome | Primary features | Additional features |
|---|---|---|
| Alpers–Huttenlocher syndrome | Encephalopathy with seizures, liver failure | Developmental delay and hypotonia |
| Chronic progressive external ophthalmoplegia | External ophthalmoplegia and bilateral ptosis | Mild proximal myopathy |
| Kearns–Sayre syndrome | Progressive external ophthalmoplegia onset before | Bilateral deafness |
| | age 20 years with pigmentary retinopathy | Myopathy |
| | Plus one of the following: cerebrospinal fluid | Dysphagia |
| | protein >1 g/L, cerebellar ataxia, or heart block | Diabetes mellitus. hypoparathyroidism |
| | | Dementia |
| Pearson's syndrome | Sideroblastic anemia of childhood | Renal tubular defects |
| | Pancytopenia | |
| | Exocrine pancreatic failure | |

**Table 17.1** (Contd.)

| Syndrome | Primary features | Additional features |
|---|---|---|
| Mitochondrial encephalomyopathy with | Stroke-like episodes before age 40 years | Diabetes mellitus |
| lactic acidosis and stroke-like episodes (MELAS) | Seizures and/or dementia | Cardiomyopathy |
| | Ragged-red fibres and/or lactic acidosis | Bilateral deafness |
| | Pigmentary retinopathy | |
| | Cerebellar ataxia | |
| Mitochondrial neurogastrointestinal | Gastrointestinal pseudoobstruction | |
| encephalomyopathy (MNGIE) | Myopathy | |
| | Leukoencephalopathy | |
| | Peripheral neuropathy | |
| Myoclonic epilepsy with ragged-red fibres (MERRF) | Myoclonus | Dementia |
| | Seizures | Optic atrophy |
| | Cerebellar ataxia | Bilateral deafness |
| | Myopathy | Peripheral neuropathy |
| | | Spasticity |
| | | Multiple lipomas |
| Leber's hereditary optic neuropathy | Subacute bilateral visual failure males:females approximately 4:1 | Dystonia |
| | | Cardiac pre-excitation syndromes |
| | Median age of onset 24 years | |
| Leigh syndrome | Subacute relapsing encephalopathy with cerebellar and brainstem signs | Basal ganglia lucencies |
| Infantile myopathy and lactic acidosis | Hypotonia | Cardiomyopathy +/– Toni–Fanconi–Debre syndrome |

# Clinical management of mitochondrial disease

There is currently no definitive treatment for patients with mitochondrial disease, except for patients with deficiency of coenzyme Q10. Management is aimed at minimizing disability, preventing complications, and providing genetic information and assisting in making informed choices.

## Supportive care and surveillance

The multi-system and chronic nature of mitochondrial disease means that many patients require integrated follow-up over many decades, involving the primary physician (often a neurologist, but sometimes a diabetologist or cardiologist, depending on the major phenotype), other specialist physicians (ophthalmology), specialist nurses, physiotherapists, and speech therapists. Management is essentially supportive, as for other phenotypically related disorders.

## Clinical genetics and genetic counselling

A major problem in clinical genetics is the lack of correlation between the phenotypic severity and level of mutant mtDNA in many mitochondrial diseases. Recurrence risks are difficult to estimate due to discrepancy of mutant and wild type mtDNA in the oocyte and secondly distribution of mutant mtDNA in respective tissues in the affected offspring. Figures for recurrence risks may vary from 5–10%, and may even be higher (~30%) in selected disorders, for example LHON, MERRF, NARP, MELAS, and Leigh disease. Recurrence risk estimates are available for selected mitochondrial disorders (Table 17.2). These are mostly empirical and should be used with caution. Specific risk assessment for cadiovascular involvement should be based on the natural history of the mitochondrial disease.

Genetic counselling for a mitochondrial condition can be complex and should be undertaken by a clinical geneticist or genetic counsellor with thorough understanding of mitochondrial genetics. A precise molecular diagnosis facilitates genetic counselling for patients and their families. However, in many cases, it is not possible to identify the underlying gene and the counselling is more speculative, and based on the family structure and likely inheritance pattern. It is important to be aware of the following observations:

- Mitochondrial disorders often display extraordinary intrafamilial variability due to different affected family members inheriting different mutant mtDNA loads.
- Most children with respiratory chain disease are compound heterozygotes with recessive nuclear gene mutations.
- Some adults may appear to have an autosomal recessive disorder or a dominantly inherited condition, for example autosomal dominant PEO.
- Affected males with a mitochondrial disease do not transmit the mutant mtDNA allele and therefore recurrence risk is negligible. Males cannot transmit pathogenic mtDNA defects.
- Patients who carry mtDNA deletions rarely have a family history suggestive of mtDNA disease.

- An affected female may trasmit the mutant mtDNA allele and therefore carries a small risk of having an affected offspring.
- Clinically asymptomatic women harbouring pathogenic mtDNA point mutations may transmit the genetic defect to their offspring.
- The mitochondrial genetic 'bottleneck' leads to a variation in the proportion of mutated mtDNA that is transmitted to any offspring. It is therefore possible for a female to have mildly affected as well as severely affected children.
- The risk of having affected offspring varies from mutation to mutation, and there does appear to be a relationship between the level of mutated mtDNA in the mother and the risk of affected offspring.
- Predictive genetic testing can be offered to maternal relatives; however, the main difficulty lies in accurately predicting the phenotype from the mutant load.

## Pharmacological treatments for mitochondrial disease

Standard doses of vitamin C and K, thiamine, riboflavin, and ubiquinone (coenzyme Q10) are reported to be of some benefit in isolated cases and open studies, particularly in patients with isolated Q10 deficiency. Dichloracetate can be used to reduce lactic acid levels but a recent clinical trial showed that the side effects of this treatment are unacceptable (a partially irreversible toxic neuropathy). Moderate exercise is important for patients with mtDNA disease to prevent or reverse deconditioning, which is common in these disorders.

Drugs to avoid in mitochondrial disorders:
- Sodium valproate—inhibits several pathways of intermediate metabolism
- Barbiturates—inhibitors of oxidative phosphorylation (OXPHOS) pathway
- Gentamicin—may cause sensorineural deafness
- Ciprofloxacin—mtDNA inhibitor
- Chloramphenicol—mitochondrial translation inhibitor
- Tetracycline—mitochondrial translation inhibitor
- Zidovudine (antiviral agent) causes mitochondrial depletion.

## Mitochondrial cardiomyopathy

The mainstay of management of mitochondrial cardiomyopathy is surveillance allowing secondary prevention and aggressive treatment of complications:
- stringent glycaemic control in diabetes associated with m.3243A>G
- using cardioprotective agents such as ACE inhibitors, beta blockers and statins
- cardiac pacing, for example in Kearns-Sayre syndrome (KSS)
- treatment of heart failure
- cardiac transplantation
    - transplantation is controversial in the field of mitochondrial disorders as a form of treatment
    - multi-organ pathology is usually regarded as a contraindication for heart transplantation in metabolic disorders because the prolongation of life achieved by restoring cardiac function could lead to long-term neurological disability.

- It is not unreasonable to consider heart transplantation in mitochondrial cardiomyopathy in cases where the clinical expression of respiratory enzyme deficiency is limited to the myocardium.
- Neuromuscular weakness can present difficulties during and after anaesthesia, but successful orthotopic cardiac transplantations have been reported in such cases.
- Successful cardiac transplantation in malignant ventricular arrythmias and Sengers syndrome has been carried out.

## Prenatal diagnosis

- Should only be undertaken in conjunction with a centre with specialist expertise in mitochondrial genetics.
- Each mtDNA mutation is unique and should be considered separately.
- The mutant load in the fetal tissue (chorionic villi or amniocytes) is generally stable. Current data suggest that the mutant load in a prenatal sample may accurately predict the mutant load in most tissues at birth.
- The main difficulty lies in accurately predicting the phenotype from the mutant load, and even with expert advice, there may be a high degree of uncertainty.
- Few women with a low recurrence risk may be suitable for prenatal diagnosis with a reasonable chance of successful outcome.

## Other treatment approaches

- Gene therapy is perhaps the most challenging and most controversial therapy. To date various attempts have been made to design a delivery system capable of delivering drugs, proteins, peptides, and genes to the site of mitochondria with varying results. Germline therapy raises ethical issues as a possible tool to prevent maternal inheritance of mutant mtDNA.
- Donor oocyte *in vitro* fertilization (IVF) may be a suitable option for women with moderate to high recurrence risk. However, this is limited due to relative shortage of potential oocyte donors.
- There is likely possibility of employing pre-implantation genetic diagnosis (PGD).
- Recent developments in techniques for nuclear and cytoplasmic transfer have provided new options in preventing mitochondrial disease. These may become available in the future. However, despite recent reports in both lay and professional media, this approach is currently not in use in the clinical practice.

## Further reading

Firth H.V. and Husrt J.A. (2005) Mitochondrial DNA diseases. In *Oxford Desk Reference*, pp. 384–387. Oxford: Oxford University Press.

Holt I. (2003) Genetics of mitochondrial disease. In *Oxford Monographs in Medical Genetics*, no. 47. Oxford: Oxford University Press.

**Table 17.2** Primary mitochondrial DNA defects causing human disease

| Rearrangements (large-scale partial deletions and duplications) | Inheritance pattern |
|---|---|
| Chronic progressive external ophthalmoplegia (CPEO) | S or M |
| Kearns–Sayre syndrome | S or M |
| Diabetes and deafness | S |
| Pearson marrow-pancreas syndrome | S or M |
| Sporadic tubulopathy | S |
| *Point mutations* | |
| Protein-encoding genes | |
| • LHON (11778G>A, 14484T>C, 3460G>A) | M |
| • NARP/Leigh syndrome (8993T>G/C) | M |
| • tRNA genes | |
| • MELAS (3243ª>G, 3271T>C, 3251A>G) | M |
| • MERRF (8344A>G, 8356T>C) | M |
| • CPEO (3243A>G, 4274T>C) | M |
| Myopathy (14709T>C, 12320A>G) | M |
| Cardiomyopathy (3243A>G, 4269A>G, 4300A>G) | M |
| Diabetes and deafness (3243A>G, 12258C>A) | M |
| Encephalomyopathy (1606G>A, 10010T>C) | M |
| rRNA genes | |
| • Non-syndromic sensorineural deafness (7445A>G) | M |
| • Aminoglycoside induced nonsyndromic deafness (1555A>G) | M |
| *Point mutations* | |
| Protein-encoding genes | |
| • LHON (11778G>A, 14484T>C, 3460G>A) | M |
| • NARP/Leigh syndrome (8993T>G/C) | M |
| tRNA genes | |
| • MELAS (3243ª>G, 3271T>C, 3251A>G) | M |

M, maternal; S, sporadic; mtDNA nucleotide positions refer to the L-chain, and are taken from the Cambridge reference sequence; LHON, Leber hereditary optic neuropathy; NARP, neurogenetic weakness with ataxia and retinitis pigmentosa; CPEO, chronic progressive external ophthalmoplegia; KSS, Kearns–Sayre syndrome; MELAS. mitochondrial encephalomyopathy with lactic acidosis and stroke-like episodes; MERRF, myoclonic epilepsy with ragged-red fibres.

# Cardiovascular disorders and inherited metabolic disease

# General issues

Inherited metabolic diseases (IMDs) are a heterogeneous group of medical conditions affecting neonates, infants, children and adults.

Each condition may be rare and clinically diverse.

The total incidence of these disorders is between 1 in 2500 to 1 in 1000.

Confirmation of diagnosis is important for effective genetic counselling of families and the recognition that there are available treatments. Patients now survive into adulthood who previously would not have survived and they require co-ordinated specialist care. In those patients who do not survive it is important to have an exact diagnosis in the index case to offer appropriate genetic counselling to the family.

There are many IMDs affecting the cardiovascular system and heart directly that contribute importantly to adverse cardiovascular outcomes. This section of the handbook deals with the general clinical approach in any IMD, including history, examination, investigations, and management. Disorders covered in other chapters include inherited lipid disorders (📖 Chapter 11) and mitochondrial disease (📖 Chapter 17).

## History

A full genetic history should be taken and genetic pedigree constructed. The majority of IMDs are autosomal recessive and therefore it is important to document any consanguinity within the family pedigree. Maternal obstetric complications—e.g. acute fatty liver of pregnancy, HELLP (haemolysis, elevated liver enzymes, low platelets) which may be associated with disorders of fatty acid oxidation. Neonates may be well initially because of placental protection and lack of exposure to a substrate load.

There is an expanding area of neonatal blood spot screening with varying numbers of disorders and methods screening babies at or soon after birth. The reader should be aware of their own local arrangements for neonatal blood spot screening and conditions screened for (this will change with time as new programmes are introduced or withdrawn). The nature of screening will depend on the local incidence of certain genetic disorders. Caution must be still be exercised as screening is not 100% complete and neither is it a substitute for accurate confirmatory diagnosis.

Patients may present in different ways:
- Acutely e.g. fatty acid oxidation disorders. Consider the previous pattern and whether Illness is associated with starvation or repeated episodes.
- As a dysmorphic syndrome (e.g. lysosomal disorders).
- Sub-acute presentation—e.g. neurological presentation with acroparesthesae in Fabry disease or evidence of developmental delay and impaired intellectual performance in homocystinuria.

## Examination

A full examination is important including the plotting of relevant growth centiles, with the occipito-frontal head circumference on appropriate growth charts.

General observation may indicate a dysmorphic appearance or skin abnormalities.

Neurological assessment will include a full ophthalmic examination including examination of the eyes for abnormalities of the cornea, lenses and retina. It is advisable to seek formal opthalmological review if an IMD is suspected.

Examination will also reveal if there is associated liver, respiratory or cardiac involvement and the need for a cardiac review with an electrocardiogram (12-lead) for conduction defects and echocardiography for cardiomyopathy.

## Investigations

The range of possible investigations is considerable and biochemical investigations may be specialized and require specific collection conditions. Liaison with the local specialized IMD laboratory/clinical service is mandatory to ensure that the appropriate samples are collected in a timely manner and transported correctly. A history of specific feeding regimes and drug history is also important in assessing biochemical samples.

Initial samples to aid and target further investigations or if a patient is not likely to survive acutely and a diagnosis of IMD is being considered include:

### First line

Full blood count, Urea and electrolytes, creatinine, anion gap, blood gases, glucose, lactate (plasma, CSF), ammonia, liver function tests, Urine ketones.

### Second line

Urine organic acids, urine amino acids, plasma amino acids, uric acid, carnitine (total and free), acylcarnitine profile, CSF lactate and amino acids.

Blood samples should also be taken to allow the storage of DNA for mutational analysis. When not available it may be possible to extract DNA (and biochemical species) from the neonatal blood spot taken at birth if this has been stored beyond the neonatal period.

If a patient is acutely unwell and not likely to survive with a strongly suspected IMD, a skin biopsy may be taken without any specific facilities (small skin ellipse collected under sterile conditions and placed in sterile normal saline, stored in normal fridge conditions—not frozen—and then transported rapidly to the appropriate laboratory for fibroblast culture, preferably within 48 hours). This can be used later for the extraction of DNA and specific enzyme analysis.

# Lysosomal storage diseases

Lysosomes are found in almost all living cells and therefore these diseases lead to a wide range of abnormalities including the brain (cognitive function), neural development, myopathy, skeletal, visceral, and skin disturbances.

Approximate incidence of these disorders may be as high as 1 in 7000.

Supportive treatment is important in providing good care to this group of patients involving paediatricians, IMD specialists, neurologists, cardiologists, ear nose and throat specialists and orthopaedic surgeons.

Enzyme replacement therapy is an important therapeutic advance for many lysosomal disorders but has significant resource issues for healthcare systems.

Substrate inhibition therapy is a relatively new but recognized treatment modality for disorders (Gaucher Disease type I, Niemann-Pick C) and currently undergoing drug trial reviews for other disorders along with the consideration of chaperone therapies.

## Mucopolysaccharidoses (MPS)

This group of disorders are a family of inheritable disorders caused by a deficiency of lysosomal enzymes that degrade glycosaminoglycans and affects predominantly connective tissue. They can affect cardiac valves and vessels, but cardiovascular disease is not usually the major initial presenting feature in these disorders.

They are transmitted in an autosomal recessive manner except for MPS II which is X-linked. Mutations underlying any one MPS disorder are very heterogeneous. Some mutant alleles may predominate in specific populations.

Specific cardiovascular problems include valvular disease (mitral and aortic), myocardial thickening, systemic and pulmonary hypertension and narrowing of the coronary arteries with ischaemia which may lead to congestive heart failure and sometimes sudden cardiovascular death. Valvular disease is commoner in MPS IH (Hurler syndrome) and MPS II (Hunter syndrome) and also recognized in MPS IH/S (Hurler–Scheie syndrome), MPS IS (Scheie syndrome), MPS IV (Morquio syndrome) and MPS VI (Maroteux–Lamy). MPS III (Sanfilippo syndrome) has severe mental deterioration but much less somatic involvement including much less cardiac involvement.

Cardiac evaluation at regular levels with echocardiography is therefore useful in these disorders. Cardiac valve replacement therapy may be considered in combination with the other features of these diseases. With the advent of enzyme replacement therapy for a number of these disorders it will be important to monitor the effect of these treatments on the cardiovascular system.

## Mucolipidoses

The mucolipidoses (including I-cell disease and pseudo-Hurler polydystrophy) are a group of rare diseases with autosomal recessive inheritance. They are characterized by significant somatic changes and require cardiac surveillance for valvular lesions.

## Anderson–Fabry disease

Also known as Fabry disease/α-galactosidase A deficiency/angiokeratoma corporis diffusum.

An X-linked lysosomal storage disorder caused by deficiency of the enzyme α-galactosidase A leading to storage of neutral glycosphingolipids in many tissues.

### Incidence
- Estimated at 1:40,000–1:117,000 live births for males.
- No ethnic predisposition.
- Prevalence probably underestimated due to its non-specific symptoms.
- Reported as the cause of 3–4% of unexplained LVH in adult males.

### Aetiology
- Mutations in the gene for α-galactosidase A located in Xq22 region of X chromosome.
- Over 400 different mutations described, the majority are missense point mutations.
- Many mutations are 'private mutations', ie. limited to a single family and there is wide phenotypical variations within families.
- Female carriers are often affected (usually with a milder form) possibly due to random X chromosome inactivation and inability of the wild-type allele to compensate for the metabolic defect.

### Clinical Features
- In males, symptom onset at an average 5–6 years and in girls 9 years.
- After 20 years disease progression results in proteinuria in men with eventual development of renal failure.
- Commonest cause of death in men is end-stage renal failure.
- Commonest cause of death in women is cardiac.
- Extra-cardiac manifestations shown in Table 18.1.

### Diagnosis
- Low or absent α-galactosidase A activity (0–4%) can be detected in serum/leucocytes/tears/tissue/cultured fibroblasts.
- Female heterozygotes may have relatively high residual activity.
- Gene sequencing and identification of disease-causing mutation is reliable for confirming the diagnosis in women.

### Cardiac features
- Intracellular accumulation of glycosphingolipids in myocardium, conduction system, valves and vascular endothelium.

*Left ventricular hypertrophy*
- Most develop concentric hypertrophy.
- Asymmetrical septal hypertrophy in 5–10% cases.
- Histologically glycosphingolipid accounts for only 1–2% of cardiac mass and other signalling pathways are activated leading to hypertrophy, apoptosis, necrosis, and fibrosis.
- Degree of hypertrophy correlates with age.
- Left ventricular outflow tract obstruction uncommmon.
- Right ventricle often affected but without major clinical consequences.

- LV systolic function is often preserved radially with reduced longitudinal function.
- Diastolic dysfunction is a common feature.

*Valvular disease*
- Thickening of papillary muscles and mitral valve leaflets with accompanying regurgitation seen in 50% patients.
- Severe valve disease requiring surgery uncommon.
- Aortic root dilatation described and can affect valve function.

*Myocardial ischaemia*
- Chest pain/angina seen in up to 50% patients.
- Angiographically normal coronary arteries in most cases.
- Accumulation of lipid in coronary endothelial cells and microvascular angina may be responsible for symptoms.

*Electrophysiological abnormalities*
- Majority of patient have an abnormal resting ECG (voltage criteria for LVH, repolarization abnormalities, short PR interval).
- Later developments include bundle branch block, AV conduction delay and progressive sinus node dysfunction.
- Various arrhythmias—commonly supra ventricular tachycardia (SVT), AF and atrial flutter.
- NSVT on Holter monitoring seen in up to 8.3%.
- Sudden cardiac death is not a predominant feature but fatal arrhythmias resistant to ICD implantation reported.

**Management**
- Cardiac management involves conventional anti-anginal and heart failure medications.
- β blockers should be used with caution as they can aggravate chronotropic incompetence and impaired AV conduction.
- Patients may not tolerate large doses of vasodilating medications due to orthostatic hypotension related to autonomic dysfunction.
- Antiplatelet therapy in patients with ischaemic symptoms.
- ACE inhibitors or angiotensin receptor blockers in heart failure and in those with proteinuria.
- In those with supraventricular arrhythmias anticoagulation should be given.
- ICD implantation should be considered in those with malignant arrhythmias unless poor life expectancy unlikely to be improved with device.
- Alcohol septal ablation and surgical myectomy have been used in outflow tract obstruction to good effect.

**Enzyme replacement therapy**
- Two recombinant enzyme preparations available in Europe.
- Both improve renal and neurological manifestations as well as quality of life.
- Some evidence for beneficial effects on heart.
- Antibodies against enzyme preparations seen in 55–80% patients but clinical effects are unclear.
- Patients should have serial renal and cardiac evaluation with creatinine clearance/24h protein excretion assessment as well as periodic ECG, echocardiogram and ambulatory ECG monitoring assessment.

**Table 18.1** Extra-cardiac features of Anderson–Fabry disease

| System | Features |
|---|---|
| Dermatological | Angiokeratoma 40% (swimming trunk distribution) |
| | Hypohydrosis 50% men/25% women |
| | Lymphoedema |
| | Coarse facial features |
| Neurological | Acroparaesthesiae (chronic pain in hands and feet) |
| | Fabry's crisis: |
| | • severe pain precipitated by stress/exertion/illness |
| | • often accompanied by fever/increased erythrocyte sedimentation rate (ESR) |
| | transient ischemic attack (TIA)/cerebro vascular accident (CVA): |
| | • rate increased 12 times in men/10 times in women |
| | Substantial hearing loss 16–54% men |
| | Tinnitus/vertigo/headache |
| Renal | Proteinuria |
| | Lipiduria |
| | Uraemia |
| | Hypertension |
| | End-stage renal failure |
| Gastrointestinal | Nausea and vomiting |
| | Abdominal pain and diarrhoea |
| | Common childhood symptom (19–52% males) |
| Pulmonary | Airways obstruction |
| | Decreased diffusion capacity |
| Ophthalmologic | Corneal opacities (cornea verticellata) |
| | Opacities posterior lens |
| | Retinal vascular tortuosity |
| | Occlusion retinal vessel infarction (rare) |
| Other | Decreased bone mineral density |
| | Azoospermia |
| | Depression |
| | Reduced saliva/tear production |
| | Anaemia |

# Fatty acid oxidation disorders

This is an important group of disorders including:
- disorders of carnitine transport and the carnitine cycle
- long chain 3 hydroxyl-acyl-CoA dehydrogenase deficiency
- mitochondrial trifunctional protein deficiency
- long-chain 3-ketoacyl-CoA thiolase deficiency
- very long-chain acyl-CoA dehydrogenase deficiency
- medium chain acyl CoA dehydrogenase deficiency.

## Pathophysiology

During periods of fasting, fatty acids are the predominant substrate for energy production via oxidation in the liver, cardiac muscle, and skeletal muscle. The brain does not directly utilize fatty acids for oxidative metabolism, but oxidizes ketone bodies derived from acetyl CoA and acetoacetyl CoA produced by $\beta$-oxidation of fatty acids in the liver. When the oxidation of fatty acids is defective, fats are still released from the adipose tissue with fasting and will reach the liver, skeletal muscle, and heart where they accumulate. The inability of the liver to metabolize them results in steatosis and decreased production of ketones.

Ketones can be used an alternate energy source by the heart, skeletal muscle, and brain, sparing glucose. If fatty acid oxidation is defective, fat cannot be utilized, glucose is consumed without regeneration via gluconeogenesis and there is a drop in glucose levels (hypoglycemia). Fats can go directly to the heart and skeletal muscle where they can accumulate and impair organ/tissue function (cardiomyopathy/myopathy). Free fatty acids and long-chain acylcarnitines can alter the electrical activity of cardiac cells resulting in arrhythmia. In certain diseases, muscle fibres can also break down during sustained exercise resulting in myoglobinuria.

## Diagnosis

The key to the diagnosis is the clinical suspicion of these disorders. Disorders may present throughout life at any age with the following:
- hypoketotic hypoglycaemic coma
- liver disease with raised ammonia
- skeletal muscle-weakness, pain or acute myolysis under strain (long chain disorders)
- cardiomyopathy.

In suspected diagnoses biochemical assessment, to elucidate a diagnosis, jointly with a specialist centre may include:
- measurement of plasma carnitine levels including total, free and acylated carnitine
- specific acylcarnitine profile
- urine organic acids
- fatty acid oxidation in skin fibroblasts.

Diagnosis may be made also from DNA mutational studies and disorders are inherited in an autosomal recessive mode.

## Disorders of carnitine transport and the carnitine cycle

Carnitine plays an essential role in the transfer of long-chain fatty acids across the inner mitochondrial membrane.

### Primary carnitine deficiency

- Primary carnitine deficiency is an autosomal recessive disorder of fatty acid oxidation due to the lack of functional carnitine transporters.
- Primary carnitine deficiency has a frequency of about 1:40,000 to 1:100,000 newborns.
- A metabolic presentation, hepatomegaly, hypoglycaemia, minimal ketones, and hyperammonaemia is more frequent before two years of age.
- Cardiomyopathy is more frequent in older patients associated sometimes with hypotonia. Cardiomyopathy can also be seen in older patients with a metabolic presentation, even if asymptomatic from a cardiac standpoint.
- Cardiac hypertrophy has been reported in heterozygotes approaching middle age. It is unclear whether this is associated with any health problem.
- Patients with primary carnitine deficiency respond to dietary carnitine supplementation.

### Carnitine palmitoyl transferase 1 deficiency

- Carnitine palmitoyl transferase 1 (CPT-1) conjugates fatty acids to carnitine allowing their subsequent transfer into the mitochondria.
- CPT-1 deficiency is usually triggered by fasting or viral illnesses.
- Affected children present, usually between birth and 18 months of age, with altered mental status and hepatomegaly.
- Laboratory evaluation indicates non-ketotic hypoglycemia, mild hyperammonemia, elevated liver function tests, and elevated free fatty acids. In this disease, plasma carnitine levels are not decreased, but usually increased. Several different mutations have been identified in patients with CPT-1 deficiency.

### Carnitine-acylcarnitine translocase deficiency

- Carnitine-acylcarnitine translocase (CACT) is located in the inner mitochondrial membrane and operates a carnitine/acylcarnitine exchange across this membrane.
- CACT deficiency presents most often in the neonatal period with seizures, irregular heart beat, and apnoea. Many times these episodes are triggered by fasting or by the physiologic birth stress.
- Patients with presentation later in life (up to 15 months of age) have been reported. In these milder cases, attacks are triggered by fever, infections and fasting as other fatty acid oxidation defects. Fasting hypoglycemia and seizures have been reported in these patients.
- The gene for this condition maps to 3p21. DNA studies have found heterogeneous mutations in different patients and can also be used for diagnostic confirmation.
- Complete deficiency of this transporter is associated with rapidly progressive disease. Residual activity has been associated with a milder phenotype and near normal development with appropriate therapy.

*Carnitine palmitoyl transferase 2 deficiency*

- Carnitine palmitoyl transferase 2 (CPT-2) deficiency presents most frequently in adolescents or young adults with predominant muscular involvement, but can also present in infancy and in the neonatal period.
- The neonatal form presents shortly after birth (few hours–4 days) with respiratory distress, seizures, altered mental status, hepatomegaly, cardiomegaly, cardiac arrhythmia, and, in many cases, dysmorphic features, renal dysgenesis, and neuronal migration defects.
- The neonatal form of CPT-2 deficiency is rapidly fatal. The infantile variety usually presents between 6 and 24 months of age with recurrent attacks of hypoketotic hypoglycemia causing loss of consciousness and seizures, liver failure and transient hepatomegaly. Several children also have heart involvement with cardiomyopathy and arrhythmia.
- The myopathic form of CPT-2 deficiency presents in young adults with muscle pain with or (in most cases) without myoglobinuria with elevation of serum creatine kinase precipitated by strenuous exercise, cold, fever or prolonged fasting. Myoglobinuria can cause kidney failure and death.
- The gene for CPT-2 maps to 1p32 and heterogenous mutations have been identified in patients with CPT2 deficiency.

**Other fatty acid oxidation disorders**

- Long chain 3 hydroxyl-acyl-CoA dehydrogenase deficiency (LCHAD).
- Mitochondrial trifunctional protein deficiency (TFP).
- Long –chain 3-ketoacyl-CoA thiolase deficiency (LKAT).
- Very long-chain acyl-CoA dehydrogenase deficiency (VLCAD).
- Multiple acyl-CoA dehydrogenase deficiency (MAD).
- Medium chain acyl CoA dehydrogenase deficiency (MCAD).

As with the carnitine defects these disorders have a wide range of presentations including neonatal presentations (malformations and facial dysmorphology are associated with MAD) and later onset in adulthood.

The presentation is characterized by hepatic, cardiac, and muscle abnormalities. In addition there may be chronic neurological presentation, and renal presentation in many but not all varients.

The cardiac presentations include:

- cardiomyopathy (hypertrophic and dilated)
- heart beat disorders (with or without cardiomyopathy)
- conduction abnormalities
- arhythmias
- sudden collapse.

Cardiomyopathy can generally be found in all of the disorders with the exception of MCAD deficiency. Also heart beat disorders and sudden collapse are not seen generally in MCAD.

# Very long chain acyl-coenzyme A dehydrogenase deficiency

- Prevalence unknown.
- Autosomal recessive inheritance.
- Infantile onset form associated with severe cardiac and hepatic symptoms.
- Severe lipid storage in heart reported to cause severe LV hypertrophy with associated heart failure.
- Often fatal in the first year of life.
- Later onset forms not associated with cardiac involvement.
- Other clinical features include exercise-induced muscle pain, rhabdomyolysis, hypoketotic hypoglycaemia, and hepatomegaly.
- Basic management goal to prevent/minimize long chain fatty acid oxidation with intravenous 10% glucose or carnitine administration.
- Long-term management is dietary avoidance of fasting and a diet low in long-chain fatty acids with increased medium-chain fatty acids.

# Glycogen storage diseases

These are a group of inherited metabolic disorders of glycogen metabolism.

There are over 14 types classified according to the enzyme deficiency and the affected tissue.

These disorders affect primarily the liver, muscle or both and their overall incidence is estimated at 1:20,000–43,000 live births.

The heart is affected in types II, III, and IV with cardiac manifestations such as severe left hypertrophy, mimicking HCM, restrictive cardiomyopathy, dilated cardiomyopathy or conduction system disease.

## Glycogen storage disease type II

- Also known as Pompe disease/acid alpha-glucosidase deficiency/acid maltase deficiency.
- Due to a deficiency of acid A glucosidase (acid maltase).
- Inherited as an autosomal recessive trait.
- Gene encoding alpha glucosidase located on chromosome 17.

### Infantile form

- Presents in infants between 8–12 weeks.
- Manifests as 'floppy baby' with failure to thrive.
- Cardiac involvement is frequent.
- Severe cardiomegaly evident on chest X-ray.
- **ECG**: short PR interval and left ventricular hypertrophy.
- **ECHO**: biventricular hypertrophy, small LV cavity, outflow tract obstruction, diastolic dysfunction.
- **CK levels** are markedly elevated.
- **Muscle biopsy:** confirms diagnosis showing vacuolated muscle fibres with a high glycogen content.
- Poor prognosis, generally fatal in first year of life, usually due to cardio-respiratory failure.
- Genetic counselling fundamental for prevention.
- Enzyme replacement therapy is promising and emphasizes the need for early recognition as is most beneficial if instituted early.

### Late onset form

- Disease develops after 12 months of age.
- Some residual acid A glucosidase activity.
- Presentation in adult life reported.
- Clinically limb girdle pattern of myopathy.
- Cardiac involvement rare, but conduction abnormalities including WPW reported.

## Glycogen storage disease type III

- Also known as Cori disease/Forbes disease/glycogen debrancher deficiency.
- Due to deficiency in glycogen debrancher enzyme activity, resulting in an excessive accumulation of abnormal glycogen.
- Gene isolated on chromosome 1.
- Accounts for 24% of all glycogen storage diseases (GSDs).

- Incidence in Europe 1:83,000 live births (1:3,600 Faroe Islands).
- Inherited as an autosomal recessive trait.
- Phenotype variability due to differences in tissue expression of the deficient enzyme.
- **Clinical features:** hepatomegaly, hypoglycaemia, short stature, dyslipdaemia, and slight mental retardation.
- Liver symptoms improve with age and usually disappear after puberty.
- **Cardiac features:** commonest is left ventricular hypertrophy resembling HCM and may be accompanied by systolic anterior motion of the mitral valve and left ventricular outflow tract obstruction.
- Patients can have clinical symptoms of heart failure also.
- Many patients have no cardiac symptoms.
- Biventricular dilation, recurrent sustained VT and sudden death reported.
- **Diagnosis:** demonstrating enzyme deficiency in liver/muscle.
- **Treatment:** primarily dietary, aimed at maintaining normoglycaemia but the effect on cardiac involvement is unknown.

## Glycogen storage disease type IV

- Also known as Anderson disease/brancher deficiency/amylopectinosis.
- Due to a deficiency of amylo-1,4 to 1,6-transglucosidase resulting in an accumulation of abnormal glycogens in liver and muscle.
- Gene located on chromosome 3.
- Accounts for 0.3% of all GSDs.
- Inherited as an autosomal recessive trait.
- **Clinical features:** extremely heterogeneous due to variation in tissue involvement.
- Classical form characterized by cirrhosis and hepatic failure in childhood.
- Rarely the hepatic disease is slowly or non-progressive.
- In these individuals, cardiac involvement usually manifests as congestive cardiac failure.
- **Treatment:** only effective therapeutic approach in progressive form is liver transplantation, which may also help muscular involvement.

# Homocystinuria (cystathionine β-synthase deficiency)

This is important to consider in the differential diagnosis of Marfan syndrome (📖 see also Chapter 10, Inherited disorders of connective tissue, p.263.).

The condition is autosomal recessive. The prevalence is varied from 1 in 344,000 based on worldwide newborn screening to about 1 in 65,000 in Ireland.

### Clinical features

Dislocation of the ocular lens (ectopia lentis) which is usually down (severe short-sightedness may also be an important clue to diagnosis), osteoporosis, lower IQ and skeletal abnormalities (pectus deformities are common) with joint stiffness.

Specific cardiovascular complications are a consequence of thromboembolism. Vascular occlusion can occur in any vessel, the majority are venous, including the portal vein, cerebrovascular accidents, peripheral arteries and a small but significant incidence of myocardial infarctions.

### Genetics

The cystathionine β-synthase gene maps to chromosome chromosome 21q22.3. Most of these mutations are missense, and the vast majority of these are private mutations. The two frequently encountered mutations are the pyridoxine-responsive I278T and the pyridoxine-non-responsive G307S.

### Diagnosis

The most consistent biochemical finding is homocystinuria. Plasma/serum analysis of amino acids will reveal a raised homocystine, raised methionine and a markedly reduced concentration of cystine. 50% of patients are sensitive to pyridoxine (B6) supplementation.

### Treatment

It is possible to significantly alter the outcome for patients with treatment which can include dietary methionine restriction, pyridoxine, folate, B12, and betaine. If patients are untreated half of the patients have a vascular event by the age of 30.

Whilst homocysteine levels may not be entirely normal on treatment there is a significant reduction in cardiovascular risk with aggressive lowering of the homocysteine levels.

# The heart and inherited haematological disorders

# Introduction

Cardiac iron overload occurs as a consequence of genetic mutations that dysregulate iron homeostasis such as the inherited haemochromatosis syndromes, or more frequently as a consequence of recurrent blood transfusions, essential in the treatment of the inherited refractory anaemias. The haemoglobinopathies are the main cause of cardiac iron overload and pose a major global public health problem. Even though these genetic disorders do not affect the heart directly, cardiac involvement through iron overload is a major cause of morbidity and mortality, as part of a complex multi-system disease with concurrent liver and endocrine involvement.

Iron overload and toxicity

- There is no dedicated and effective iron excretion pathway in humans making us vulnerable to iron overload if the supply exceeds the demand.
- Approximately 1–2mg/day of iron is absorbed by the small intestine and bound to transferrin in plasma. It is used primarily by erythrocytes in the bone marrow for heme production.
- Iron in excess of the body's metabolic requirements overwhelms the carrying capacity of transferrin, and free non-transferrin bound iron (NTBI) appears in plasma.
- Circulating NTBI is taken up by the heart, liver and many other tissues including the endocrine organs.
- NTBI catalyses the formation of reactive oxygen species which damage cellular proteins, lipids and DNA.
- Cardiac dysfunction arises as hydroxyl radicals formed by NTBI interfere with the mitochondrial respiratory chain.
- Iron deposits are greatest in the epicardium>subendocardium and papillary muscles>middle third of the ventricular myocardium>atria>conduction system.

# The pathophysiology of thalassaemia

Haemoglobin is a tetrameric molecule composed of two globin dimers, each made up of an α-like and a β-like globin chain. Thalassaemia is caused by mutations leading to reduced expression of one or more globin chains. The difference in the rate of expression between the affected and the normally expressed globin genes leads to an excess of the unaffected globin chains. The excess globin chains are toxic and cause both ineffective erythropoiesis and haemolysis.

The combined effects of reduced and imbalanced globin production cause the anaemia seen in the thalassaemias. In severe cases the anaemia, which is exacerbated by hypersplenism, is profound and the extreme metabolic demands of the ensuing massive bone marrow expansion lead to premature morbidity and mortality.

In general, ineffective erythropoiesis is more severe in β-thalassaemia since the excess α chains are more toxic than the excess β and γ chains encountered in α thalassaemia. This leads to significantly less dependence to blood transfusions and hence less aggressive iron loading in the α-thalassaemia syndromes.

The thalassaemia syndromes are genetically classified according to the globin gene involved. They are also classified clinically by the severity of the haematological phenotype. The haematological phenotype is a major determinant of the cardiac manifestations:

• Thalassaemia major: Severe anaemia requiring lifelong regular blood transfusions for survival
• Thalassaemia minor: Asymptomatic carriers
• Thalassamia intermedia. This group includes a wide range of phenotypes that lie between the two extremes.
  • Some patients with thalassaemia intermedia may require blood transfusion at times of stress such as infections.
  • With increasing age some intermedia patients become transfusiondependent and behave like thalassaemia major.

# The genetics of thalassaemia

Thalassaemia alleles are common with a heterozygote frequency of 3–30%. There is geographical overlap with regions endemic for malaria through the survival advantage of heterozygotes who are protected from severe malaria. Immigration from endemic areas to Europe no longer confines these diseases to particular localities.

### $\alpha$-Thalassaemia

- The $\alpha$-like globin genes form a cluster on chromosome 16.
- There are two $\alpha$ globin genes per chromosome and the normal genotype is $\alpha\alpha/\alpha\alpha$.
- Pathogenic mutations lead to:
  - $\alpha^0$-thalassaemia haplotypes with no $\alpha$ chain production.
  - $\alpha^+$-thalassaemia haplotypes with residual $\alpha$ globin production.
- In general, inheritance of the normal $\alpha\alpha$ haplotype with any of the $\alpha^0$ or $\alpha^+$ thalassaemia haplotypes leads to $\alpha$ thalassaemia trait.
- Inheritance of two $\alpha^0$ alleles results in haemoglobin Bart's hydrops fetalis syndrome which is not compatible with life.
- Inheritance of $\alpha^0$ with $\alpha^+$ alleles causes mostly Haemoglobin H (HbH) disease, which is characterized by the excess $\beta$-globin forming tetramers ($\beta_4$ = HbH). HbH has a very high oxygen affinity and does not contribute to gas exchange in a meaningful manner.
- Coinheritance of two $\alpha^+$ alleles causes a spectrum of phenotypes that ranges mostly between $\alpha$-thalassaemia trait and Hb H disease.
- These above patterns of inheritance are generalizations and many exceptions exist.

### $\beta$-Thalassaemia

- The $\beta$-like globin genes form a cluster on chromosome 11 and include one $\beta$ and $\delta$ globin gene per chromosome.
- Pathogenic mutations lead to:
  - $\beta^0$-thalassaemia haplotypes with no $\beta$-globin chain production
  - $\beta^+$-thalassaemia haplotypes with residual $\beta$-globin chain production.
- $\beta$-thalassaemia major is the most severe form and the underlying genotype is the compound heterozygote or more rarely the homozygote state($\beta^0/\beta^+$, $\beta^0/\beta^0$, $\beta^+/\beta^+$).
- $\beta$-thalassaemia minor is an asymptomatic state and is caused by the inheritance of one abnormal $\beta$ globin gene ($\beta^0/\beta$ or $\beta+/\beta$).
- $\beta$-thalassaemia intermedia includes a wide range of phenotypes that range between the major and minor forms($\beta^0/\beta$, $\beta^+/\beta^+$).
- The above patterns of inheritance are generalizations and exceptions exist.

# Iron overload in thalassaemia

## The mechanism of iron overload

- Parenteral iron:
  - Thalassaemia major patients require lifelong blood transfusions, approximately once a month, to maintain a pre-transfusion haemoglobin of 9–10.5g/dl
  - each unit of blood contains 200mg of iron, and since the human body lacks an effective excretion pathway for excess iron, transfusion therapy leads to iron overload by the second decade of life
  - transfusional iron overload is also seen in a variety of severe heamatologic conditions such as sideroblastic anaemia, congenital or acquired aplastic anaemia, Blackfan–Diamond anaemia and the myelodysplastic syndromes. The management of iron overload in these patients is the same as in thalassaemia major.
- Enteral iron:
  - there is an unexplained paradoxical increase in intestinal iron absorption despite an overall increase in total body iron. This appears to be related to the degree of bone marrow expansion.

Blood transfusion is the primary source of excess iron in thalassaemia major, whilst increased intestinal iron absorption plays a more important role in the non-transfusion-dependant thalassaemia intermedia syndromes.

## Chelation

- Chelation reduces tissue iron concentrations by removing labile intracellular iron and transit iron released by macrophages.
- Chelated iron is excreted in faeces or urine.
- Controlling iron overload takes months or years since only a small portion of body iron is available at any one time for chelation.
- Chelating agents prevent free radical formation limiting tissue damage until iron concentrations are controlled.
- Deferoxamine:
  - the mainstay of chelation treatment
  - requires prolonged infusions(sc/iv)
  - expensive, burdensome and many patients comply poorly.
- Deferiprone:
  - oral administration
  - effective in preventing and treating cardiac iron overload
  - less effective in removing hepatic iron.
- Desferasirox:
  - a newer oral agent with od regimen
  - efficacy data are limited.

The properties of each chelation treatment are summarized in Table 19.1.

**Table 19.1** Chelation treatments

|  | Deferoxamine | Deferiprone | Deferasirox |
| --- | --- | --- | --- |
| Mode of administration | s/c, iv | po | po |
| Regiment | 20 to 50mg/kg/day infused over 8 to 24h on at least 5 to 7 days per week | 75mg/kg/day tds<br><br>Combination treatment with deferoxamine also possible | 20 to 30mg/kg/day od<br><br>Combination treatment with deferoxamine also possible |
| Half life | 0.5hrs | 3–4hrs | 12–16hrs |
| Side effects | Potentially irreversible auditory and retinal toxicity, impaired growth, bony abnormalities, local reactions, increased risk of yersinia infection, localized reactions | Deranged liver enzymes, arthropathy, nausea, neutropenia and agranulocytosis, zinc deficiency, possible liver fibrosis, immune dysregulation | Gastrointestinal disturbances<br><br>Rash, mild non-progressive creatinine increase, elevated liver enzymes |

# Cardiac disease in β-thalassaemia

β-thalassaemia major
- Untreated patients:
  - in the absence of regular blood transfusions, patients develop a hyperdynamic circulation as a consequence of severe anaemia and the high metabolic demands of erythroid expansion
  - high output cardiac failure during the first decade of life is amongst the leading causes of death.
- Patients receiving regular blood transfusions but no chelation:
  - transfusional cardiac iron overload causing left +/− right ventricular dilation and systolic dysfunction become a major cause of death in the second and third decade of life
  - ventricular dysfunction is often complicated by atrial arrhythmias, conduction system disease, a high ventricular ectopic burden and ventricular tachycardias
  - restrictive physiology sometimes dominates the clinical picture
  - once heart failure develops, the 3-month mortality rate is 58%.
- Patients receiving transfusions with chelation:
  - chelating agents developed in the 1960s have reduced cardiac complications and improved survival
  - chelation can not only prevent cardiac dysfunction secondary to iron overload, but intensification of treatment in severely affected patients can reverse the cardiomyopathy
  - about 50% of UK patients with β-thalassaemia major still die before the age of 35 years primarily because of poor compliance with iron-chelation therapy.
- Viral myocarditis/pericarditis may be an important modulator of the clinical course in some patients.

β-thalassaemia intermedia
- Pulmonary hypertension and right heart failure with preserved left ventricular function dominate the clinical picture.
- Pulmonary hypertension develops as a result of chronic tissue hypoxia and haemolysis which causes vasoconstriction by reducing nitric oxide levels. *In situ* thrombosis in the pulmonary vasculature also plays a role as thalassaemia intermedia is a prothrombotic state.
- Transfusional iron overload is not encountered since regular high-volume blood transfusions are not required.
- Iron overload through intestinal absorption is found in approximately a fifth of thalassaemia intermedia patients but its contribution to the development of cardiac disease in these circumstances appears to be limited. The role of chelation in these patients is not known.

β-thalassaemia minor
An asymptomatic carrier state with no cardiac manifestations.

# Cardiac disease in α-thalassaemia

### Haemoglobin H disease

As most patients with HbH disease do not require regular blood transfusions, transfusional iron overload is not a feature of this syndrome. However, with increasing age hepatic iron overload is frequently encountered, but cardiac iron overload is rare. The role of chelation in HbH disease is not known. Even though the haematological phenotype is similar to β-thalassaemia intermedia pulmonary hypertension, and right ventricular failure are not commonly seen.

### α-thalassaemia trait

This is an asymptomatic condition with no cardiac manifestations.

### The heart in thalassaemia

Chronic tissue hypoxia leads to a number of compensatory haemodynamic responses:
- to improve oxygen delivery cardiac output increases primarily by an increase in stroke volume
- the ventricles are volume loaded but the ejection fraction appears to be similar to sex- and age-matched controls
- the resting heart rate is not increased
- the peripheral resistance is low and associated with low diastolic blood pressure
- the 'normal' values of commonly measured haemodynamic parameters in non-iron loaded thalassaemia patients have not been systematically studied. The variations in haemoglobin, the volume load of blood transfusions and concurrent medical illnesses make the study of such haemodynamic parameters difficult.

# The pathophysiology of haemochromatosis

Haemochromatosis is an inherited disease characterized by the constellation of diabetes, bronze pigmentation of the skin, arthritis, hepatic cirrhosis, and cardiac disease secondary to iron overload. The *HFE* gene responsible for the disease was first identified in 1996 and since then mutations in other non-HFE genes involved in iron metabolism have been identified. In contrast to thalassaemia and other refractory anaemias where the iron overload is primarily a consequence of treatment of another disease process, haemochromatosis is a disease of iron metabolism itself and caused by mutations of genes that modulate iron regulatory pathways.

# The genetics of haemochromatosis

*HFE*-related haemochromatosis
- Autosomal recessive.
- Caused by mutations of the *HFE* gene on chromosome 6.
- The HFE protein is expressed on the surface of cells involved in iron metabolism and modulates the uptake of transferrin-bound iron.
- Two point mutations have been described but the exact mechanism by which these mutations result in iron overload is not fully understood.
- C282Y:
  - the substitution of cysteine to tyrosine at position 282 of the HFE protein prevents the interaction with transferrin receptor 1.
  - in Europe the average prevalence of C282Y heterozygosity is 9.2% whilst the homozygous state is found in 0.4% of the general population.
- H63D:
  - the substitution of histidine by aspartic acid at position 63 does not prevent the interaction of the HFE protein with transferrin receptor 1 and its pathogenic implications are less clear.
  - H63D is commoner in southern Europe.

Non-*HFE*-related haemochromatosis
A minority of cases of haemochromatosis are not related to mutations in the *HFE* gene. These include:
- Juvenile haemochromatosis, an autosomal recessive disease with more aggressive features than the classic HFE form. Mutations in two genes have been implicated, the haemojuvelin (*HJV*) gene on chromosome 1 and less frequently the hepcidin antimicrobial peptide (*HAMP*) gene on chromosome 19.
- Mutations in the transferrin receptor-2 (*TFR2*) gene on chromosome 7 have been implicated in an autosomal recessive form haemochromatosis with similar clinical features to the classic HFE-related disease.
- An autosomal dominant form of haemochromatosis caused by mutations of the *SLC40A1* gene on chromosome 2 has also been described. This gene encodes for ferroportin, a transmembrane iron transporter which is found on enterocytes, hepatocytes and the reticuloendothelial system and transports iron into the bloodstream. The clinical course of ferroportin disease is variable.

Mutations in other unidentified genes probably contribute for unexplained cases.

# Iron overload in haemochromatosis

### The mechanism of iron overload

Two processes contribute to iron overload in haemochromatosis:
- enhanced gastrointestinal absorption of iron
- excessive release of iron into the circulation from macrophages.

Both processes are thought to be caused by low hepcidin levels found in all of the haemochromatosis syndromes. Hepcidin is an iron regulatory hormone and inhibits iron release in the circulation from the intestine and macrophages by interacting with the main iron export protein, ferroportin. It is thought that haemojuvelin, transferrin receptor 2, and HFE modulate the hepcidin–ferroportin axis and thus mutations in these genes cause haemochromatosis.

### Venesection

- Venesection appears to improve survival and limit cardiac involvement.
- Approximately 500ml removed every 1 to 2 weeks until ferritin normalizes or patient becomes anaemic.
- Use of chelation to clear iron stores quickly and avoid complications of cardiac failure in haemochromatosis has not been systematically examined.

# Cardiac disease in haemochromatosis

- Haemochromatosis has a low penetrance.
- Disease expression is affected by sex, age, and other genetic and environmental factors which modulate the primary genetic abnormality.
- The introduction of venesection in the early 1950s has reduced the incidence of end organ disease.
- Prior to the era of venesection 15% of patients with haemochromatosis presented with cardiac disease and 33% eventually developed cardiomyopathy.
- Cardiac involvement includes:
  - biventricular dilation and dysfunction
  - isolated right or left ventricular impairment
  - diastolic dysfunction
  - restrictive cardiomyopathy
  - arrhythmias (about a third of patients)

## The heart in cirrhosis

The haemodynamic effects of cirrhosis, another common complication of haemoachromatosis, should be considered when evaluating the cardiac status of patients with haemochromatosis. The presence of cirrhosis is associated with:

- hyperdynamic circulation
- high cardiac output
- diastolic dysfunction
- low systemic vascular resistance
- blood pressure tends to be low
- sinus tachycardia.

These changes are not related to cardiac iron overload.

# Evaluation of patients

### History

The evaluation is complicated as cardiac involvement is rarely found in isolation. Anaemia, endocrine abnormalities—e.g. hypothyroidism, liver disease—are also present and contribute to symptomatology. Past transfusion history and compliance to treatment provide clues to the degree of iron overload.

### Examination

There are no specific signs for cardiac iron overload.

### Serum ferritin

This is elevated in both thalasaemia and haemochromatosis.

The relationship between cardiac iron overload and serum ferritin levels is not good enough to guide the management of cardiac disease.

### Electrocardiography

Non-specific findings.

### Echocardiography

This is useful in the evaluation of cardiac morphology and function, as well as screening for pulmonary arterial hypertension. However, echocardiography is unreliable in recognizing patients with significant cardiac iron overload before the onset of cardiac dysfunction and cardiac failure.

### Cardiac magnetic resonance imaging

- Iron in tissues causes CMR images to decay and become darker faster. The decay of CMR images as quantified by T2* reflects tissue iron concentration.
- Low T2* values (<20ms) reflect high cardiac iron content and are associated with ventricular dysfunction. All patients presenting with heart failure secondary to iron overload have abnormal myocardial T2*, and almost 90% have T2*<10ms.
- Patients with preserved function but high cardiac iron deposition (T2*<20ms) who are at high risk of developing cardiac complications can be identified. This provides a unique opportunity to intensify chelation treatment and prevent cardiac morbidity and mortality.
- Intensification of chelation treatment progressively normalizes T2* with an associated improvement in cardiac function.

# Management of patients at risk of cardiac iron overload

- Prevention:
  - adequate chelation in patients with high transfusion requirements and venesection in the haemochromatosis syndromes reduces cardiac morbidity and mortality
  - patients at risk of cardiac iron overload should be reviewed frequently for cardiac involvement
  - Serial CMR T2* measurements are invaluable in identifying high-risk patients requiring more intensive treatment
  - preventative strategies commonly fail because of poor compliance.
- Treatment of heart failure:
  - conventional treatment for heart failure and asymptomatic left ventricular dysfunction is recommended but this strategy has never been systematically examined in this subgroup of patients
  - extrapolation from other cardiac conditions guides the management of other cardiac complications such as atrial fibrillation
  - conventional medical treatment is usually a holding measure until cardiac function improves with specific treatment.
- Treatment of cardiac iron overload:
  - cardiac dysfunction secondary to cardiac iron overload is largely reversible with aggressive treatment to remove excess iron
  - patients with thalassaemia major require continuous intravenous chelation, often in combination with another agent, for many months or years to reverse the cardiomyopathy. The progress is monitored with echocardiography and T2* measurements
  - with the advent of T2* measurement, patients with cardiac iron overload at risk of developing cardiac dysfunction can be identified. This allows intensification of chelation treatment before the deleterious effects of iron become apparent
- Pulmonary hypertension:
  - best managed by treatments that suppress haemolysis
  - in the thalassaemias this involves intensification of transfusion (as well as chelation)
  - Sildenafil and inhaled nitric oxide have also been used, but they have not been systematically studied.

Finally, cardiac iron overload is part of a complex disease process that spans across multiple medical specialties. A multidisciplinary approach is therefore the most effective approach in achieving the best management of these patients.

# Therapeutic approaches in cardiovascular genetics

# Pharmacogenetics

Pharmacogenetics is the use of genetic information to predict the likelihood of response to medication (efficacy) or the likelihood of a significant side effect (adverse drug reaction) to that medication.

Pharmacogenomics, an allied discipline, is the use of genetic information in a broader sense, for example the use of gene expression profiles to predict drug response or the identification of therapeutic targets.

Both inherited (germline) genetic changes or acquired (somatic) genetic changes can influence response to medication. Somatic changes are more relevant to cancer treatment. Changes in genes that alter the absorption, distribution, metabolism and elimination (ADME) of a drug are potentially important, as they alter the available concentration of an active drug (pharmacokinetics). In some patients, the same available dose leads to a difference in response (pharmacodynamics) due to potential genetic differences in the drug receptors or other pathways which feed into the complex drug-effector mechanism.

As we have seen in a previous chapter (📖 Chapter 9, Inherited arrhythmias and conduction disorders) certain drugs can prolong the QT interval e.g. phenytoin, sotalol. Prolongation of the QT interval is a very important reason why some drugs do not progress past phase 1 trials and do not come to market. Pharmaceutical companies spend considerable efforts in drug development to ensure that drugs do not prolong the QT interval or predispose patients to arrythmias.

Howver, some drugs, like cisapride, a serotonin 5-HT$_4$ receptor agonist for use in gastrooesophageal reflux disease, have progressed to market and been used widely before being withdrawn, due to precipitation of fatal cardiac arrythmias secondary to a prolonged QT interval in a small number of patients.

In 10–15% of patients with drug-induced torsades de pointes (TdP) variants in ion channel genes including *KCNQ1* and *KCNE2* have been identified.

The use of pharmacogenetics in clinical practice in cardiac disorders has been limited so far. A few examples are emerging where knowledge of a patient's genotype may predict drug efficacy or avoid a potential adverse reaction.

# Warfarin

Warfarin is a widely used oral anticoagulant in the prevention of thromboembolic events, for example in patients with atrial fibrillation or with a prosthetic heart valve. Over 30 million prescriptions per year are written in the USA for warfarin. It is the second most common cause of adverse drug reactions. The major risks associated with warfarin relate to haemorrhagic events within the first six weeks of starting treatment as the international normalized ratio (INR) is often outside the normal range with standard dose initiation.

Clinical algorithms including patient age, gender, weight, smoking status, co-morbidity, and co-medication have been established to improve the risk profile by predicting personalized dosing regimens.

Warfarin acts as a vitamin K antagonist by inhibiting the enzyme vitamin K epoxide reductase complex, subunit 1 (VKORC1). VKORC1 acts to recycle vitamin K from its inactive epoxide form.

Pharmacogenetic studies have defined that common variants in the cytochrome P450 genes, CYP2C9 and CYP4F2 and VKORC1 alter the dose of warfarin required to achieve anti-coagulation. Of these three genes, a common variant in the promoter of VKORC1 has the biggest effect.

These gene variants have been incorporated into warfarin dosing algorithms with clinical parameters, e.g. ℗ http://www.warfarindosing.org to generate a predicted starting dose to reduce the likelihood of adverse events. Recent studies suggest that the use of pharmacogenetic information plus clinical parameters is the optimum way to reduce adverse reactions to warfarin.

In 2007, pharmacogenomic information for warfarin was approved by the Food and Drug Administration (FDA) to be included in the product label stating that VKORC1 and CYP2C9 genotypes may be useful in determining the optimal initial dose of warfarin. A number of randomized controlled trials are being undertaken to determine the optimum use of genotype information in reducing adverse events due to warfarin.

Rarely, patients may be resistant to warfarin, requiring very high doses (on average >9mg/day) to achieve anticoagulation. Warfarin resistance is due to mutations in the VKORC1 gene.

**Table 20.1** Drugs and the variants in genes which predict altered drug response in cardiovascular medicine

| Drug | Genetic variant(s) | Drug response |
|------|-------------------|---------------|
| Warfarin | *VKORC1*–1639G>A | Sensitivity to lower dose |
| | *CYP2C9*2* and *\*3* | Sensitivity to lower dose |
| | *CYP4F2* (Val433Met and others) | Sensitivity to lower dose |
| Warfarin | *VKORC1*—rare mutations | Resistance to high doses |
| Clopidogrel | *CYP2C19*2* | Standard dose less effective |

# Clopidogrel

Clopidogrel is an oral antiplatelet agent used to inhibit blood clots in coronary artery disease, peripheral vascular disease, and cerebrovascular disease. It is also indicated with aspirin to prevent thrombosis after intra-coronary artery stent. It acts by irreversibly inhibiting the $P2Y_{12}$ receptor.

Variants in the cytochrome P450, family 2, subfamily C, polypeptide 19 (CYP2C19) can alter the response to clopidrogel. Approximately 30% of individuals carry reduced function *CYP2C19* alleles e.g. *CYP2C19\*2*. Individuals with variant *CYP2C19* alleles have low plasma concentrations of the active clopidogrel metabolite and higher risk for adverse events such as death, myocardial infarction, stroke and coronary stent thrombosis compared with non-carriers. Trials to establish if alternative antiplatelet agents or higher doses of clopidogrel should be used in individuals with CYP2C19 variants should be undertaken.

P-glycoprotein (Pgp) encoded by the multi-drug resistance (*MDR1*) gene is an important transporter of molecules across cell membranes. Digoxin, a cardiac glycoside drug, frequently used in the treatment of atrial fibrillation is transported by Pgp. Variants in the *MDR1* gene have been associated with expression of the transporter and digoxin uptake. However, testing for MDR1 variants is not used in clinical practice to predict digoxin toxicity. Importantly though, many drugs, e.g. amiodarone, quinidine, verapamil, itraconazole, and erythromycin inhibit Pgp activity and their concomitant use with digoxin can lead to toxicity.

As digoxin acts on the sodium–potassium adenosine tri-phosphatase (ATPase) pump, inherited forms of arrhythmia that alter intracellular calcium control, such as catecholaminergic polymorphic ventricular tachycardia (CPVT) due to *RYR2* mutations or long QT syndrome due to ankyrin-B mutations may also predispose to digoxin toxicity.

# β-blockers

β-blockers are among the most widely prescribed of all drugs, with more than 120 million prescriptions in the United States in 2004. They are recommended as first-line treatment of numerous cardiovascular diseases such as heart failure, hypertension, and angina, as well as treatment after myocardial infarction. In addition, they are prescribed as a preventative measure in patients with long QT and to reduce the risk of aortic dilatation in patients with Marfan syndrome. Responses to β-blockers have been extensively studied and many genetic variants have been associated with treatment outcome. However, the results are conflicting and translation of pharmacogenetics into clinical practice for has not followed. The most promising association has been between the Arg389Gly variant in *ADRB1* and better response to β-blockers relating to hypertension and heart failure treatment.

Losartan is a selective, competitive angiotensin II receptor type 1 (AT$_1$) antagonist, has been shown to reduce aortic dilation in some patients with Marfan syndrome. Trials are being undertaken to establish the effectiveness of this treatment in Marfan syndrome. *In vitro* studies indicate that two cytochrome P450 enzymes, CYP2C9 and CYP3A4, are predominantly involved in the biotransformation of losartan to its metabolites. It is suggested that patients with *CYP2C9\*2* or *CYP2C9\*3* variants are less likely to respond to losartan, but further studies are required.

# Index

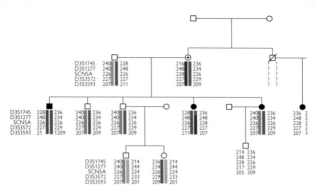

**Plate 1** Linkage analysis of a Brugada family.

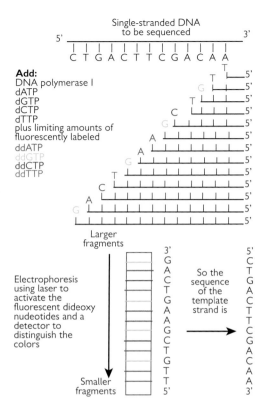

**Plate 2** PCR products are denatured to create single-stranded DNA. Taq polymerase enzyme copies the single-stranded DNA template incorporating the 4 complementary nucleotides (A, C, G, and T). Limiting amounts of modified, fluorescently labelled nucleotides are also incorporated. The incorporation of modified nucleotides causes the extension of the DNA copy to halt. The process continues cyclically, like PCR, to produce different-sized DNA fragments corresponding to each position of the DNA sequence within the original PCR product. Each of the fragments has a fluorescently labelled tag corresponding to its final nucleotide of the DNA sequence. The fluorescently-labelled fragments are separated by size on an automated DNA sequencer, and the colour and size of each tagged fragment recorded to determine the DNA sequence.

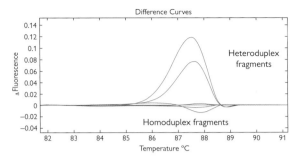

**Plate 3** High-resolution melt (HRM) analysis. Heteroduplexes and homoduplexes are melted at differing temperatures as detected by emitted fluoresence, and giving characteristic melt curves related to specific DNA variants. Heteroduplex DNA melts at lower temperatures as it comprises double-stranded DNA that is not perfectly matched. Homoduplex (normal) DNA melts at a higher temperature. Heteroduplex samples are simply identified as having different melt curves (in red).

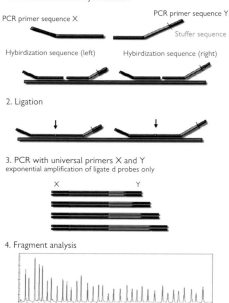

**Plate 4** Multiple ligation probe amplification (diagram courtesy of MRC Holland). Synthetic DNA probes are designed to hybridize and ligate on specific DNA fragments throughout a gene (generally one per exon). Hybridization is limited by the copy number of each gene fragment in the starting material. The ligated sequences are then amplified by PCR and separated by size. Subsequent fragment analysis includes the quantification of each PCR product, and comparison of patient samples with normal controls to determine if a deletion or duplication is present.

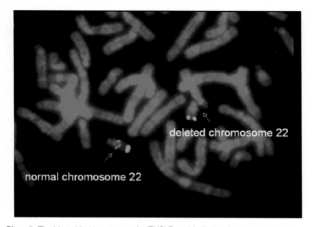

**Plate 5** The Vysis 22q11 region probe TUPLE1 is labelled with spectrum orange, the control probe ARSA which maps to 22q13.3 is labelled with spectrum green and DAPI has been used as a counterstain for the chromosomes.

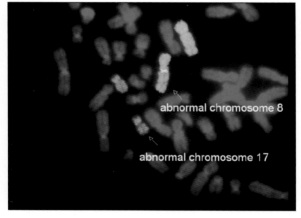

**Plate 6** The whole chromosome 8 paint is labelled with spectrum green, the whole chromosome 17 paint is labelled with spectrum orange, and DAPI has been used as a counterstain for the chromosomes.

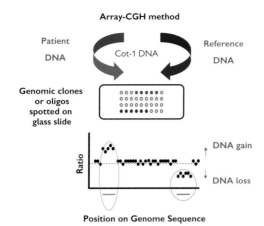

**Plate 7** Laboratory process for array CGH.

Reprinted from Kumar and Elliott (eds) *Principles and Practice of Clinical Cardiovascular Genetics.*, Oxford University Press, New York, 2010; Figure 5.3, page 70.

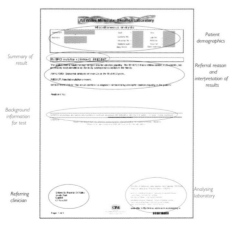

**Plate 8** Molecular genetics report.

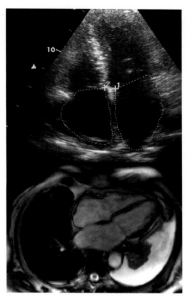

**Plate 9** Two-dimensional echocardiogram (upper panel) and cardiac magnetic resonance scan showing typical bilateral enlargement.

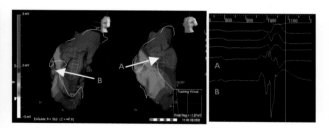

**Plate 10** Non-contact mapping of the right ventricle in a patient with ARVC. This is a voltage map recording the activation of the ventricle from a ventricular ectopic arising in the RVOT. At site A in the anterior RV the electrograms are fractionated and low in amplitude compared to an adjacent site where they are narrower and larger in amplitude indicating the patchy distribution of the disease.

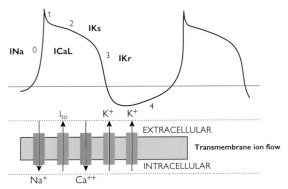

**Plate 11** Principle ion channel currents responsible for the monophasic action potential.